2004 Report on the global AIDS epidemic

4th global report

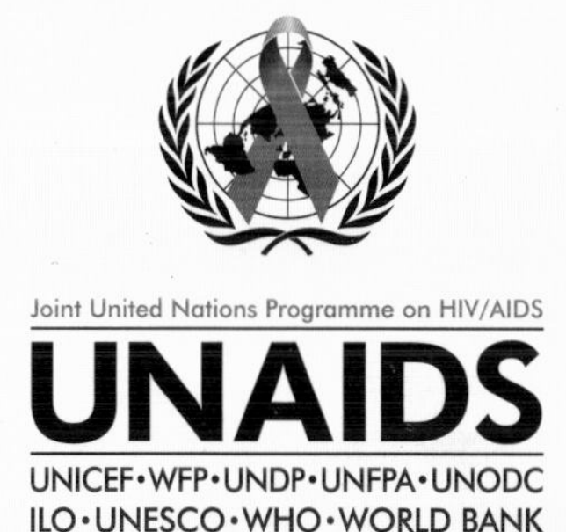

Joint United Nations Programme on HIV/AIDS

UNAIDS

UNICEF • WFP • UNDP • UNFPA • UNODC
ILO • UNESCO • WHO • WORLD BANK

Contents

Acknowledgements

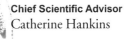

Managing Editor/Production Coordinator
Sandra Woods

Principal writers:
Sue Armstrong
Chris Fontaine
Andrew Wilson

Chief Scientific Advisor
Catherine Hankins

Editorial/Research Assistant
Susan Squarey

Project Supervisor
Marika Fahlen

Major editorial contributions:
Michael Bartos, Sandy Beeman, Anindya Chatterjee, Paul De Lay, Julian Fleet, Robert Greener, Alec Irwin, Mike Isbell, Lesley Lawson, Miriam Maluwa, Aurorita Mendoza, Lisa Regis

Editorial guidance:
Peter Ghys, Peter Piot, Francoise-Renaud Thery, Michel Sidibe, Karen Stanecki, Brian Williams

Production team:
Heidi Betts, Alistair Craik, Efren Fadriquela, Nathalie Gouiran, Marie-Laure Granchamp, Lon Rahn, Elena Sannikova, Olga Sheean and Elizabeth Zaniewski

This report would not have been possible without the support and valuable contributions of our colleagues in UNAIDS' Cosponsor organizations, the UNAIDS Secretariat, national AIDS programmes and research institutions around the world. The following people are among those who made significant contributions and deserve our special gratitude:

Angeline Ackermans, Peter Aggleton, Calle Almedal, Peter Badcock-Walters, Andrew Ball, Heidi Bazarbachi, Julia Benn, Elizabeth Benomar, Alina Bocai, Ties Boerma, Raul Boyle, Don Bundy, Angela Burnett, Alexandra Calmine, Michel Caraël, Pedro Chequer, Mark Connolly, Kieran Daly, Ernest Darkoh, Michel de Groulard, Getachew Demeke, Isabelle de Zoysa, Mandeep Dhaliwal, Neelam Dhingra-Kumar, Rebecca Dodd, Enide Dorvily, Alexandra Draxler, René Ehounou Ekpini, Olavi Elo, José Esparza, Tim Farley, Nina Ferencic, Nathan Ford, Edwige Fortier, Michael Fox, Vidhya Ganesh, Geoffrey Garnett, Amaya Gillespie, Aida Girma, Nick Goodwin, Ian Grubb, Lenin Guzman, Laura Hakokongas, Keith Hansen, Mary Haour-Knipe, Lyn Henderson, Alison Hickey, Wolfgang Hladik, Gillian Holmes, Dagmar Horn, Lee-Nah Hsu, Enida Imamovic, José Antonio Izazola, Jantine Jacobi, Noerine Kaleeba, Pradeep Kakkattil, Mohga Kamal Smith, Carol Kerfoot, Brigitte Khair-Mountain, Robert Kihara, Alexander Kossukhin, Christian Kroll, Amna Kurbegovic, Robin Landis, Susan Leather, Jean-Louis Ledecq, Seung-hee Lee, Ken Legins, Gael Lescornec, Jon Liden, Tony Lisle, Carol Livingston, Ruth Macklin, Bunmi Makinwa, Valerie Manda, Geoff Manthey, Tim Marchant, Hein Marais, William McGreevey, Henning Mikkelsen, David Miller, Jadranka Mimica, Hi-Mom, Roeland Monasch, Erasmus Morah, Rosemeire Munhoz, Elizabeth Mziray, Warren Naamara, Alia Nankoe, Francis Ndowa, Paul Nunn, Philip Onyebujoh, Gorik Ooms, Victor Ortega, Jos Perriens, Eduard Petrescu, Jean-Pierre Poullier, Elizabeth Pisani, Ben Plumley, Joel Rehnstrom, Chen Reis, Sinead Ryan, Marcos Sahlu, Roger Salla Ntounga, Karin Santi, George Schmid, Kristan Schoultz, Geeta Sethi, Ismail Shabbir, Catherine Sozi, Paul Spiegel, Susan Stout, Inge Tack, Miriam Temin, Kate Thomson, Georges Tiendrebeogo, Susan Timberlake, Warren Tiwonge, Stephanie Urdang, Mirjam van Donk, Bob Verbruggen, Anna Vohlonen, Neff Walker, Bruce Waring, Alice Welbourn, Caitlin Wiesen, Alan Whiteside, Desmond Whyms, Brian Williams (WHO), Kenneth Wind-Andersen, Anne Winter, Soumaya Yaakoubi, and Alti Zwandor

Figures

Preface

The global AIDS epidemic is one of the greatest challenges facing our generation. AIDS is a new type of global emergency—an unprecedented threat to human development requiring sustained action and commitment over the long term. As this report shows, the epidemic shows no sign of weakening its grip on human society.

The AIDS crisis continues to deepen in Africa, while new epidemics are growing with alarming speed in Asia and Eastern Europe. No region of the world has been spared.

While there is a pressing need for additional resources and commitment, this report also documents some of the success stories that have been achieved—by groups of people living with or affected by HIV, as well as by governments, nongovernmental organizations, business people and religious leaders.

AIDS has been with us for more than 20 years. It will continue to challenge us for many decades to come. The most important lesson we have learned so far is that we can make a difference: we can prevent new infections, and we can improve the quality of care and treatment for people living with HIV.

Our greatest challenge is to extend the extraordinary examples of leadership recorded in this report to the mainstream of everyday life. In the absence of a cure, the mass mobilization of every sector of society remains our only weapon.

Kofi A. Annan

Secretary-General of the United Nations

Foreword

Every two years, on the occasion of the International Conference on AIDS, this Global Report sets out our current knowledge on the state of the epidemic based on the experiences of the Joint United Nations Programme on HIV/AIDS (UNAIDS), which comprises nine United Nations system agencies. It makes for sobering reading.

Far from levelling off, rates of infection are still on the rise in many countries in Sub-Saharan Africa. Indeed, in 2003 alone, an estimated 3 million people in the region became newly infected. Most alarmingly, new epidemics appear to be advancing unchecked in other regions, notably Eastern Europe and Asia.

Countries in Eastern Europe and East Asia are experiencing the fastest growing HIV epidemic in the world. The large, populous countries of China, India and Indonesia are of particular concern. General prevalence is low there, but this masks serious epidemics already under way in individual provinces, territories and states.

AIDS is the most globalized epidemic in history, and we are witnessing its growing 'feminization'. Every year brings an increase in the number of women infected with HIV. Globally, nearly half of all persons infected between the ages of 15 to 49 are women. In Africa, the proportion is reaching 60%. Because of gender inequality, women living with HIV or AIDS often experience greater stigma and discrimination.

Yet this is a problem with a solution. As our report indicates, we know what works—successful approaches are evolving locally, nationally and globally. They are being helped by the growing momentum of international political leadership, by business workplace programmes, and by the dynamic mobilization of affected communities themselves—a key element that remains at the heart of our global response.

The good news is that the world is significantly increasing its commitments and resources. Yet as the number of governments, financial institutions and partners responding to AIDS increases, there is an urgent need for greater support for, and collaboration with, heavily affected countries. There is also a need to avoid duplication and fragmentation of resources.

Building on commitments made by leading donors in April 2004, we must not only raise more resources, but make sure that they are spent wisely to help countries mount sustainable and effective AIDS strategies. In particular, we must join forces to help countries strengthen their capacity to deliver these strategies.

A particularly welcome development is that the world has increasingly recognized the need to improve access to antiretroviral treatment for all people infected with HIV, regardless of the country in which they live. Treatment must be at the heart of every comprehensive AIDS strategy. However, prevention is equally important. We must never lose sight of doing everything we can to prevent people from becoming infected in the first place.

Over 20 years of AIDS provides us with compelling evidence that unless we act now we will be paying later—a trenchant message for the countries of Asia and the Pacific. AIDS demands that we do business differently; not only do we need to do more and do it better, we must transform both our personal and our institutional responses in the face of a truly exceptional global threat to security and stability.

AIDS is likely to be with us for a very long time, but how far it spreads and how much damage it does is entirely up to us.

Peter Piot
Executive Director
Joint United Nations Programme on HIV/AIDS

Global estimates of HIV and AIDS as of end 2003

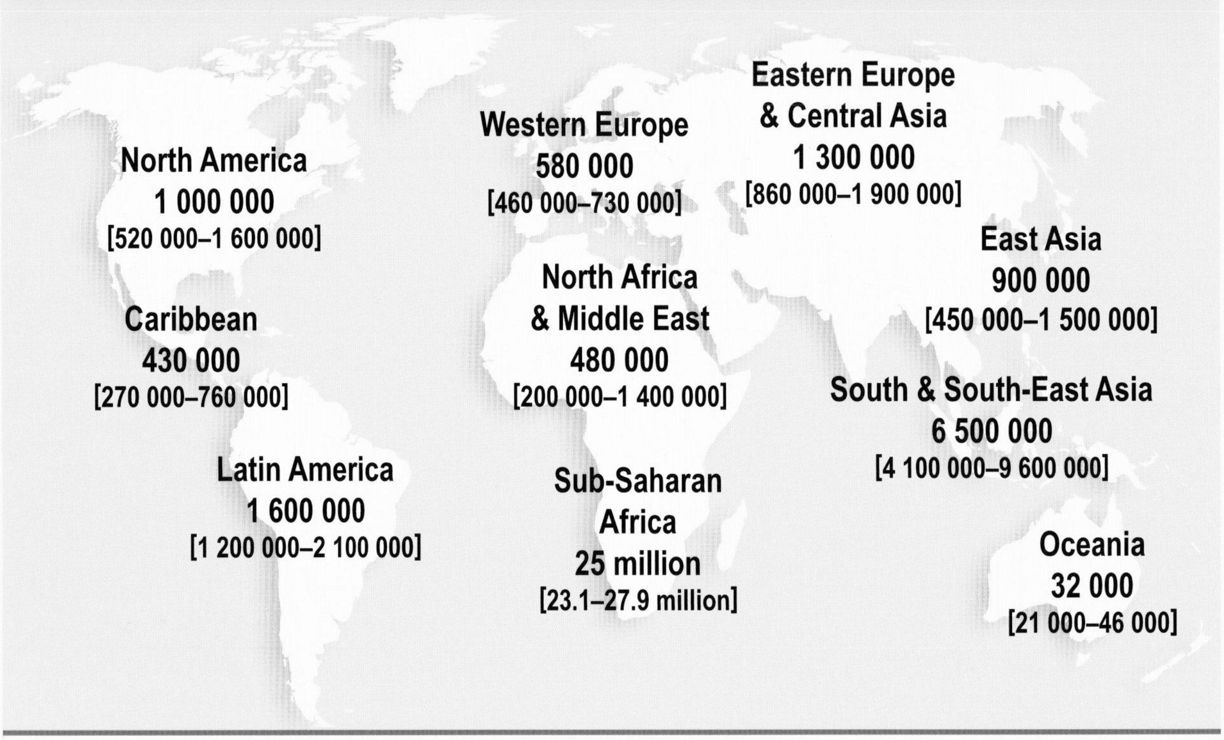

Total number of adults and children living with HIV: 38 million [35-42 million]

Number of people living with HIV	**Total**	**37.8 million**	**[34.6–42.3 million]**
	Adults	**35.7 million**	**[32.7–39.8 million]**
	Women	**17 million**	**[15.8–18.8 million]**
	Children <15 years	**2.1 million**	**[1.9–2.5 million]**
People newly infected with HIV in 2003	**Total**	**4.8 million**	**[4.2–6.3 million]**
	Adults	**4.1 million**	**[3.6–5.6 million]**
	Children <15 years	**630 000**	**[570 000–740 000]**
AIDS deaths in 2003	**Total**	**2.9 million**	**[2.6–3.3 million]**
	Adults	**2.4 million**	**[2.2–2.7 million]**
	Children <15 years	**490 000**	**[440 000–580 000]**

Overcoming AIDS: the 'Next Agenda'

1

The gender factor

Women are more physically susceptible to HIV infection than men. Data from a number of studies suggest that male-to-female transmission during sex is about twice as likely to occur as female-to-male transmission, if no other sexually transmitted infections are present. Moreover, young women are biologically more susceptible to infection than older women before menopause.

Women's increased risk is also a reflection of gender inequalities. Gender refers to the societal beliefs, customs and practices that define 'masculine' and 'feminine' attributes and behaviour. In most societies, the rules governing sexual relationships differ for women and men, with men holding most of the power. This means that for many women, including married women, their male partners' sexual behaviour is the most important HIV-risk factor.

The epidemic also has a disproportionate impact on women. Their socially defined roles as carers, wives, mothers and grandmothers means they bear the greatest part of the AIDS-care burden. When death and illness lead to household or community impoverishment, women and girls are even more affected due to their low social status and lack of equal economic opportunities.

Women and girls' special vulnerability

Challenging negative gender roles is critical to the global AIDS response. The 2001 UN Declaration of Commitment on HIV/AIDS recognized that gender inequality is fuelling the epidemic. In the Declaration, governments pledged to create multisectoral strategies to reduce girl's and women's vulnerabilities. Its 2003–2005 benchmarks include:

- addressing the epidemic's gender dimensions (article 37);
- accelerating national strategies that promote women's advancement and their full enjoyment of all human rights; the sharing of responsibility by men and women to ensure safer sexual behaviour and empowering women to make decisions about their sexuality and protect themselves from HIV (article 59);
- eliminating discrimination against women, including violence against women, harmful traditional practices, trafficking and sexual exploitation (articles 61–2);
- reducing mother-to-child HIV transmission by increasing women's access to antenatal care, information, counselling and testing, other prevention services, and treatment (article 54); and
- reviewing the epidemic's social and economic impact, especially on women in their role as caregivers (article 68).

Since 2001, a variety of regional, national and international initiatives have emerged. The United Nations Development Fund for Women launched a programme to intensify gender and human rights activities within 10 highly affected countries' national responses (Barbados, Brazil, Cambodia, India, Kenya, Nigeria, Rwanda, Senegal, Thailand, and Zimbabwe). Among other activities, the programme aims to enhance national capacity to review legislation or policies with implications for the epidemic's gender dimensions.

"Too often I have listened to women describe how their experiences are not part of the policy discussion. Whether talking about the unequal impact of globalization, the ravages of war and armed conflict, or the reality of living with HIV/AIDS, they feel marginalized and excluded from decision-making and resources that affect their lives. And yet, it is well-known that the most effective policy approaches come from listening to those who have experienced such problems first hand, who can provide needed perspectives, improve understanding and offer creative solutions so that resources may be used creatively". —Noeleen Heyzer, Executive Director, the United Nations Development Fund for Women

HIV-positive women's organizations are becoming increasingly visible. Globally, the International Community of Women Living with HIV and AIDS helps positive women's organizations to share their experiences. One of the organization's recent initiatives is the Voices and Choices project. It includes participatory research and advocacy for improved policy and practices. In 12 francophone African countries, it also currently researches support, treatment and care provision for HIV-positive women.

A new coalition

In 2003, the Global Coalition on Women and AIDS was launched. It brings together HIV-positive persons, civil society leaders, celebrity activists, nongovernmental organization (NGO) representatives, and UN figures to facilitate collaboration and to support innovative scaling up of efforts that have an impact on women's and girls' lives. The Global Coalition will work on: preventing HIV infection among girls and young women; reducing violence against women; protecting girls' and women's property and inheritance rights; ensuring women's and girls' equal access to treatment and care; supporting community-based care with a special focus on women and girls; promoting women's access to new prevention technologies and supporting ongoing efforts towards girls' universal education.

Overcoming AIDS: the 'Next Agenda'

AIDS is an extraordinary kind of a crisis. To stand any chance of effectively responding to the epidemic we have to treat it as both an emergency *and* a long-term development issue. This means resisting the temptation to accept the inevitability of AIDS as just another of the world's many problems. The AIDS epidemic is exceptional; it requires an exceptional response that remains flexible, creative, energetic and vigilant.

AIDS is unique in human history in its rapid spread, its extent and the depth of its impact. Since the first AIDS case was diagnosed in 1981, the world has struggled to come to grips with its extraordinary dimensions. Early efforts to mount an effective response were fragmented, piecemeal and vastly under-resourced. Few communities recognized the dangers ahead, and even fewer were able to mount an effective response. Now, more than 20 years later, 20 million people are dead and 37.8 million people (range: 34.6–42.3 million) worldwide are living with HIV. And still, AIDS expands relentlessly, destroying people's lives and in many cases seriously damaging the fabric of societies.

But experience has shown that the natural course of the epidemic can be changed with the right combination of leadership and comprehensive action. Two decades of tackling AIDS have yielded important successes and have taught crucial lessons about which approaches work best, although a cure remains elusive. We now know that comprehensive approaches to prevention bring the best results. Forthright national leadership, widespread public awareness and intensive prevention efforts have enabled entire nations to reduce HIV transmission. In Africa, Uganda remains the pre-eminent example of sustained success. In Asia, comprehensive action in Thailand averted some five million HIV infections during the 1990s. Cambodia too has managed to curb rapid growth of its epidemic. On every continent we can point to cities, regions or states where concerted efforts have kept the epidemic at bay.

At the same time, we now have antiretroviral medicines that can prolong life and reduce the physical effects of HIV infection. Coordinated national and international action has slashed the prices of these medicines in low- and middle-income countries, and sustained efforts are now under way to make access a reality for people living with HIV across the world who desperately need antiretroviral therapy.

Furthermore, the veil of silence and stigma that has crippled efforts to respond to AIDS is finally lifting in many countries. Leaders of governments, businesses and religious and cultural institutions are increasingly coming forward to take action against AIDS. The movement of people living with HIV has become a global force in the vanguard of social

1

Progress update on the global response to the AIDS epidemic, 2004

The AIDS epidemic: dynamic and diverse

- The epidemic remains extremely dynamic, growing and changing character as the virus exploits new opportunities for transmission.
- Girls and young women are at greatest risk. As of December 2003, women accounted for nearly 50% of all people living with HIV worldwide, and for 57% in sub-Saharan Africa.
- Young people (15–24 years old) account for half of all new HIV infections worldwide; more than 6000 contract the virus each day.
- The 2001 UN Declaration of Commitment on HIV/AIDS envisions major progress in delivering comprehensive care services by 2005. However, only minimal coverage has been achieved for care and treatment of HIV-related disease. Current prevention efforts in most low- and middle-income countries come nowhere near the scale of the epidemic.
- Achieving the 2005 targets will require urgent, innovative and expanded efforts to strengthen and accelerate the response.

change in responding to the epidemic. The impact of AIDS on development prospects in the worst-affected regions is being increasingly recognized, and action is under way to make necessary fundamental shifts in development practice.

Despite these signs of progress, more sophisticated monitoring and evaluation of the epidemic's behaviour reveal the scale of the challenge: fewer than one in five people who need prevention services and tools have access to them. Globally, five to six million people need antiretroviral medicines now; yet only 7% in low- and middle-income countries have access to these drugs—fewer than 400 000 people at the end of 2003. Many national leaders are still in denial about the impact of AIDS on their people and societies.

An unprecedented level of financial resources is now available to tackle the disease, but it is still less than half of what is really needed. Even these funds are not being applied in a fully effective, coordinated manner. In some instances, AIDS funding sits idle, blocked in government bank accounts or stalled by rules of international funders.

The result: the AIDS epidemic is now at a true crossroads. If the world's response to AIDS continues in its well-meaning but haphazard and ineffectual fashion, then the global epidemic will continue to outpace the response. But there is an alternative: to embark boldly upon the 'Next Agenda'—an agenda for future action that adopts the essential, radical and innovative approaches needed for countries to reverse the course of the epidemic.

A few home truths…

Women now the most affected

In the early days of the epidemic, men vastly outnumbered women among people infected with HIV. Indeed, it initially took the medical establishment some time and a great deal of evidence before it accepted the very idea that HIV was a threat to women. The proportion of females infected by HIV worldwide steadily grew until by 2002 about half of all people infected were women and girls.

In Southern Africa, where almost every family has been touched by AIDS, infected females outnumber males by as much as two to one

Assessing global and national progress in scaling up responses to AIDS

As part of follow-up activities to the 2001 UN Declaration of Commitment on HIV/AIDS, the UNAIDS Secretariat and Cosponsors collaboratively developed a series of global, regional and national indicators to measure the world's progress in reaching the Declaration's targets.

In 2003, 103 Member States of the UN provided UNAIDS with national reports on their progress, which formed the basis of a comprehensive assessment of global, regional and national responses to AIDS. It was called 'Progress report on the global response to the HIV/AIDS epidemic, 2003'.

In 2004, key elements of this material have been further updated by a study called *'Coverage of selected services for HIV/AIDS prevention and care in low- and middle-income countries in 2003'* (Policy Project, 2004). These two reports present progress on key global and national indicators in areas such as national response scale up, resources, eliminating stigma and discrimination, and prevention and treatment programmes.

Examples of key findings include the following: since 2002 global funding available to respond to AIDS almost tripled, but remains seriously inadequate, and—due to various blockages—is not reaching those who need it most; 38% of countries still have not adopted AIDS-related anti-discrimination legislation; and nearly one-third of countries lack policies that ensure women's equal access to critical prevention and care services.

The UNAIDS report's goal was to spur all stakeholders to generate even greater commitment towards achieving the 2001 UN Declaration of Commitment targets. Updated indicators in each area are spread throughout this global report and can be found in boxes called 'Progress update on the global response to the AIDS epidemic'.

in some age groups. Besides being the majority of those infected, women and girls are now bearing the brunt of the epidemic in other ways too: it is they who principally take care of sick people, and they are the most likely to lose jobs, income and schooling. Women may even lose their homes and other assets if they are widowed. To bring the concerns of women and girls into sharp focus, gender sections can be found in each chapter.

Young people: harsh impact

The epidemic is also affecting young people disproportionately: 15–24-year-olds account for half of all new HIV infections worldwide; more than 6000 contract the virus every day. This trend is especially alarming because this is the largest youth generation in history. Today's 15–24-year-olds have never known a world without AIDS, and have no 'folk memory' of the shocking early days of the 'new' disease. Yet it is today's young people who will be responsible for sustaining responses to the epidemic—they are tomorrow's leaders, thinkers and decision-makers, and it is vital that they play an integral part in responding to the epidemic (see 'Young People' focus).

The epidemic's dimensions and the task ahead

No other infectious disease in history has been so intensively studied. In the two decades since AIDS was first recognized, an enormous amount has been learned about HIV and the forces that drive the epidemic around the world.

Factors that influence HIV transmission: vulnerability and risk

Given the increases in the number of women infected with HIV, there is a special need to address the specific factors that contribute to women's vulnerability and risk. These include ensuring adolescent girls have access to information and services, that violence against women is not tolerated, that women can enforce property rights, that they do not miss out on treatment and that prevention options are expanded (for example, through developing a microbicide). However, in seeking to empower women, it is important to recognize that cultural and social expectations for boys and men can be just as much of a trap; they too need to be empowered to recognize and reject pressures to treat women and girls badly.

HIV transmission is not a random event; the spread of the virus is profoundly influenced by the surrounding social, economic and political environment. Wherever people are struggling against adverse conditions, such as poverty, oppression, discrimination and illiteracy, they are especially vulnerable to being infected by HIV. Efforts to prevent the spread of HIV need to focus both on individual risk behaviour, and on the broad structural factors underlying exposure to HIV—so as to help people control the risks they take and thereby protect themselves.

Vulnerability, risk and the impact of AIDS coexist in a vicious circle. Vulnerability can be reduced by providing young people with schooling, supporting protective family environments and extending access to health and support services population-wide. Addressing vulnerability at the structural level includes reforming discriminatory laws and policies, monitoring practices and providing legal protections for people living with HIV.

Challenges in scaling up antiretroviral treatment

Since 2002, the feasibility of providing antiretroviral therapy in resource-poor settings has become almost universally recognized. Governments and donors worldwide are increasingly committed to expanding access as quickly as possible to the many people who need life-prolonging antiretroviral treatment.

Scaling up antiretroviral treatment requires assured long-term political support and funding. Any lapse in support could result in collapsed antiretroviral programmes, with resultant interruptions in treatment giving HIV the opportunity to become drug resistant. Not only would this be an individual tragedy, it would also create a grave social threat, since drug-resistant strains of the virus can spread and render entire treatment programmes useless.

Health staffing is also crucial to the prospects of extending antiretroviral access. Already, Africa has a major shortage of nurses, midwives and doctors, as they leave their native countries for better salaries, working conditions and opportunities in higher-income countries. For example, 70% of doctors trained in South Africa currently live abroad. The gap is partially filled with health professionals from other African countries, which then widens the gap there. The cycle of out-migration leaves the lowest-income countries on the continent in dire need.

It is important to avoid the kind of chaos reported from some countries, where desperate patients buy antiretrovirals without medical advice and often without prescriptions. Treatment literacy should be an integral part of all treatment programmes, and people with HIV can play an important role since they speak with the authority of their own experience. In addition, community members can be trained to support treatment adherence and can assume some of the duties of health-care workers. This will help make more efficient use of all available resources.

AIDS-related stigma hampers the response and accelerates transmission

AIDS-related stigma and discrimination directly hamper the effectiveness of AIDS responses. Stigma and concerns about discrimination constitute a major barrier to people coming forward to have an HIV test, and directly affect the likelihood of protective behaviours. For example, the silence around HIV can prevent the use of condoms or can lead to HIV-positive women breastfeeding their infants for fear of being identified.

Stigma is not only directed towards people living with HIV. In many cases, HIV stigma has attached itself to pre-existing stigmas—to racial and ethnic stereotypes and to discrimination against women and sexual minorities. At the same time, long-standing patterns of racial, ethnic and sexual inequality increase vulnerability to HIV. In many countries stigma and discrimination remain important barriers to understanding how marginalized groups of society are coping with the epidemic.

Data now show that relatively new epidemics in East Asia, Eastern Europe and Central Asia are spreading fast. Despite the overwhelming evidence that AIDS is everywhere, the impulse to say AIDS is only a problem 'somewhere else' is still strong. In such a climate, people who are stigmatized and live on the margins of society, such as injecting drug users and men who have sex with men, are often badly served by prevention programmes. In some countries, their care and support needs are systematically ignored.

Developing a comprehensive approach to HIV prevention

Current HIV-prevention coverage is extremely low. Only a fraction of people at risk of HIV exposure have meaningful access to basic prevention services, although most countries have developed strategic frameworks for prevention activities. In low- and middle-income countries in 2003, only one in ten pregnant women was offered services for preventing mother-to-child HIV transmission, and an even smaller proportion of adults aged 15–49 years had access to voluntary counselling and testing.

Closing this prevention gap will require major recommitment of resources as well as a commitment to full-scale programming—too many efforts today are still at the 'demonstration project' level. It should be stressed that efforts to expand coverage of prevention services should avoid 'more of the same'. They need to take account of what experience has shown works best. For example, evidence suggests that messages and activities developed at the grassroots level are much more effective than those developed by remote 'professionals,' and that to make a difference, prevention messages need to be focused and go beyond simply raising awareness of AIDS.

Full-scale and comprehensive prevention efforts will need to be sensitive to the different contexts of the epidemic. For example, where overall HIV prevalence remains low, the relative importance of measures addressing particularly vulnerable sections of the population—such as sex workers, men who have sex with men, or migrant populations—increases. Where population-wide prevalence is high, efforts still need to be tailored to particular populations, but reducing HIV transmission will depend on achieving and sustaining a broad range of safe behaviours across wide population sectors, such as all young people. Evidence-informed decisions about effective prevention require knowledge of local epidemics, how they are changing over time, and who is currently at greatest risk of HIV exposure.

The changing nature of the epidemic requires prevention efforts to be constantly renewed. For example, it has become clear that the overwhelming emphasis on more effective treatment in high-income countries since the latter half of the 1990s was to the detriment of renewed prevention efforts. Prevention gains stalled and, in many cases, rises in HIV transmission were experienced for the first time in a decade. Similarly, in Thailand, outstanding success in reducing transmission associated with sex work in the 1990s changed the shape of the epidemic; now, the area of greatest need is within marriages and regular relationships.

Impact alleviation

The first signs of the full-scale societal impact of AIDS are becoming apparent in Southern and Eastern Africa, with the exacerbation of food crises, increases in the number of orphans, and relentless weakening of human capacity in both government and private sec-

The UN system: active on all fronts

The United Nations system has remained committed to the effective implementation of the 2001 Declaration of Commitment on HIV/AIDS. The Joint UN response to the AIDS epidemic continues to gather pace, especially with the addition of the World Food Programme (WFP) as the ninth UNAIDS Cosponsor.

Twenty-nine individual UN agencies take global leadership roles in their areas of specialization. Among UNAIDS Cosponsors these are: United Nations Office on Drugs and Crime (UNODC) on injecting drug users; United Nations Population Fund (UNFPA) on gender and young people; United Nations Educational, Scientific and Cultural Organization (UNESCO) on education; United Nations Children's Fund (UNICEF) on orphans and mother-to-child transmission; International Labour Organization (ILO) on HIV and the workplace; United Nations Development Programme (UNDP) on HIV, governance and development; and the World Bank through its Multi-Country AIDS Programme. With the joint World Health Organization and UNAIDS '3 by 5' Treatment Initiative, the WHO has increased its role in the global expansion of access to antiretroviral treatment.

The United Nation's Secretary-General's four Special Envoys on HIV/AIDS have increased HIV-related political, donor, civil society and media attention. For example, Nafis Sadik, the Special Envoy for Asia, has boosted Nepal's human-rights approach to AIDS. In several Caribbean countries, Dr George Alleyne, the Special Envoy for the Caribbean, encouraged legal reforms and steps to reduce AIDS-related stigma and discrimination. Meanwhile, the UN Special Envoy for Eastern Europe and Central Asia, Dr Lars Kalling, is raising awareness of how injecting drug use is a key factor in HIV spread.

In Africa, Stephen Lewis, the Special Envoy for that region, has joined with James T. Morris, Executive Director of WFP and the UN Secretary-General's Special Envoy for Humanitarian Needs in Southern Africa, to raise awareness about Southern Africa's deadly combination of AIDS, drought and shrinking human capacity.

tors. AIDS is fundamentally changing the fabric and functioning of societies. One way in which the epidemic creates a vicious circle is by striking hardest at those countries with the weakest capacity to implement responses. In many nations, AIDS is now depleting capacity faster than it can be replenished.

Given the deep and lasting effects of the epidemic, the most-affected countries need to review and adapt policies and investments across a wide range of areas to cope with the coming impact. AIDS calls for a complete re-thinking of how skills will be built, retained and sustained. In low-prevalence countries, aggressive prevention efforts are important in order to preserve investments in human and institutional development. A long-term perspective on retaining or rebuilding development capacity needs to be adopted. The immediate pressures of responding to the epidemic and keeping people alive will have immediate returns, but must also be accompanied by forward-looking measures that restore social resilience (see 'Impact' chapter).

More commitment needed to help orphans

An issue of particular concern is the neglect of orphaned children. AIDS has killed one or both parents of an estimated 12 million children in sub-Saharan Africa. Yet less than half of the countries with the most acute crisis have national policies in place to provide essential support to children orphaned or made vulnerable by the epidemic. To limit the impact of AIDS on the social and economic life of communities and countries, it is a political imperative that orphaned and vulnerable children be cared for.

Challenges of the 'Next Agenda'

It will take some extraordinary efforts to make the leap from the current piecemeal approaches to AIDS to the dynamic requirements of the 'Next Agenda'. The world's foremost national and international leaders, scientists, policy-makers, business and community leaders and the UN system all need to create new concepts and embrace key challenges in order to revolutionize and harmonize the global AIDS response.

Resources and funding

In financing, the 'Next Agenda' will require innovations that enhance country capacity to determine resource needs in prevention, care and impact alleviation. It requires countries and the international community to respond with unprecedented commitment and political will. Important progress has been made in raising additional funds, but global spending in 2003 was less than half of what will be needed in 2005, and only one-quarter of the amount needed in 2007 (see 'Finance' chapter). National and community-level civil society organizations require support to access and effectively use funds. For their part, donors and the international community need to carefully determine their fair share of contributions to the AIDS response.

Efforts to track resources and to prove they are being used efficiently also need strengthening, since this evidence is key to continuing financial support for programmes.

Building and rebuilding capacity

In addition to mobilizing still more funds, a great deal of work is needed to seriously scale up country programming capacity, and to clear blockages and bottlenecks in the system to ensure the money gets to where it is needed to support activities. AIDS itself has seriously depleted response capacity, and in many cases its impact has been worst in those communities and nations where capacity was already weakest as a result of decades of inadequate development.

Bold new approaches are required to reinvest in human and community resources, starting with preserving lives to the greatest extent possible, including through the roll-out of antiretroviral therapy. Long- and short-term strategies are needed in equal measure. In the immediate term, most countries possess untapped human capacity reserves (for example, in trained work-forces that have retired or moved away from their professions). In the longer term, strategies that reverse the worst effects of 'brain drain' need to be devised.

Harmonization and coordination

At the national level, all stakeholders need to accept that an effective AIDS response can only be achieved if countries own and drive it within their own borders. International assistance is important, but it only works effectively if it is embedded within a national response. The concepts of national ownership, multisectorality, mainstreaming, harmonization and coherence need to be based on guiding principles called the 'Three Ones': one agreed AIDS action framework that provides the basis for coordinating the work of all partners; one national AIDS coordination body, with a broad-based multisectoral mandate; and one agreed country-level monitoring and evaluation system.

Action informed by science

The threat posed by AIDS is now widely recognized. More resources than ever before have been pledged to respond; and more than ever, evidence is available about what works in response to the epidemic. Unfortunately at times, a willingness to be guided by scientific evidence and to develop consensus on effective approaches is put aside in favour of preconceived prejudices or sectoral interests, to the detriment of a concerted global response to AIDS. Time costs lives and it is vital that the world unites with a common understanding of what is needed to mount a rapid and effective response.

The exceptionality of AIDS

AIDS is an exceptional disease with exceptional and wide-ranging impact; it requires an exceptional response. It has the characteristics of both a short-term emergency and of a long-term development crisis. New and hybrid forms of response are needed. International financial institutions need to create mechanisms which alleviate countries' debt-service payments so they can devote additional resources to their AIDS response. Potential short-term inflationary effects of increased and additional resources applied to the HIV epidemic can be managed, and in any event, pale in comparison with what will be the long-term effects of half-hearted responses to AIDS on the economies of hard-hit countries.

The world has new tools and a new opportunity to beat the scourge of AIDS. This is the moment for a bold new agenda to tackle AIDS; we must not let it pass.

2

A global overview of the AIDS epidemic

Women increasingly infected by HIV

In recent years, the overall proportion of HIV-positive women has steadily increased. In 1997, women were 41% of people living with HIV; by 2002, this figure rose to almost 50%. This trend is most marked in places where heterosexual sex is the dominant mode of transmission, particularly the Caribbean and sub-Saharan Africa. Women also significantly figure in many countries with epidemics that are concentrated in key populations such as injecting drug users, mobile populations, and prisoners.

Sub-Saharan Africa

Nowhere is the epidemic's 'feminization' more apparent than in sub-Saharan Africa, where 57% of adults infected are women, and 75% of young people infected are women and girls. Several social factors are driving this trend. Young African women tend to have male partners much older than themselves—partners who are more likely than young men to be HIV-infected. Gender inequalities in the region make it much more difficult for African women to negotiate condom use. Furthermore, sexual violence, which damages tissues and increases the risk of HIV transmission, is widespread, particularly in the context of violent conflict.

In countries where the general population's prevalence is high and women's social status is low, the risk of HIV infection through sexual violence is high. A survey of 1366 women attending antenatal clinics in Soweto, South Africa, found significantly higher rates of HIV infection in women who were physically abused, sexually assaulted or dominated by their male partners. The study also produced evidence that abusive men are more likely than non-abusers to be HIV-positive (Dunkle et al., 2004).

Asia

Similar factors are threatening women in South and South-East Asia, but the overall impact in the region is much lower because the epidemic in most countries is concentrated among injecting drug users and other key populations. At the end of 2003, women accounted for 28% of infections, a slight increase compared to end-2001 estimates. In South Asia, women's low economic and social position has profound implications. Congruence between indicators of women's poor status and their HIV vulnerability suggests a close link between patriarchy and HIV in South Asia (UNDP, 2003). Women typically have limited access to reproductive health services and are often ignorant about HIV, the ways in which it can spread and prevention options. Social and cultural norms often prevent them from insisting on prevention methods such as use of condoms in their relations with their husbands.

Global increases, global inequality

Increases in the percentage of HIV-infected women also appear to be rising in: North America (25% in 2003, compared to 20% in 2001); Oceania (19% in 2003, compared to 17% in 2001); Latin America (36% in 2003, compared to 35% in 2001); the Caribbean (49% in 2003, compared to 48% in 2001), and Eastern Europe and Central Asia (33% in 2003, compared to 32% in 2001). While it is difficult to compare all the regional factors causing this increase, it is clear that gender inequalities—especially the rules governing sexual relationships for women and men—are at the heart of the matter.

A global overview of the AIDS epidemic

In 2003, an estimated 4.8 million people (range: 4.2–6.3 million) became newly infected with HIV. This is more than in any one year before. Today, some 37.8 million people (range: 34.6–42.3 million) are living with HIV, which killed 2.9 million (range: 2.6–3.3 million) in 2003, and over 20 million since the first cases of AIDS were identified in 1981.

The epidemic remains extremely dynamic, growing and changing character as the virus exploits new opportunities for transmission. There is no room for complacency anywhere. Virtually no country in the world remains unaffected. Some countries that have let down their guard are seeing a renewed rise in numbers of people infected with HIV. For example, in some industrialized countries, widespread access to antiretroviral medicines is fuelling a dangerous myth that AIDS has been defeated. In sub-Saharan Africa, the overall percentage of adults with HIV infection has remained stable in recent years, but the number of people living with HIV is still growing.

The epidemic is not homogeneous within regions; some countries are more affected than others. Even at country level there are usually wide variations in infection levels between different provinces, states or districts, and between urban and rural areas. In reality, the national picture is made up of a series of epidemics with their own characteristics and dynamics.

Since 2002, there has been a resurgence of energy and commitment in responding to the epidemic. Finances have increased considerably, and donors are exploring ways of channelling AIDS resources more quickly and efficiently to where they are most needed. The cost of antiretroviral medicines has tumbled, and concerted efforts are being made to extend treatment to millions of people in low- and middle-income countries whose lives depend on it. There is now also more funding available for prevention.

Together, all these approaches are making a difference in curbing the spread of HIV and in restoring quality of life to infected people and their families. But they are doing so on a scale that is nowhere near the level required to halt or reverse the epidemic. At the rate it is currently spreading, HIV will have an increasingly serious impact into the foreseeable future, unravelling the fabric of societies in its path.

Trends of global HIV infection

The number of people living with HIV continues to rise, despite the fact that effective prevention strategies exist. All the estimates in this report are based on updated estimation methodologies and the latest available data. Hence current estimates cannot be compared directly with previously published estimates. UNAIDS and the World Health Organization (WHO) have produced country-specific estimates for HIV every two years since 1998. During that time, the methods and assumptions used to make these estimates have been continually evolving. The UNAIDS Reference Group on Estimates, Modelling and Projections (scientists and researchers from a variety of institutions, convened by UNAIDS) meets annually to guide this process and refine the research tools, drawing on work carried out through smaller technical groups over the course of the year. Updated assumptions and methods are then applied to the subsequent round of estimates.

UNAIDS and WHO have revised their global estimates of the number of adults living with HIV, particularly in the sub-Saharan region. These new estimates are the result of more accurate data from country surveillance, additional information from household surveys, and steady improvements in the modelling methodology used by UNAIDS, WHO and their partners. This has led to lower global HIV estimates for 2003, as well as for previous years. Although the global estimates are lower, this does not mean the AIDS epidemic is easing off or being reversed. The epidemic continues to expand.

There are massive challenges in determining the exact prevalence levels of any disease—all figures are estimates based on available data. While the facts on HIV have been more accurate than many infectious diseases, there are those who would argue that UNAIDS and WHO have sometimes underestimated the epidemic, and at other times inflated the HIV numbers. The reality is more complex since global estimates are based on country estimates which themselves are derived from country surveillance systems. These systems collect data on HIV infection levels in different groups, but data are incomplete and their quality has varied.

In many countries, vast populations in rural areas are not well covered by surveillance. Because of social and political prejudice, many surveillance systems also bypass the population groups most likely to be exposed to HIV, such as injecting drug users, sex workers and men who have sex with men. By 2002, only 36% of low- and middle-income countries had a fully implemented surveillance system; however, 58% of countries with a generalized epidemic (where HIV prevalence is above 1%) had such a system.

The three most-commonly-used sources of data are sentinel surveillance systems that undertake periodic surveys among specific population groups; national population-based surveys; and case reports from health facilities. Each type of data has strengths and weaknesses. If more sources can be tapped, a more detailed picture can be pieced together and more accurate estimates achieved. In sub-Saharan Africa, the virus is spreading throughout the general population in many countries, and estimates are based largely on information gathered from pregnant women attending selected antenatal clinics. Recently, several countries have conducted national population-based surveys with HIV testing, some of which have been Demographic and Health Surveys. Examples include Burundi, Kenya, Mali, Niger, South Africa, Zambia and Zimbabwe. The data from these surveys have suggested that previous estimates based on sentinel surveillance were too high. However, all data are subject to possible biases. For example:

- The assumption that HIV prevalence among pregnant women is equivalent to the prevalence among both men and women in the surrounding communities may not be valid in all countries.
- Data from antenatal clinics do not fully represent remote rural populations, and there are few data to help adjust for this bias.
- In household surveys in some countries, people who refuse to participate, and those who are not at home when the survey team passes, may well have higher levels of HIV infection.

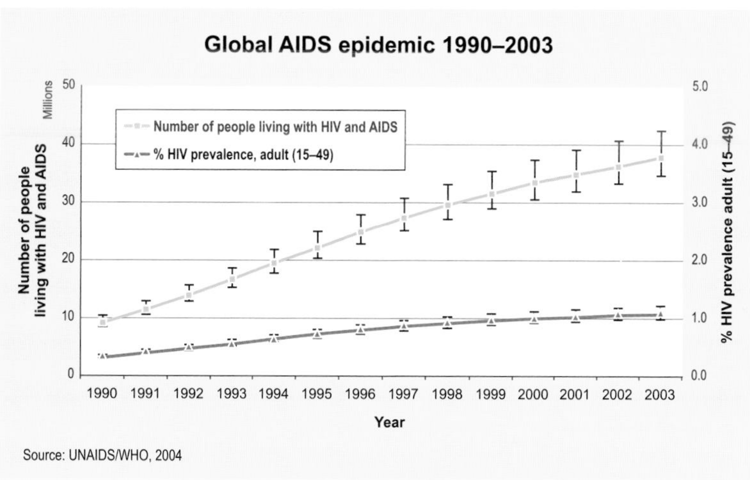

Figure 1

2

Difficulties in reconciling different estimates based on data from health facilities and population-based surveys are not applicable solely to HIV. For many conditions and diseases, including micronutrient deficiencies, noncommunicable disorders, and infectious diseases, estimates are improved through surveys collecting clinical and biological data. Even when non-disease indicators, such as poverty levels, are used, reconciling national household accounts with household surveys has become a difficult technical issue. But most experts agree that both should be used and that the truth about global poverty and inequality lies somewhere between the extremes suggested by the two methodologies.

An accurate picture of the epidemic is vital for directing national responses. Some countries may exaggerate estimates if they believe that doing so will increase their chances of obtaining international funding support. Or they may understate estimates to disguise poor political leadership, or because they fear high HIV levels will scare off tourists or business investors. However, much of the difference in interpreting the data does not stem from purposeful misrepresentation, but from the simple fact that there are important data gaps.

Even before the latest household survey results were released, more sophisticated sentinel surveillance and improved analysis resulted in lower estimates for a number of African countries. This is good news in that it means that fewer people than previously thought will suffer the horror of AIDS, but it should not be cause for undue optimism. For Africa, AIDS remains a catastrophe, and unrelenting commitment is required to turn the epidemic around and alleviate its tremendous impact.

Good intelligence is the key to appropriate action

Almost universally, mainstream society disapproves of, and sometimes harshly punishes, behaviour such as illicit drug use, sex between men, and sex work. This societal disapproval has meant that people engaged in these behaviours are frequently ignored by epidemiological surveillance systems, even though they are among the most likely to be exposed to HIV. Failure to monitor what is going on among them inevitably means that efforts to respond to the epidemic will be out of step with what is required, and HIV will retain the upper hand. Countries that conduct comprehensive surveillance are more likely to have an accurate picture of their epidemic, and can better plan an effective response.

Progress update on the global response to the AIDS epidemic, 2004

AIDS epidemic continues to expand; vulnerable populations at greatest risk

2

- Country data indicate that the number of people living with HIV continues to rise in all parts of the world despite the fact that effective prevention strategies exist. Sub-Saharan Africa remains the hardest-hit region with extremely high HIV prevalence among pregnant women aged 15–24 reported in a number of countries.
- In Asia, the HIV epidemic remains largely concentrated in injecting drug users, men who have sex with men, sex workers, clients of sex workers and their immediate sexual partners. Effective prevention programming coverage in these populations is inadequate.
- Diverse epidemics are under way in Eastern Europe and Central Asia. Injecting drug use is the main driving force behind epidemics across the region.
- In many high-income countries, sex between men plays an important role in the epidemic. Drug injecting plays a varying role. In 2002, it accounted for more than 10% of all reported HIV infections in Western Europe and was responsible for 25% of HIV infections in North America.
- In Latin America and the Caribbean, 11 countries have an estimated national HIV prevalence of 1% or more.

Source: UNAIDS

Asia

An estimated 7.4 million people (range: 5.0–10.5 million) in Asia are living with HIV. Around half a million (range: 330 000–740 000) are believed to have died of AIDS in 2003, and about twice as many—1.1 million—(range: 610 000–2.2 million) are thought to have become newly infected with HIV. Among young people 15–24 years of age, 0.3% of women (range: 0.2–0.3%) and 0.4% of men (range: 0.3–0.5%) were living with HIV by the end of 2003. Epidemics in this region remain largely concentrated among injecting drug users, men who have sex with men, sex workers, clients of sex workers and their sexual partners.

China and India: large epidemics

The region includes the world's most populous countries—China and India—with 2.25 billion people between them. National HIV prevalence in both countries is very low: 0.1% (range: 0.1–0.2%) in China and between 0.4% and 1.3% in India. But a closer focus reveals that both have extremely serious epidemics in a number of provinces, territories and states.

In China, 10 million people may be infected with HIV by 2010 unless effective action is taken. The virus has spread to all 31 provinces, autonomous regions and municipalities, yet each area has its own distinctive epidemic pattern. In some, injecting drug use is fuelling HIV spread. Among injecting drug users, HIV prevalence is 35–80% in Xinjiang, and 20% in Guangdong. In other areas, such as Anhui, Henan, and Shandong, HIV gained a foothold in the early 1990s among rural people who were selling blood plasma to supplement their meagre farm incomes. Infection levels of 10–20% have been found, rising to 60% in certain communities. As a result, many people have already died of AIDS.

India has the largest number of people living with HIV outside South Africa—estimated at 4.6 million in 2002. Most infections are acquired sexually, but a small proportion is acquired through injecting drug use. Injecting drug use dominates in Manipur and Nagaland in the north-east of the country, bordering Myanmar and close to the Golden Triangle. In this area, HIV infection levels of 60–75% have

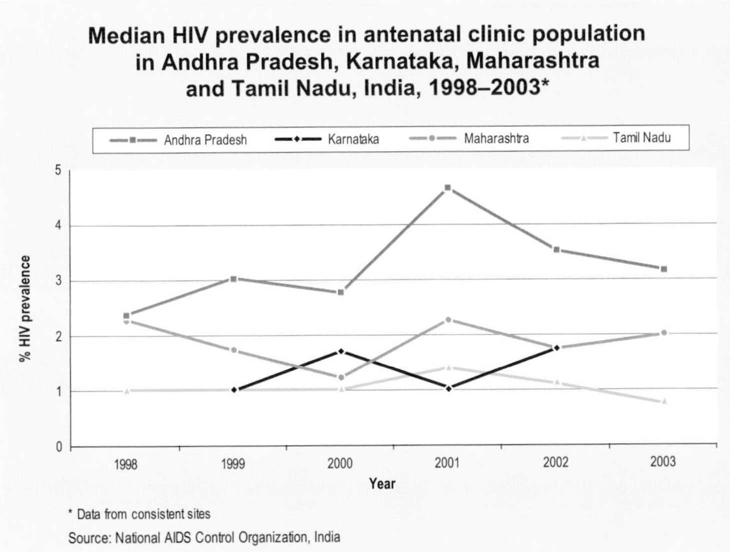

Figure 2

HIV transmission through sex between men is also a major cause for concern in many areas of India. Recent research shows that many men who have sex with men also have sex with women. In 2002, behavioural surveillance in five cities among men who have sex with men found that 27% reported being married, or living with a female sexual partner. In a study conducted in a poor area of Chennai in 2001, 7% of men who have sex with men were HIV-positive. Attention currently focuses on areas with high recorded prevalence, but there is concern about what might be happening in the vast areas of India for which there are little data.

been found among injecting drug users using non-sterile injecting equipment.

In the southern states of Andhra Pradesh, Karnataka, Maharashtra, and Tamil Nadu, HIV is transmitted mainly through heterosexual sex, and is largely linked to sex work. Indeed, according to selected surveys, more than half of sex workers have become infected with HIV. In all four states, infection levels among pregnant women in sentinel antenatal clinics have remained roughly stable at over 1%, suggesting that a significant number of sex workers' clients may have passed on HIV to their wives (see Figure 2).

In India, knowledge about HIV is still scant and incomplete. In a 2001 national behavioural study of nearly 85 000 people, only 75% of respondents had heard of AIDS and awareness was particularly low among rural women in Bihar, Gujarat and West Bengal. Less than 33% of all respondents had heard of sexually transmitted infections and only 21% were aware of the links between sexually transmitted infections and HIV.

Risk behaviour on the rise

Elsewhere in South Asia, behavioural information suggests that conditions are ripe for HIV to spread. For example, in Bangladesh, national adult prevalence is less than 0.1%, but there are significant levels of risky behaviour. Large numbers of men continue to buy sex in greater proportions than elsewhere in the region. Moreover, most of these men do not use condoms in their commercial sex encounters and female sex workers report the lowest condom use in the region.

Among injecting drug users, 71% of those who do not participate in needle-exchange programmes use non-sterile injecting equipment, compared with 50% of attendees in central Bangladesh programmes, and 25% in north-west Bangladesh programmes. Drug use in south-east Bangladesh appears to be on the rise (Dhaka, 2003). Surveys show that only about 65% of young people, fewer than 20%

2

of married women, and just 33% of married men have even heard of AIDS.

In Pakistan, 2001 country-level studies of populations more likely to be exposed to HIV revealed very low prevalence. Pakistan has an estimated adult HIV prevalence of 0.1%. It also has about three million heroin users, many of whom started injecting drugs in the 1990s. The first outbreak of HIV infection among injecting drug users happened in 2003. In Larkana, a small rice-growing town in Sindh province, 10% of 175 injecting drug users tested HIV-positive. A behavioural survey in Quetta found that a high proportion of respondents used non-sterile injecting equipment; and over half of them said they visited sex workers. Few had heard of AIDS, and even fewer had ever used a condom.

In South-East Asia, three countries in particular—Cambodia, Myanmar and Thailand—are experiencing particularly serious epidemics. Cambodia's national HIV prevalence is around 3%—the highest recorded in Asia. Data suggest that there have been some dramatic changes in the shape of Cambodia's epidemic. For instance, infection among brothel-based sex workers fell from 43% in 1998 to 29% in 2002 (see Figure 3).

There have also been sustained declines in prevalence among their customers, who include urban policemen, military conscripts and motorcycle taxi riders. This is believed to be due to increased condom use, as well as fewer visits to sex workers. However, the picture is incomplete: little has been done to monitor the epidemic among drug users, or

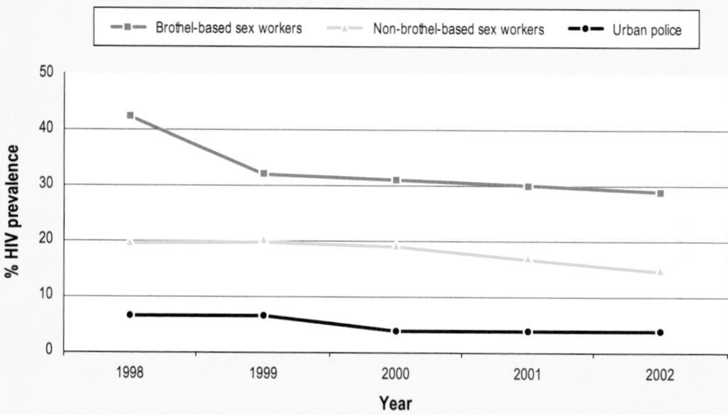

Figure 3

men who have sex with men, even though HIV prevalence among male sex workers in the capital was above 15% when last measured in 2000 (Girault et al., 2004).

Thailand: progress is lagging

In Thailand, the number of new infections has fallen from a peak of around 140 000 a year in 1991, to around 21 000 in 2003. This remarkable achievement came about mainly because men used condoms more, and also reduced their use of brothels. However, Thailand's epidemic has been changing over the years (see Figure 4). There is mounting evidence that HIV is now spreading largely among the spouses and partners of clients of sex workers and among marginalized sections of the population, such as injecting drug users and migrants.

Despite Thailand's indisputable success, coverage of prevention activities is inadequate. This is especially the case among men who have sex with men, and injecting drug users; their infection levels remain high. In Bangkok, over 15% of men who have sex with men who were tested in a 2003 study were HIV-positive, and 21% had not used a condom with their last casual partner.

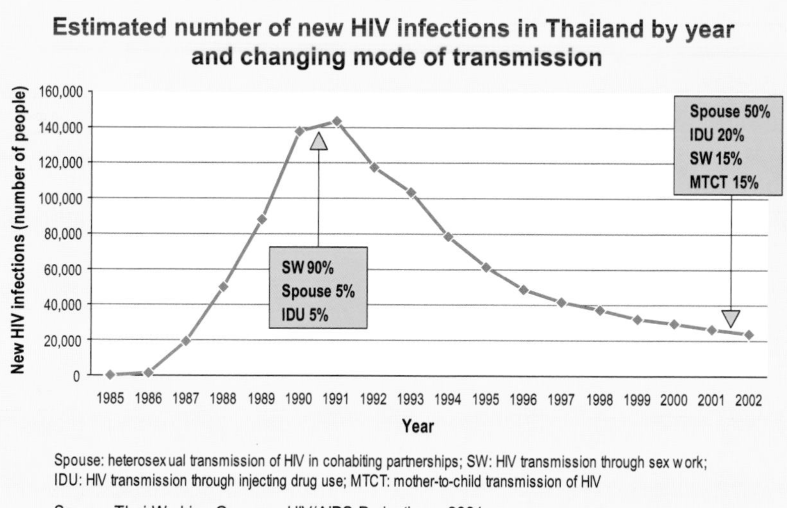

Figure 4

Many young Thai men avoid brothels because they are afraid of contracting HIV. However, the drop in commercial sex patronage appears to have been accompanied by an increase in extramarital and casual sex. Young Thai women also appear more likely to engage in premarital sexual relationships than earlier generations (VanLandingham and Trujillo, 2002). In Chiang Rai province, a study among vocational students revealed that only 7% of males surveyed said they had ever bought sex, but that almost half the students (male and female) were sexually active. Behavioural surveillance between 1996 and 2002 shows a clear rise in the proportion of secondary-school students who are sexually active. It also shows consistently low levels of condom use.

One of the newest epidemics in the region is in Viet Nam. National prevalence is still well below 1%, but, in many provinces, sentinel surveillance has revealed HIV levels of 20% among injecting drug users. Although HIV prevalence among injecting drug users increased significantly in some provinces in the late 1990s, recent outbreaks are now occurring in other provinces such as Can Tho, Hue, Nam Dinh, Thai Nguyen, and Thanh Hoa. Use of contaminated drug injecting equipment is believed to be responsible for two-thirds of HIV infections, but unsafe sex is also a concern in Viet Nam. In major cities in 2002, prevalence levels of 8–24% were reported among sex workers.

Indonesia's epidemic is currently unevenly distributed across this archipelago nation of 210 million people; six of the 31 provinces are particularly badly affected. The country's epidemic is also driven largely by the use of contaminated needles and syringes for drug injection. HIV prevalence among its 125 000–196 000 injecting drug users has increased threefold—from 16% to 48% between 1999 and 2003. In 2002 and 2003, HIV prevalence ranged from 66% to 93% among injecting drug users attending testing sites in the capital city, Jakarta. Indonesia's drug users are regularly arrested and sent to jail. In early 2003, 25% of inmates in Jakarta's Cipinang prison were HIV-positive.

Among Indonesia's more than 200 000 female sex workers, HIV prevalence varies widely. In many areas, recent serosurveillance shows that HIV infection in this population group is still rare. But some areas of the country have recorded sharp rises in the past year or two, with reported levels as high as 8–17%. Among transgender sex workers, known as *waria,* data show a sharp increase in HIV prevalence—from 0.3% in 1995 to nearly 22% in 2002 in Jakarta. There is strong evidence that various sexual and injecting-drug-user networks in Indonesia overlap significantly, thus creating an ideal environment for HIV to spread.

2

Oceania

In Australia, following a long-term decline, the annual number of new HIV diagnoses has gradually increased over a five-year period, from around 650 cases in 1998 to around 800 in 2002. HIV transmission continues to occur mainly through sexual contact between men. Among men diagnosed with newly acquired HIV infection between 1997 and 2002, more than 85% were found to have had a history of sex with another man. Relatively small percentages of newly acquired infections were attributed to a history of injecting drug use (3.4%), or heterosexual contact (8.5%). Similarly, the principal form of HIV transmission in New Zealand continues to be sexual contact between men.

Papua New Guinea, which shares an island with one of Indonesia's worst-affected provinces, Irian Jaya, has the highest prevalence of HIV infection in Oceania. Prevalence is over 1% among pregnant women in the capital, Port Moresby, and in Goroka and Lae. Papua New Guinea's epidemic appears largely heterosexually driven. High levels of other sexually transmitted infections indicate behavioural patterns that would also facilitate HIV transmission beyond sex workers and their clients.

In other islands in Oceania, HIV infection levels are still very low, but levels of sexually transmitted infections are high. A person with a sexually transmitted infection faces a higher risk of contracting and transmitting HIV during sexual encounters. In Vanuatu, pregnant women have chronically high levels of some sexually transmitted infections: 28% have *Chlamydia* and 22% have *Trichomonas* infection. Some 6% of pregnant women are infected with gonorrhoea, and 13% with syphilis. About 40% of the women had more than one sexually transmitted infection. Similarly, in Samoa, 31% of pregnant women had *Chlamydia* and 21% had *Trichomonas* infection. Overall, 43% of pregnant women had at least one sexually transmitted infection.

Sub-Saharan Africa

Sub-Saharan Africa has just over 10% of the world's population, but is home to close to two-thirds of all people living with HIV—some 25 million (range: 23.1–27.9 million). In 2003 alone, an estimated 3 million people (range: 2.6–3.7 million) in the region became newly infected, while 2.2 million (range: 2.0–2.5 million) died of AIDS. Among young people 15–24 years of age, 6.9% of women (range: 6.3–8.3%) and 2.1% of men (range: 1.9–2.5%) were living with HIV by the end of 2003.

Figure 5

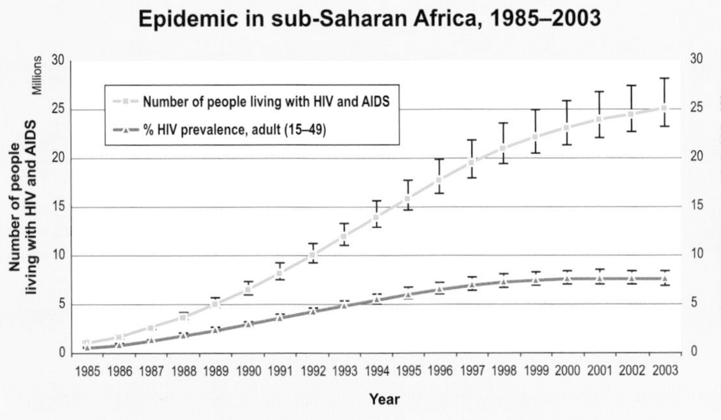

Source: UNAIDS/WHO, 2004

Many African countries are experiencing generalized epidemics. This means that HIV is spreading throughout the general population, rather than being confined to populations at higher risk, such as sex workers and their clients, men who have sex with men, and injecting drug users. In sub-Saharan Africa, as the total adult population is growing, the number of people living with HIV is increasing, with the result that adult prevalence has remained stable in recent years (see Figure 5). However, this overall stabilization of prevalence in the sub-Saharan region conceals important regional variations.

Although prevalence is stable in most countries, it is still rising in a few countries, such as Madagascar and Swaziland, and is declining nationwide in Uganda and in smaller areas in several other countries. Stabilized infection levels in an epidemic often result from rising death rates from AIDS, which conceal a continuing high rate of new infections. Even when HIV prevalence falls, as in Uganda, the number of new infections can remain high.

Within countries, there can be variations in prevalence by region. It has long been recognized that in most countries HIV infection levels are higher in urban than in rural areas. A review of national community-based studies shows that HIV prevalence in urban areas is about twice as high as in rural areas (see Figure 6).

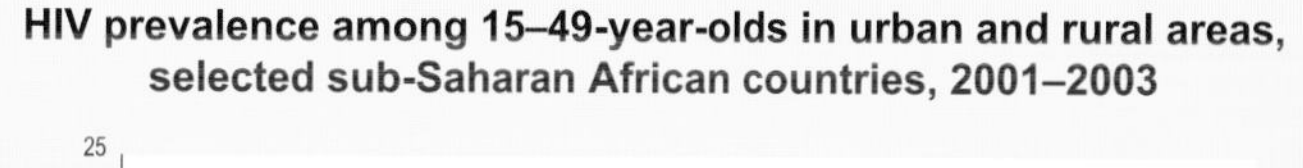

HIV prevalence among 15–49-year-olds in urban and rural areas, selected sub-Saharan African countries, 2001–2003

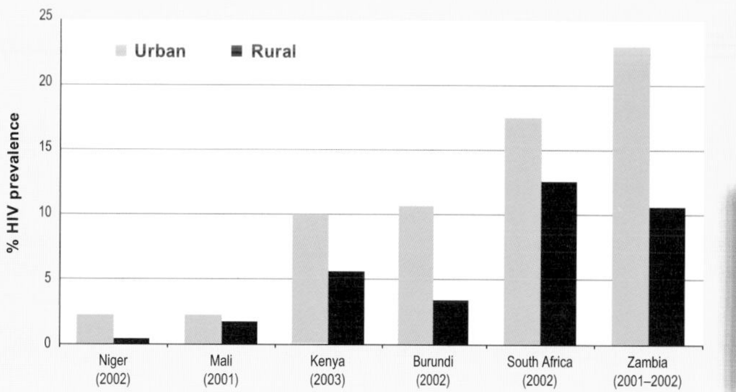

Notes

(1) *Burundi*: population age is 15–54. (2) *Mali*: population age for men is 15–59. (3) *South Africa:* Urban data from urban formal and urban informal and rural data from tribal areas and farms.

Sources: *Burundi* (Enquête Nationale de Séroprévalence de l'Infection par le VIH au Burundi. Bujumbura, Décembre 2002). *Kenya* (Kenya Demographic and Health Survey 2003). *Mali* (Enquête Démographique et de Santé. Mali 2001). *Niger* (Enquête Nationale de Séroprévalence de l'Infection par le VIH dans la population générale âgée de 15 à 49 ans au Niger 2002). *South Africa* (Nelson Mandela/HSRC Study of HIV/AIDS. South African National HIV Prevalence, Bahavioural Risks and Mass Media. Household Survey 2002). *Zambia* (Zambia Demographic and Health Survey 2001–2002).

Figure 6

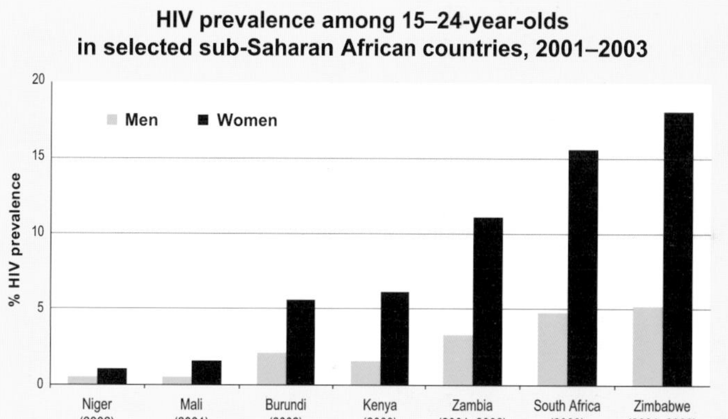

Sources: *Burundi* (Enquête Nationale de Séroprévalence de l'Infection par le VIH au Burundi. Bujumbura, Décembre 2002). *Kenya* (Kenya Demographic and Health Survey 2003. *Mali* (Enquête Démographique et de Santé. Mali 2001). *Niger* (Enquête Nationale de Séroprévalence de l'Infection par le VIH dans la population générale âgée de 15 à 49 ans au Niger (2002). *South Africa* (Pettifor AE, Rees HV, Steffenson A, Hlongwa-Madikizela L, MacPhail C, Vermaak K, Kleinschmidt I: HIV and sexual behaviour among young South Africans: a national survey of 15–24 year olds. Johannesburg: Reproductive Health Research Unit, University of Witwatersrand, 2004). *Zambia* (Zambia Demographic and Health Survey 2001–2002). *Zimbabwe* (The Zimbabwe Young Adult Survey 2001–2002)

Figure 7

Women face greater risk

African women are being infected at an earlier age than men, and the gap in HIV prevalence between them continues to grow. At the beginning of the epidemic in sub-Saharan Africa, women living with HIV were vastly outnumbered by men. But today there are, on average, 13 infected women for every 10 infected men—up from 12 infected women for every 10 infected men in 2002. The difference between infection levels is more pronounced in urban areas, with 14 women for every 10 men, than in rural areas, where 12 women are infected for every 10 men (Stover, 2004).

The difference in infection levels between women and men is even more pronounced among young people aged 15–24. A review of HIV-infection levels among 15–24-year-olds compared the ratio of young women living with HIV to young men living with HIV (see Figure 7). This ranges from 20 women for every 10 men in South Africa, to 45 women for every 10 men in Kenya and Mali.

In sub-Saharan Africa, heterosexual transmission is by far the predominant mode of HIV transmission. Unsafe injections in health-care settings are believed to be responsible for around 2.5% of all infections. Recently, it

2

has been suggested that unsafe medical injections account for most HIV transmission in the region (Gisselquist et al., 2002). However, a recent thorough review of the evidence concluded that, while a serious issue, unsafe injections are not common enough to play a dominant role in HIV transmission in sub-Saharan Africa (Schmid et al., 2004).

The 'unsafe injections' theory does not take into account the possibility that people sick with HIV-related disease might receive more injections. Moreover, the pattern of injections in health-care settings does not match sub-Saharan Africa's HIV-infection distribution pattern by age and sex. Although the safety of injections must be assured in all health-care settings, effective strategies addressing sexual transmission have the largest potential to turn the epidemic around in this region.

Diverse levels and trends

There is tremendous diversity across the subcontinent in the levels and trends of HIV infection (see Figure 8). Southern Africa remains the worst-affected region in the world, with data from selected antenatal clinics in urban areas in 2002 showing HIV prevalence of over 25%, following a rapid increase from just 5% in 1990. Prevalence among pregnant women in urban areas was 13% in Eastern Africa in 2002, down from around 20% in the early 1990s. During this period, prevalence in West and Central Africa remained stable.

There is no single explanation for why the epidemic is so rampant in Southern Africa. A combination of factors, often working in concert, seems to be responsible. These factors include poverty and social instability that result in family disruption, high levels of other sexually transmitted infections, the low status of women, sexual violence, and ineffective leadership during critical periods in the spread of HIV. An important factor, too, is high mobility, which is largely linked to migratory labour systems.

Median HIV prevalence (%) in antenatal clinics in urban areas, by subregion, in sub-Saharan Africa, 1990–2002

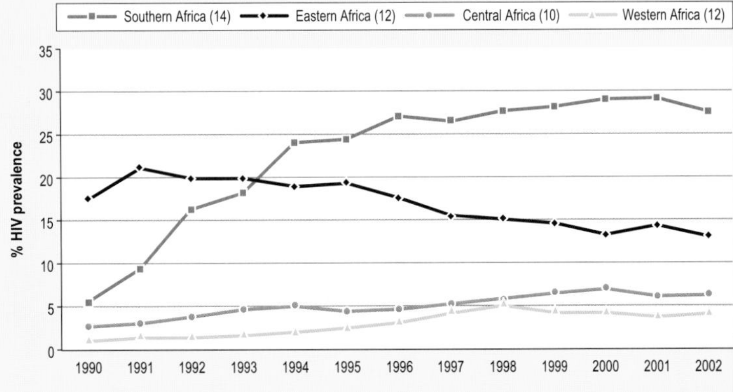

Source: Adapted from WHO AFRO 2003 Report

Figure 8

The epidemics in Southern Africa have grown rapidly. For example, in Swaziland, the average prevalence among pregnant women was 39% in 2002—up from 34% in 2000 and only 4% in 1992. Moreover, in a number of countries, the penetration of the virus into the general population has exceeded what was considered possible. In Botswana, weighted antenatal clinic prevalence has been sustained at 36% in 2001, 35% in 2002, and 37% in 2003. In South Africa, prevalence among pregnant women was 25% in 2001 and 26.5% in 2002.

In parts of East and Central Africa, there are signs of real decline in infections in some countries. This is most notable in Uganda, where national prevalence dropped to 4.1% (range: 2.8–6.6%) in 2003. In Kampala, prevalence was around 8% in 2002—down from 29% 10 years ago. But even Uganda cannot afford to relax: surveys suggest that today's young people may be less knowledgeable about AIDS than their counterparts in the 1990s.

Mobility and the spread of HIV

Human mobility has always been a major driving force in epidemics of infectious disease. Two recent studies have examined its role in the spread of HIV.

One study on the relationship between mobility, sexual behaviour and HIV infection in an urban population interviewed a representative sample of 1913 men and women in Yaoundé, Cameroon. The study measured mobility over a one-year period. It found HIV prevalence of 7.6% among men who had been away from home for periods longer than 31 days. Prevalence among those who had been away for less than 31 days in the year was 3.4%, while prevalence among those who had not been away from home in the previous 12 months was 1.4%. The association between men's mobility and HIV was apparently related to risky sexual behaviour and remained significant after controlling for other important variables. There was no association between women's mobility and HIV infection (Lydié et al., 2004).

Across Southern Africa, the phenomenon of men migrating to urban centres in search of work and leaving their partners and children at home in rural areas is widespread and has complex historical roots. Researchers interested in the role migration plays in spreading HIV in South Africa studied the pattern of infection in couples in Hlabisa, a rural district of KwaZulu-Natal, in which nearly two-thirds of adult men spent most nights away from home.

The study confirmed that migration does play an important role in spreading HIV but revealed a more complex picture than had been expected, which challenged some basic assumptions. Looking at discordant couples (that is, couples in which just one partner is HIV-positive), the study found that, in nearly 30% of cases, the infected person was the female partner who stayed home in the rural area, while her migrant partner was HIV-negative. In other words, migration may create vulnerability to HIV exposure at both ends of the trail, and the virus may be spread in both directions (Lurie et al., 2003).

The association of mobility with HIV infection may also affect the findings of household surveys. Mobile men, who generally have higher levels of HIV infection, are less likely to be found at home for these surveys. This is especially important in countries with high levels of mobility or migration, and for surveys with a high proportion of absentees.

No other country in the region has so dramatically reversed the epidemic as Uganda, but HIV prevalence among pregnant women has declined in several other places. For example, in the Ethiopian capital, Addis Ababa, prevalence has fallen from a peak of 24% in 1995 to 11% in 2003. Prevalence has also dropped in several sites in Kenya, including in Nairobi, while prevalence in many other sites appears stable. However, not all countries in the region show stabilized levels. In Madagascar, there has been an alarming rise in prevalence among pregnant women; it increased by almost fourfold since 2001, to reach 1.1% in 2003.

In West Africa, the epidemic is diverse and changeable. National prevalence has remained relatively low in the Sahel countries, with prevalence around 1%. However, the overall figures can conceal very high infection levels among certain population groups. In Senegal, for example, national HIV prevalence is below 1% (range: 0.4–1.7%); yet, among sex workers in two cities, prevalence rose from 5% and 8% respectively in 1992, to 14% and 23% in 2002.

2

Prevalence levels are highest in Côte d'Ivoire at 7% (range: 4.9–10%), although Abidjan recorded its lowest level (6%) in a decade in 2002.

Benin and Ghana show HIV prevalence in the 2–4% range, with little change over time. Nigeria, with a population of over 120 million, has the highest number of people living with HIV in West Africa. The national prevalence in 2003 was 5.4% (range: 3.6–8%). HIV prevalence among pregnant women ranges from 2.3% in the south-west region to 7% in the north-central region. Variation between states is even larger—from 1.2% in Osun to over 6% in Kaduna and to 12% in Cross River. HIV prevalence among pregnant women is over 1% in all states and is over 5% in 13 states.

North Africa and the Middle East

With the exception of a few countries, systematic surveillance of the epidemic is not well developed in North Africa and the Middle East. Furthermore, there is inadequate monitoring of the situation among populations at higher risk of HIV exposure, such as sex workers, injecting drug users and men who have sex with men. This means that potential epidemics in these populations are being overlooked.

In many countries, available information is based only on case reporting, and suggests that around 480 000 people (range: 200 000–1.4 million) are living with HIV in the region, which has a prevalence of 0.2% of the adult population (range: 0.1–0.6%). Some 75 000 people (range: 21 000–310 000) are believed to have become newly infected in 2003, and AIDS killed about 24 000 (range: 9900–62 000) that year. Among young people aged 15–24, 0.2% of women (range: 0.2–0.5%) and 0.1% of men (range: 0.1–0.2%) were living with HIV by the end of 2003.

Sudan is by far the worst-affected country in the region. Its overall HIV prevalence is nearly 2.3% (range: 0.7–7.2%); the epidemic is most severe in the southern part of the country. Heterosexual intercourse is the principal mode of transmission. The virus is spreading in the general population, infecting women more rapidly than men. Among pregnant women in the south, HIV prevalence is reported to be six-to-eight times higher than around Khartoum in the north. In Somalia, the epidemic is believed to have similar dynamics, but few surveillance data are available.

Morocco has expanded its surveillance system based on pregnant women and patients attending clinics for sexually transmitted infections, to also include sex workers and prisoners. In 2003, prevalence was 0.13% among pregnant women, 0.23% among patients at sexually-transmitted-infection clinics, 0.83% among prisoners and 2.27 % among female sex workers.

In some countries in the region, HIV infection appears concentrated among injecting drug users. Substantial transmission through contaminated injecting equipment has been reported in Bahrain, Libya and Oman. However, there is insufficient behavioural and serosurveillance among injecting drug users, resulting in an incomplete picture of HIV spread.

Unsafe blood transfusion and blood-collection practices still pose a risk of HIV transmission in some countries of the region, although efforts are being made to expand blood screening and sterile procedures in health-care systems to full coverage. In addition, there is concern that the virus may be spreading undetected among men who have sex with men. Male-to-male sexual behaviour is illegal and widely condemned in the region and the lack of surveillance means that knowledge of the epidemic's path in this population is poor.

Eastern Europe and Central Asia

Diverse HIV epidemics are under way in Eastern Europe and Central Asia. About 1.3 million people (range: 860 000–1.9 million) were living with HIV at the end of 2003, compared with about 160 000 in 1995. During 2003, an estimated 360 000 people (range: 160 000–900 000) in the region became newly infected, while 49 000 (range: 32 000–71 000) died of AIDS. Among young people aged 15–24, 0.6% of women (range: 0.4–0.8%) and 1.3% of men (range: 0.9–1.8%) were living with HIV by the end of 2003.

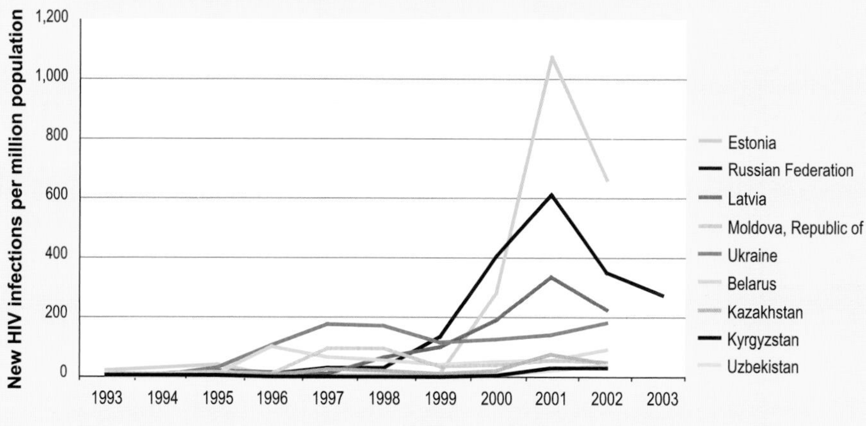

Figure 9

Estonia, Latvia, the Russian Federation and Ukraine are the worst-affected countries in this region, but HIV continues to spread in Belarus, Kazakhstan and Moldova (see Figure 9). For example, in Russia, the number of new cases registered in 2000 (56 630) was almost twice the cumulative number of cases registered since 1987 (French, 2004). However, the number of reported cases was down in 2002 and 2003, possibly due to testing saturation among injecting drug users, and changes in testing patterns.

The main driving force behind epidemics across the region is injecting drug use—an activity that has spread explosively in the years of turbulent change since the demise of the Soviet regime. A striking feature is the low age of those infected. More than 80% of HIV-positive people in this region are under 30 years of age. By contrast, in North America and Western Europe, only 30% of infected people are under 30.

The Russian Federation has the largest number of people living with HIV in the region, estimated at 860 000 (range: 420 000–1.4 million). The picture is uneven; well over half of all reported cases of HIV infection come from just 10 of the 89 administrative territories. Most drug users in Russia are male. But the proportion of females among new HIV cases is growing fast—up from one in four in 2001, to one in three just a year later. The trend is most obvious in parts of Russia where the epidemic is oldest, and this suggests that sexual intercourse has been playing an increasing role in transmission. From 1998 to 2002, HIV infection levels among pregnant women in Russia increased from less than 0.01% to 0.1%—a 10-fold increase. However, in St Petersburg, HIV seroprevalence increased from 0.013% in 1998 to 1.3% in 2002—a 100-fold increase.

In Ukraine, drug injecting remains the principal mode of transmission, but sexual transmission is becoming increasingly common, especially among injecting drug users and their partners. However, an increasing proportion of those who become infected through unsafe sex have no direct relationship with drug users.

Recently, several Central Asian countries—notably, Kazakhstan, Kyrgyzstan and Uzbekistan—have reported growing numbers of people diagnosed with HIV, most of them injecting drug users. Central Asia is at the crossroads of the main drug-trafficking routes between East and West and, in some places, heroin is said to be cheaper than alcohol.

Throughout the region, estimates and trends are based almost exclusively on case reporting by the health services and the police, since there is little money or infrastructure for systematic surveillance. This raises concerns that HIV may be spreading among people who rarely come into contact with the authorities or testing services. For example, very little is known about how the epidemic affects men who have sex with men, since sex between men is widely stigmatized and rarely acknowledged. However, in Central Europe, sex between men is clearly the predominant mode of HIV transmission in the Czech Republic, Hungary, Slovenia and the Slovak Republic.

Latin America

Around 1.6 million people (range: 1.2–2.1 million) are living with HIV in Latin America. In 2003, around 84 000 people (range: 65 000–110 000) died of AIDS, and 200 000 (range: 140 000–340 000) were newly infected. Among young people 15–24 years of age, 0.5% of women (range: 0.4–0.6%) and 0.8% of men (range: 0.6–0.9%) were living with HIV by the end of 2003. In Latin America, HIV infection tends to be highly concentrated among populations at particular risk, rather than being generalized. In most South American countries, almost all infections are caused by contaminated drug-injecting equipment or sex between men. Low national prevalence is disguising some very serious epidemics. For example, in Brazil—the most populous country in the region, and home to more than one in four of all those living with HIV—national prevalence is well below 1%. But infection levels above 60% have been reported among injecting drug users in some cities. Moreover, the picture varies considerably from one part of the country to another. In Puerto Rico, more than half of all infections in 2002 were associated with injecting drug use, and about one-quarter were heterosexually transmitted.

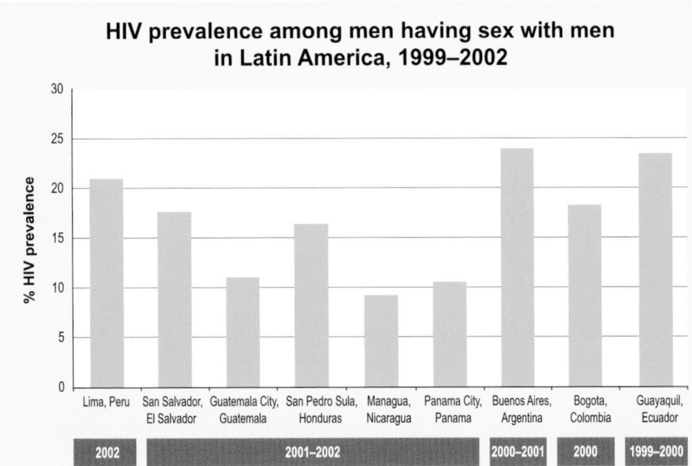

Sources: (1) Lima data: HIV Infection and AIDS in Americas: lessons and challenges for the future. Provisional Report MAP/Epi 2003 (2) San Salvador, Guatemala City, San Pedro Sula, Managua and Panama City data: Multicenter study of HIV/STD prevaler and socio-behavioral patterns, PASCA/USAID (3) Buenos Aires data: Avila, M., M. Vignoles, S. Maulen, et al., HIV Seroincidence Population of Men Having Sex with Men from Buenos Aires, Argentina (4) Bogota data: MS/INS/LCLCS/NMRCD 2000 study Guayaquil data: Guevara J., Suarez P., Albuja C. y col. Seroprevalencia de infección por VIH e Grupos de Riesgo en Ecua Revista medica del Vozandes. Vol 14, No.1:7-10, 2002

Figure 10

In Central America, injecting drug use plays less of a role, and the virus is spread predominantly through sex. A recent international study shows that HIV prevalence among female sex workers ranges from less than 1% in Nicaragua, 2% in Panama, 4% in El Salvador and 5% in Guatemala, to over 10% in Honduras.

Among men who have sex with men, levels of HIV infection appear to be uniformly high, ranging from 9% in Nicaragua to 24% in Argentina (see Figure 10).

Sex between men is the predominant mode of transmission in several countries, notably Colombia and Peru. However, conditions appear ripe for the virus to spread more widely, as large numbers of men who have sex with men also have sex with women. Peru is a case in point: in a survey of young men and women (aged 18–29), 9% of men indicated that at least one of their last three sexual partners was a man and that condoms were not used in 70% of those contacts.

Caribbean

Around 430 000 people (range: 270 000–760 000) are living with HIV in the Caribbean. In 2003, around 35 000 people (range: 23 000–59 000) died of AIDS, and 52 000 (range: 26 000–140 000) were newly infected. Among young people 15–24 years of age, 2.9% of women (range: 2.4–5.8%) and 1.2% of men (range: 1.0–2.2%) were living with HIV by the end of 2003.

Figure 11

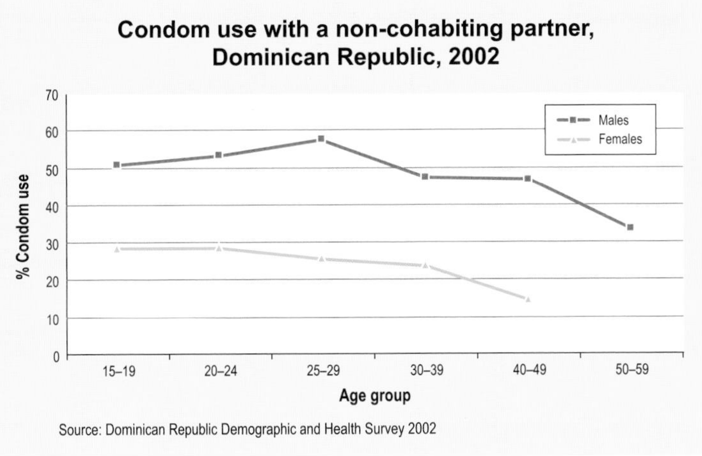

Source: Dominican Republic Demographic and Health Survey 2002

Of the seven countries in the Caribbean region, three have national HIV prevalence levels of at least 3%: the Bahamas, Haiti, and Trinidad and Tobago. Barbados is at 1.5% (range: 0.4–5.4%) and Cuba's prevalence is well below 1%. The Caribbean epidemic is predominantly heterosexual, and is concentrated among sex workers in many places. But the virus is also spreading in the general population. The worst-affected country is Haiti, where national prevalence is around 5.6% (range: 2.5–11.9%). However, HIV spread is uneven: sentinel surveillance reveals prevalence ranging from 13% in the north-west of the country, to 2–3% in the south.

Haiti shares the island of Hispaniola with the Dominican Republic, which also has a serious HIV epidemic. However, in the Dominican Republic, previously high prevalence has declined, due to effective prevention efforts that encouraged people to reduce the number of sexual partners and increase condom use (see Figure 11). Over 50% of males aged 15–29 used a condom with a non-cohabiting partner. In the capital, Santo Domingo, prevalence among pregnant women declined from around 3% in 1995 to below 1% at the end of 2003. But high levels are still reported elsewhere, and range from under 1% to nearly 5%. In 2000, HIV prevalence among female sex workers ranged from 4.5% in the eastern province tourist centre of La Romana, to 12.4% in the southern province of Bani.

High-income countries

An estimated 1.6 million people (range: 1.1–2.2 million) are living with HIV in these countries. Around 64 000 (range: 34 000–140 000) became newly infected in 2003, and 22 000 (range: 15 000–31 000) died of AIDS. Among young people 15–24 years of age, 0.1% of women (range: 0.1–0.2%) and 0.2% of men (range: 0.2–0.3%) were living with HIV by the end of 2003.

In high-income countries, unlike elsewhere, the great majority of people who need antiretroviral treatment do have access to it. This means that they are staying healthy and surviving longer than infected people elsewhere. In the United States, deaths due to AIDS have continued to decline because people have broad access to antiretroviral therapy. There were 16 371 reported deaths in 2002, down from 19 005 in 1998. In Western Europe, the number of reported deaths among AIDS patients also continued to decline—from 3373 in 2001 to 3101 in 2002.

In the United States, about half of newly reported infections in recent years have been among African Americans. They represent 12% of the population, but their HIV prevalence is 11 times higher than among whites.

In New York City, a new system for tracking the epidemic began in June 2000. It added HIV infection reporting to the previously existing system of AIDS case reporting. A recently published analysis of the first full year of data from 2001 has revealed that over 1% of the city's adult population, and almost 2% of Manhattan's, are HIV-positive.

In many high-income countries, sex between men plays an important role in the epidemic. For example, it is the most common route of infection in Australia, Canada, Denmark, Germany, Greece, New Zealand and the United States.

In recent years, heterosexual transmission in the industrialized world has sharply increased. In several western European countries, including Belgium, Norway and the United Kingdom, the increase in heterosexually transmitted infections is dominated by people from countries with generalized epidemics, predominantly sub-Saharan Africa. Because the countries with the largest epidemics in Western Europe (Italy and Spain) do not yet have national HIV-reporting systems, it is unclear whether this trend is occurring in other regions of Western Europe.

Drug injecting plays a varying role in spreading HIV in high-income countries. In 2002, it accounted for more than 10% of all reported HIV infections in Western Europe (in Portugal it was responsible for over 50% of cases). In Canada and the United States, about 25% of HIV infections are attributed to drug injecting. Infections transmitted through contaminated injecting equipment are particularly frequent among indigenous people, who are often among the poorest and most marginalized inhabitants of the industrialized world.

3

The impact of AIDS on people and societies

3

Women: more vulnerable to HIV than men

The impact of AIDS on women is severe, particularly in areas of the world where heterosexual sex is the dominant mode of HIV transmission. In sub-Saharan Africa, women are 30% more likely to be HIV-positive than men. The difference in infection levels between women and men is even more pronounced among young people. Population-based studies say that 15–24-year-old African women, on average, are 3.4 times more likely to be infected than their male counterparts.

Risk from husbands and lovers

Marriage and other long-term, monogamous relationships do not protect women from HIV. In Cambodia, recent studies found 13% of urban and 10% of rural men reported having sex with both a sex worker and their wife or steady girlfriend. Meanwhile, the country's 2000 Demographic and Health Survey found only 1% of married women used condoms during their last sexual intercourse with their husbands (Cambodian National Institute of Statistics/Orc International, 2000).

The risk of this behaviour to wives and girlfriends is clear. In Thailand, a 1999 study found 75% of HIV-infected women were likely infected by their husbands. Nearly half of these women reported heterosexual sex with their husbands as their only HIV-risk factor (Xu et al., 2000). In some settings, it appears marriage actually increases women's HIV risk. In some African countries, adolescent, married 15–19-year-old females have higher HIV-infection levels than non-married sexually active females of the same age (Glynn et al., 2001).

Violence and the virus

HIV-transmission risk increases during violent or forced-sex situations. The abrasions caused by forced vaginal or anal penetration facilitate entry of the virus—a fact that is especially true for adolescent girls. Moreover, condoms are rarely used in such situations. In some countries, one in five women report sexual violence by an intimate partner, and up to 33% of girls report forced sexual initiation (WHO, 2001).

Impact of HIV on women and girls in the community and at home

Women may hesitate to seek HIV testing or fail to return for their results because they are afraid that disclosing their HIV-positive status may result in physical violence, expulsion from their home or social ostracism. Studies from many countries, especially in sub-Saharan Africa, have found these are well-founded fears (Human Rights Watch, 2003). In Tanzania, a study of voluntary counselling and testing services in the capital found, after disclosure, only 57% of women who tested HIV-positive reported receiving support and understanding from partners (Maman et al., 2002).

Young girls may drop out of school to tend to ailing parents, look after household duties or care for younger siblings. After a spouse's death, a mother is more likely than a father to continue caring for his/her children, and a woman is more willing to take in orphans. Older women often shoulder the burden of care when their adult children fall ill. Later they may have to become surrogate parents to their bereaved grandchildren (HelpAge, 2003). AIDS-related stigma and discrimination often lead to the social isolation of older women caring for orphans and ill children, and deny them psychosocial and economic support.

When their partners or fathers die of AIDS, women may be left without land, housing or other assets. For example, in a Ugandan survey, one in four widows reported their property was seized after their partner died (UNICEF, 2003). A woman may also be prevented from using her property or inheritance for her family's benefit, which in turn hurts her ability to qualify for loans or agricultural grants. The denial of these basic human rights increases women's and girls' vulnerability to sexual exploitation, abuse and HIV.

The impact of AIDS on people and societies

"Human development is about creating an environment in which people can develop their full potential and lead productive, creative lives in accord with their needs and interests... The most basic capabilities for human development are to lead long and healthy lives, to be knowledgeable, to have access to the resources needed for a decent standard of living and to be able to participate in the life of the community. Without these, many choices are simply not available, and many opportunities in life remain inaccessible" (UNDP, 2001).

In both low- and high-prevalence settings, HIV and AIDS hinder human development. Consequently, the epidemic's dynamics need to be explored in human development terms. This focuses analysis and policy recommendations on people rather than the virus.

Globally, the epidemic continues to exact a devastating toll on individuals and families. In the hardest-hit countries, it is erasing decades of health, economic and social progress, reducing life expectancy by decades, slowing economic growth, deepening poverty, and contributing to and exacerbating chronic food shortages.

In high-prevalence countries in sub-Saharan Africa, the epidemic has a serious impact on households and communities. Most studies indicate a seemingly modest macroeconomic impact, with these countries losing on average between 1% and 2% of their annual economic growth. But the resulting effects on government revenue and expenditure will significantly weaken their capacity to mount an effective response, or indeed make progress towards the Millennium Development Goals.

Southern African countries are facing a growing human-capacity crisis. They are already losing skilled staff essential for governments to deliver vital public services, and AIDS is exacerbating this crisis. Increasingly, countries cannot meet existing social service commitments, let alone mobilize the necessary staff and resources to respond effectively.

In some Southern African countries, HIV prevalence continues to rise beyond levels previously thought possible. This means extraordinary multisectoral responses in affected countries are needed more urgently than ever. To visualize the future, UNAIDS and partners have undertaken 'AIDS in Africa: Scenarios for the Future'—an innovative project that draws on the expertise in scenario building offered by the Global Business Environment Division of Shell International Limited, and involves 50 Africans from all walks of life. Alternative scenarios for the year 2025 are being developed considering the underlying dynamics of AIDS that shape economies and societies. The project aims to help policy-makers test their current assumptions and actions, and adjust their course to more positively shape the future.

Progress update on the global response to the AIDS epidemic, 2004

Impact on countries to get worse before it improves

- More than 40% of countries with generalized epidemics have yet to evaluate the socioeconomic impact of AIDS. This hinders essential efforts to mitigate the epidemic's consequences for families, communities and society in general, as well as for human development.
- Of countries with generalized HIV epidemics, 39% have no national policy in place to provide essential support to children orphaned or made vulnerable by AIDS. In low- and middle-income countries, less than 3% of all orphans and vulnerable children receive publicly supported services.
- In sub-Saharan Africa's worst-affected countries, the epidemic's demographic impact on population structure means that if current infection rates continue and there is no large-scale treatment programme, up to 60% of today's 15-year-olds will not reach their 60th birthday.

Source: *Progress Report on the Global Response to the HIV/AIDS Epidemic,* UNAIDS, 2003; *Coverage of selected services for HIV/AIDS prevention and care in low- and middle-income countries in 2003,* Policy Project, 2004; Timaeus and Jassen, 2003.

The impact on population and population structure

Sub-Saharan Africa has the world's highest HIV prevalence and faces the greatest demographic impact. In the worst-affected countries of Eastern and Southern Africa, the probability of a 15-year-old dying before reaching age 60 has risen dramatically. In some countries, up to 60% of today's 15-year-olds will not reach their 60th birthday (Timaeus and Jassen, 2003).

HIV's impact on adult mortality is greatest on people in their twenties and thirties, and is proportionately larger for women than men. In low- and middle-income countries, mortality rates for 15–49-year-olds living with HIV are now up to 20 times greater than death rates for people living with HIV in industrialized countries. This reflects the stark differences in access to antiretroviral therapy. In low- and middle-income countries, mortality generally varies between two and five deaths per 1000 person years (PY) for people in their teens and twenties. However, HIV-infected individuals in these age groups experience death rates of 25–120 per 1000 PY, rising to 90–200 per 1000 PY for people in their forties (Porter and Zaba, 2004).

Until recently, low- and middle-income countries had extended life expectancy significantly. However, since 1999, primarily as a result of AIDS, average life expectancy has declined in 38 countries. In seven African countries where HIV prevalence exceeds 20%, the average life expectancy of a person born between 1995 and 2000 is now 49 years—13 years less than in the absence of AIDS. In Swaziland, Zambia and Zimbabwe, the average life expectancy of people born over the next decade is projected to drop below 35 years in the absence of antiretroviral treatment (UN Population Division, 2003).

Figure 12

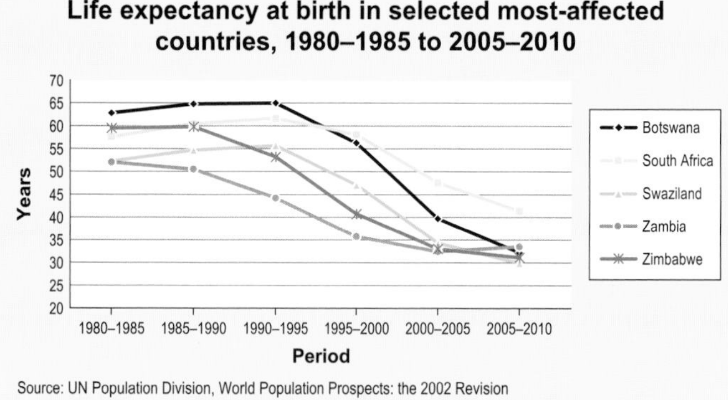

Population size with and without AIDS, South Africa, 2000 and 2025

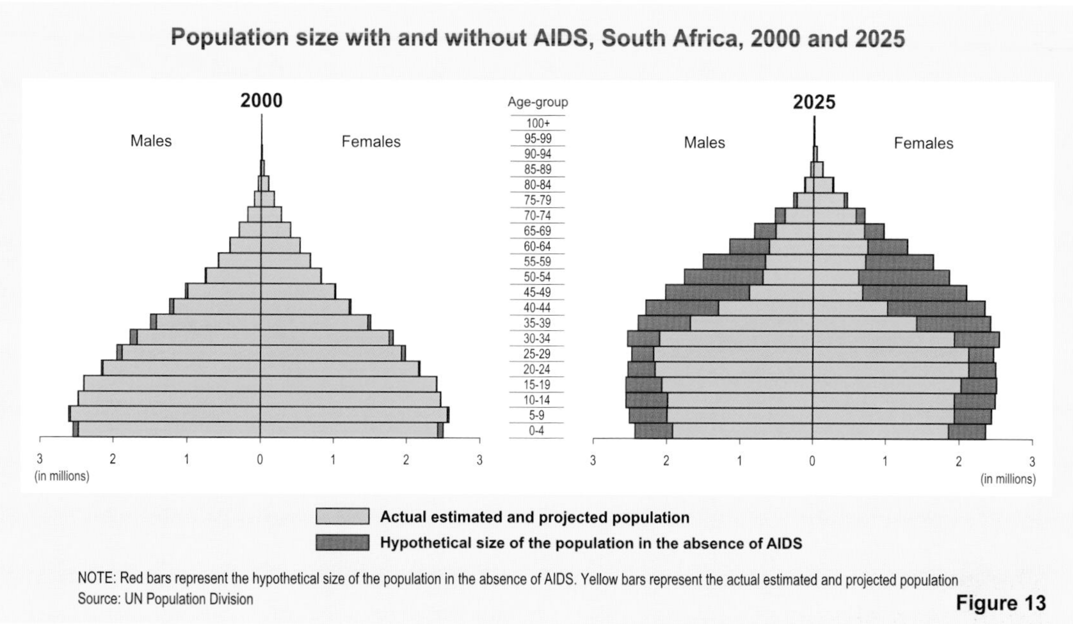

NOTE: Red bars represent the hypothetical size of the population in the absence of AIDS. Yellow bars represent the actual estimated and projected population
Source: UN Population Division

Figure 13

Unless the AIDS response is dramatically strengthened, by 2025, 38 African countries will have populations which will be 14% smaller than predicted in the absence of AIDS. In the seven countries where prevalence exceeds 20%, the population is projected to be more than one-third smaller due to the epidemic (UN Population Division, 2003).

HIV is not evenly distributed throughout national populations. Instead it primarily affects young adults, particularly women. This means the epidemic is dramatically altering heavily affected countries' demographic and household structures. Normally, national populations can be graphically depicted as pyramids. As epidemics mature in high-prevalence countries, new patterns emerge. For example, if South Africa's epidemic remains the same, its population structure will distort; there will be far fewer people in mid-adult years, and fewer women than men aged 30–50.

Women affected more than men

The epidemic's impact on women and girls is especially marked. Most women in the hardest-hit countries face heavy economic, legal, cultural and social disadvantages which increase their vulnerability to the epidemic's impact. (see boxes on gender beginning each chapter).

In many countries, women are the carers, producers and guardians of family life. This means they bear the largest AIDS burden. Families may withdraw young girls from school to care for ill family members with HIV. Older women often shoulder the burden of care when their adult children fall ill. Later they may become surrogate parents to their bereaved grandchildren. Young women widowed by AIDS may lose their land and property after their husbands die—whether or not inheritance laws are designed to protect them. Widows are often responsible for producing their families' food and may be unable to manage alone. As a result, some are driven to transactional sex in exchange for food and other commodities.

When the male head of a household becomes ill, women invariably take on the additional care duties. Providing care to an AIDS patient is arduous and time-consuming; even more so when it is done on top of other household

3

duties. A caregiver's burden is especially heavy when water must be fetched from a distance, and sanitation and washing chores cannot be carried out in or near the home. South Africa aptly illustrates this. It is one of the most developed countries on the continent. Yet, a 2002 survey of AIDS-affected households found fewer than half had running water in the dwelling and almost a quarter of rural households had no toilet (Steinberg et al., 2002).

Stigma has concrete repercussions for people living with HIV. Family support and solidarity cannot be assumed. A woman who discloses her HIV status may be stigmatized and rejected by her family. In most cases, women are the first in the family to be diagnosed with HIV and may be accused of being the source of it in the family.

The impact of AIDS on poverty and hunger

At the national level, the epidemic's economic and demographic effects have received substantial media and academic attention. However, the epidemic's often-catastrophic impact on HIV-affected households deserves greater analysis and policy effort. In some of the worst-affected countries, before the AIDS epidemic even started having an impact, the living standards of the poor were already deteriorating markedly. The epidemic drives these households to destitution.

For example, in Zambia's foundering economy, per capita Gross Domestic Product shrank by more than 20% between 1980 and 1999 (from US$ 505 to US$ 370). Over the same period, average daily calorie intake per person fell from 2273 to 1934 (UNCTAD, 2002). Amid such steady impoverishment, a poor household has limited abilities to overcome new adversities. It also has no resources to help others. Many of these households break up. After the death of one or both parents, children are parcelled out to relatives or community members.

The nature and severity of HIV on a household depends on the surrounding epidemic's extent and intensity. At the moment, sub-Saharan African households are most heavily affected by AIDS. But the epidemic does not discriminate. It devastates households and communities everywhere, even in countries with comparatively low national prevalence. For example, a study conducted for China's UN Theme Group on HIV/AIDS found significant economic and emotional impacts on AIDS-affected households. It also indicated the need for rapid increases in health-sector spending (Yuan et al., 2002).

Over the past 10–15 years, many of the worst-affected countries' social services have withered or become less affordable, incomes and formal employment levels have plunged and wars and large-scale population migration have disrupted social stability. Throughout sub-Saharan Africa, life-threatening diseases other than AIDS, such as tuberculosis and malaria, are on the rise. In this deteriorating context, poor households and communities are struggling to cope with the epidemic (Mutangadura, 2000).

How do households feel the impact of AIDS?

In recent years, many Southern African countries' prevalence levels have increased. Furthermore, the impact of East Africa's long-term, high-prevalence level is also now becoming visible, often representing an extreme shock for affected households dealing with these crises.

- AIDS causes the loss of income and production of a household member. If the infected individual is the sole breadwinner, the impact is especially severe.

- AIDS creates extraordinary care needs that must be met (usually by withdrawing other household members from school or work to care for the sick).
- AIDS causes household expenditures to rise as a result of medical and related costs, as well as funeral and memorial costs (Food and Agricultural Organization, 2003a).

Poor households are particularly in danger of losing their economic and social viability, and of eventually being forced to dissolve, with the children migrating elsewhere (Rugalema, 2000; Akintola and Quinlan, 2003). AIDS-affected households also appear more likely to suffer severe poverty than non-affected households, and older parents who lose adult children to AIDS are exceptionally prone to destitution (Rugalema, 1998).

(UN Population Division, 2003). In South Africa and Zambia, studies of AIDS-affected households—most of them already poor—found monthly income fell by 66%–80% due to coping with AIDS-related illness (Steinberg et al., 2002; Barnett and Whiteside, 2002). In Thailand, a 1997 study showed when a person with steady employment died of AIDS, the household's lifetime income loss was more than 20% greater than a household with non-AIDS-related deaths (Pitayanon et al., 1997).

Food insecurity

Between 1999 and 2001, 842 million people worldwide were undernourished—95% of them in low- and middle-income countries. Sub-Saharan Africa accounts for 11% of the world's population. It is also home to 24% of the world's undernourished people. This means the epidemic is unfolding in a setting dominated by chronic malnutrition and food insecurity.

Increasing needs in the 'care economy'

The 'care economy' is the term used to describe unpaid work in the home, usually done by women. As the epidemic becomes ever more severe, women's unpaid care workload increases dramatically. In sub-Saharan Africa, an estimated 90% of AIDS care occurs in the home, placing extraordinary strains on women who must take care of the children and produce an income or food crops. To help them cope, carers need support programmes, as well as national and macroeconomic policies designed to mitigate these impacts. The care burden should also be redistributed between men and women (Ogden and Esim, 2003) (see 'Finance' chapter).

Lost income

In the 1990s, a comparative study tracked 300 AIDS-affected households in Burundi, Côte d'Ivoire and Haiti. It found a steady decline in the number of economically active members per household. This was usually followed by a drop in per capita household consumption

In fact, AIDS is intensifying chronic food shortages. It causes farm labour losses and depletes family income that would normally purchase food. In Zambia, research shows the poorest economically active households rely heavily on cash income for food (Food Economy Group, 2001). When the price of food increases, poor families are hit hardest.

3

In high-prevalence countries, a vicious cycle exists between food shortages, malnutrition and AIDS (Food and Agriculture Organization, 2001). In Zimbabwe, adult HIV prevalence is around 25%. By 2000, AIDS had robbed the country of between 5%–10% of its agricultural workforce. By 2020, FAO projects farm labour losses will approach 25%. In Malawi, households that lost females under age 60 were twice as likely to experience a food deficit as households in which men in the same age bracket had died (SADC, 2003). In Uganda, 1990s research demonstrated food insecurity and malnutrition were the most serious problems for many female-headed AIDS-affected households.

Food insecurity is especially damaging for people living with HIV because they need more calories than uninfected individuals. Furthermore, malnourished HIV-infected people progress more quickly to AIDS (Harvey, 2003). HIV prevention, nutritional care, and AIDS mitigation measures need to be incorporated into general food security and nutrition programmes (Food and Agriculture Organization, 2003c).

Southern Africa's food crisis

Southern Africa's 2002–2003 food crises illustrated the epidemic's potential future impact on heavily affected countries. In six of the 10 highest-prevalence countries—Lesotho, Malawi, Mozambique, Swaziland, Zambia and Zimbabwe—more than 15 million people required emergency food aid due to widespread chronic and acute food shortages. In essence, Southern Africa's epidemic provided a vivid example of the magnifying effect of AIDS on poverty, gender inequities and weak national institutions.

Initially, the food shortages were triggered by aberrant weather conditions and a series of policy- and governance-related failures that seriously affected food production in advance of the food crisis (Harvey, 2003; Wiggins, 2003). AIDS made the situation worse. In Malawi, Zambia and Zimbabwe, households with chronically ill adults, recent deaths and orphans suffered marked reductions in agricultural production and income generation (SADC, 2003).

"Throughout the region people are walking a thin tightrope between life and death. The combination of widespread hunger, chronic poverty and the HIV/AIDS pandemic is devastating and may soon lead to a catastrophe. Policy failures and mismanagement have only exacerbated an already serious situation."

– James Morris, World Food Programme's Executive Director, July 2002.

How households respond

Households cope with the epidemic's devastation in various ways. In Kagera, Tanzania, households that experienced a death added at least one member, perhaps because extended family members stepped in to help out (World Bank, 1999). Elsewhere, in Rakai, Uganda, households became considerably smaller, possibly because children were sent to relatives, or adults left to search for employment (World Bank, 1999).

The household impact of AIDS can be especially severe when the infected individual is an adult woman. In all low- and middle-income countries, women and girls perform the lion's share of social reproduction work. They raise and nurture children, perform domestic labour and take care of the sick. In societies defined by extensive labour migration systems—including

Food crisis exacerbated by AIDS: a different kind of shock

Famine or food shortages are felt differently by AIDS-affected households and families. Normally there is ample forewarning before an impending food shortage. Within the limits of their resources and opportunities, most families can draw on past experiences and knowledge handed down from previous generations to safeguard their future viability.

By contrast, AIDS-affected households have reduced coping capacity. For instance, AIDS tends to cluster in households, generally striking individuals in their working and nurturing prime. Then, partners and children become infected, and are unable to compensate for the illness of the prime breadwinner or care-givers (Baylies, 2002). Due to a family's illness, less labour-intensive, non-cash crops may be planted and therefore cash may be less available than normally to purchase food. Stored food may be less nutritious. Caring for sick household members may further reduce the capacity to seek other food sources.

many of those hardest hit by the AIDS epidemic in Southern Africa—women head the majority of households, especially in rural areas. In South Africa, one survey has found almost three-quarters of AIDS-affected households were female-headed. A significant proportion of these women were battling AIDS-related illnesses themselves (Steinberg et al., 2002).

In Manicaland, Zimbabwe, when a woman died from AIDS, in two out of three cases households dissolved (Mutangadura, 2000). Much of the burden generated when an adult woman dies shifts to other, usually older, women who step in to foster the children. Often, the new foster mother has limited employment options and depends on low-paying, informal activities to generate income for the newly expanded household (Mutangadura, 2000).

In Cambodia, a recent study by the Khmer HIV/AIDS NGO Alliance and Family Health International found that an estimated one in five children in AIDS-affected families reported they were forced to start working in the previous six months to support their family. One in three had to provide care and take on major household work. Many had to leave school, forego necessities such as food and clothes, or were sent away from their home. Furthermore, all the children were exposed to high levels of stigma and psychosocial stress. Girls were more vulnerable to this than boys.

An AIDS-affected household's response depends on the resources it can gather together. When possible, families liquidate savings, borrow money or seek extended-family support (Food and Agriculture Organization, 2003a). Often, though, these households have limited savings and a lack of credit or insurance options. This means they must rely solely on their labour power to make up their lost income (Beegle, 2003).

> **"AIDS undercuts the resilience which households and communities draw upon to cope during periods of difficulty. In the face of an external shock, poor households respond with a variety of strategies, including altering income-generating activities and consumption patterns as well as calling upon family and community support. AIDS strikes at productive adults, the asset most likely to help during a crisis."**
>
> (UNAIDS, 2003)

Household responses can also differ between urban and rural settings. In urban settings, households often resort to informal borrowing and using their savings. Rural households tend to sell assets, migrate or rely on child labour (Mutangadura, 2000).

During planting and harvesting seasons, economic considerations often force poor families to suspend or postpone care-giving to earn income or grow food for the household. When such short-term economic considerations take precedence over continuing health concerns, it can compromise a household's long-term viability (Sauerborn et al., 1996).

Some studies indicate families may partially recover their earlier consumption levels. This suggests households can gradually develop coping mechanisms. Nevertheless, such coping occurs within a broader context of household impoverishment and social exclusion (Barnett and Whiteside, 2002).

Frequently, AIDS-affected households shuffle tasks and duties among surviving members (Barnett and Whiteside, 2002). In Tanzania, women with sick husbands spend up to 45% less time doing agricultural or income-earning work than they did before illness struck (UN Population Division, 2003).

Increased spending needs

To cover increased AIDS-related medical costs, households often reduce spending on food, housing, clothing and toiletries (World Bank, 1999). On average, AIDS care-related expenses can absorb one-third of a household's monthly household income (Steinberg et al., 2002). A South African study found more than 5% of AIDS-affected households were forced to spend less on food to cover these increased costs. This finding is even more distressing because almost 50% of the households had already reported experiencing food shortages (Steinberg et al., 2002). In South Africa's Free State province, a long-term study reported AIDS-affected households maintain food, health and rent expenses by reducing spending on clothing and education (Bachmann and Booysen, 2003). Furthermore, families often spend more on funerals and memorials than on medical care (World Bank, 1999).

To make matters worse, many households sell assets to cover the costs associated with AIDS. Asset liquidation usually begins with the sale of non-essential items, but can quickly progress to selling key productive assets. In Chiang Mai, Thailand, 41% of households affected by AIDS reported having sold land, and 24% were in debt. Among rural households in Burkina Faso, selling livestock and reorganizing household labour were the usual responses to serious illness (Sauerborn et al., 1996). Once rid of productive assets, the chances diminish that households can recover and rebuild their livelihoods. This leads to the threat of a terminal slide toward destitution and collapse.

Community support

AIDS-affected households rely heavily on relatives and community support systems to weather the epidemic's economic impact. These networks lend money, provide food and assist with labour and child care. When rural families confront the twin challenges of AIDS and food shortages, urban household members often send money or food. Conversely, rural relatives provide food to urban counterparts or invite them to rejoin the rural household.

Community support structures include savings clubs, burial societies, grain-saving schemes, loan clubs and labour-exchanging schemes (Mutangadura, 2000). But relatives and community support systems are sometimes not available to poor households that lack the means and time to invest sufficiently in reciprocal arrangements (Adams, 1993). In particular, poor female-headed households lack access to these networks.

In general, wealthier households have greater access to reciprocal networks than their poorer counterparts (Baylies, 2002). But, even when they function well, relatives and community networks seldom have the capacity to meet a vulnerable, AIDS-affected household's needs. For example, in Zimbabwe's Manicaland, poorer households report receiving help with food, clothing and labour, but no assistance with paying school and health-care fees, or rent (Mutangadura, 2000).

Taking action

A combination of initiatives is needed to strengthen the coping capacity of AIDS-affected households to address the complex and interrelated challenges they face (Nalugoda et al., 1997; Lundberg et al., 2000). Development experts have long debated the relative merits of targeted versus broad-based poverty reduction measures. The epidemic affects both aspects: many household emergency conditions require targeted action, while impoverishment results in long-term development challenges.

The 2003 report to the UN Chief Executives Board (UNAIDS CEB, 2003) recommended eleven programmatic actions for UN agencies in Eastern and Southern Africa. These were:

- Action 1: Implement community safety-net programmes;
- Action 2: Improve data collection on community impact and dynamics;
- Action 3: Strengthen livelihoods in highly affected communities and for key groups;
- Action 4: Undertake dedicated programmes for women's empowerment;
- Action 5: Undertake dedicated programmes to assist the growing orphan population;
- Action 6: Undertake urgent capacity building to fight AIDS, especially in the health sector;
- Action 7: Undertake urgent capacity building to deal with the impacts of AIDS;
- Action 8: Mainstream AIDS into development planning;
- Action 9: Build leadership to lead participatory programme reviews;
- Action 10: Advocate and support partnership forums;
- Action 11: Invest in monitoring, tracking and evaluation systems.

Welfare programmes can help, and should be specially targeted towards the most deprived and vulnerable households and communities. Local institutions, such as health clinics, could identify and obtain help for impoverished households struggling with serious illness. Special care could include home visits, food and nutritional support, and waiving school user fees, etc. (Sauerborn et al., 1996). Other necessary targeted initiatives include community-based programmes to provide families with direct financial assistance so they do not have to sell productive assets to cope with AIDS costs.

Reducing stigma and discrimination goes hand-in-hand with providing help to HIV-affected households. Stigma sometimes causes shame or fear of ostracism, and deters household members from seeking and receiving community-based assistance. In South Africa, one survey found that only one-third of respondents who had revealed their HIV-positive status received a supportive response in their communities. One in ten said they met with outright hostility and rejection (Steinberg et al., 2002).

Programmes are necessary to build and strengthen basic infrastructure, especially water and sanitation; reduce caregivers' day-to-day burdens; and increase households' abilities to cope with AIDS burdens. Other broad-based strategies include programmes providing child support payments or school lunches. Furthermore, social welfare support programmes for the elderly are needed, especially for those raising their grandchildren.

Income-generating initiatives that address women's particular economic vulnerability are integral to the AIDS response. First, women's circumstances within impoverished AIDS-affected households require readily available emergency relief. Then, microfinance programmes that offer reasonable interest rates need to be expanded. Other strategies that benefit women include: death insurance to cover funeral costs for terminally-ill patients; flexible saving arrangements and emergency loans. These initiatives support the entire household, a necessity since research indicates women in low- and middle-income countries devote any additional income to meeting their children's needs (Hunter and Williamson, 1997).

The epidemic's deep and multifaceted impact on households and communities makes it crucially important to address AIDS within a poverty-reduction context. To date, few countries have incorporated meaningful AIDS components into their poverty-reduction plans (see 'Finance' chapter).

Impact on agriculture and rural development

A healthy agricultural sector is central to the well-being and self-sufficiency of low- and middle-income countries. Agriculture affects food security, the fate of national economies and the sustainability of environmental assets. It accounts for 24% of Africa's gross domestic product, 40% of its foreign exchange earnings and 70% of its employment. In 2000, about 56% of Africans (more than 430 million people) were engaged in agriculture.

Unfortunately, especially in the hardest-hit countries, the epidemic attacks the agricultural base—it infects and then kills many agricultural workers prematurely. This causes a loss of labour, reduced farming income and household assets and lowered household-level food security (Topouzis, 2003). The UN's Food and Agriculture Organization estimates AIDS will have claimed one-fifth or more of agricultural workers in most countries in Southern Africa by 2020 (Villareal, 2003; Food and Agriculture Organization, 2003b).

This loss of workers is critical. When one or two key crops must be planted and harvested at specific times, losing even a few workers during these periods can scuttle production (Bollinger and Stover, 1999). Households try to adapt by farming smaller plots of land, cutting back on weeding, repairing fences and tending irrigation channels, or livestock husbandry. Often land must be left fallow, becoming affected by erosion and degradation, while livestock that can't be tended become more vulnerable to disease, predators and thieves (Barnett and Whiteside, 2002). In a Ugandan study, almost half the respondents said AIDS-related labour shortages forced them to reduce the variety of crops they farmed (Asingwire, 1996).

In rural communities, gender inequality also increases the epidemic's agricultural impact. In Tanzania, women with seriously ill husbands spend up to 50% less time doing farm work (Rugalema, 1998). Following the male adult's death, households frequently turn to subsistence crops, avoiding the high-value crops usually managed by men (Yamano and Jayne, 2002). In many societies, women lack legal or even customary title to land, livestock and other key assets, and widows may lose what they helped develop and maintain.

Taking action

In heavily-affected countries, the causes of food insecurity are multiple, complex and interrelated. Critical factors include: agricultural, trade and macroeconomic policies; land tenure and inheritance systems; climate patterns; and the state's capacity to provide rural areas with vital support services (Barnett and Whiteside, 2002). As the epidemic progresses, chronic food insecurity will likely grow worse. Any response must derive from an understanding of how households obtain their livelihoods, targeting as many aggravating factors as possible and integrating AIDS into policies and programmes to achieve food security and rural development. These will create a long-term defence against both famine and AIDS.

Urgent priorities include initiatives that enable people living with HIV to stay healthy for as long as possible—such as antiretroviral therapy, tuberculosis treatment, and nutritional assistance. Such initiatives help AIDS-affected households preserve or recover their livelihoods (Baylies, 2002). Other valuable responses would encourage planting less labour-intensive crops that still provide nutritious food, strengthening school food programmes, and securing women's and children's rights to retain land and assets, thereby improving the security of land tenure. Accordingly, laws should be reformed to recognize women's rights to inherit land. Also, effective local-level enforcement mechanisms need to ensure adherence to these laws (Food and Agriculture Organization, 2003a).

Impact on the supply, demand and quality of education

The epidemic's impact on education has far-reaching implications for long-term development. Globally, AIDS is a significant obstacle to children achieving universal access to primary education by 2015—a key target of both the Education for All Initiative (UNESCO, 2000) and the Millennium Development Goals (United Nations, 2001). UNESCO estimates 55 nations are unlikely to reach universal primary enrolment by 2015; 28 of these are among the 45 most AIDS-affected countries (UNESCO, 2002). An estimated US$ 1 billion per year is the net additional cost to offset the results of AIDS (i.e. the loss and absenteeism of teachers and incentives to keep orphans and vulnerable children in school).

The epidemic weakens the quality of training and education, which means fewer people benefit from good standard school and university education. It also accelerates the impact of a pre-existing professional 'brain drain'. However, responses to these issues are piecemeal; overstretched ministries with limited resources are overwhelmed by the need. Many education ministries are adding HIV prevention to their curricula—a valuable part of a successful AIDS response. However, too few are examining the epidemic's impact on the education system itself and taking appropriate action.

Supply of teachers

Teachers and lecturers belong to the most HIV-affected age group, although vulnerability patterns differ between countries. For example, in Botswana, Malawi and Uganda, teacher mortality rates were broadly compatible with general population rates, although they were higher among both primary school and male teachers (Bennell et al., 2002). In Zimbabwe, male and female teachers have infection rates similar to those of the general population—about 19% for males and 28% for females (Gregson et al., 2001). In South Africa's KwaZulu-Natal, teacher mortality varied significantly by age group (Badcock-Walters et al., 2003).

In Kenya, Uganda, Swaziland, Zambia and Zimbabwe, the epidemic is expected to significantly contribute to future shortages of primary teachers (Goliber, 2000; Malaney, 2000; Swaziland Ministry of Education, 1999). Without forward long-term planning, these countries will have great difficulty meeting their school enrolment targets. For example, if Namibia continues to train teachers at its current rate of 1000 per year and maintains a desired pupil-to-teacher ratio of one teacher for every 34 primary students, the teacher shortfall will increase from 1000 in 2001 to more than 7000 by 2010 (Malaney, 2000).

This has important implications for planners and reinforces the need for educational systems to collect precise data on the epidemic's impact on personnel. These data are needed to plan training and recruitment strategies, and create staff health-care budgets when treatment options and funding sources increase.

But AIDS is not the sole cause of teacher losses. One recent study noted that low pay and morale—already a serious problem in Malawi, Namibia, South Africa and Uganda—are contributing to overall teacher attrition (Bennell et al., 2002). Clearly, multifaceted strategies need to address the impact of the epidemic, as well as other factors depriving school systems of the teachers needed to maintain and ultimately increase school enrolment.

School attendance

Many AIDS-affected families may withdraw children from school to compensate for labour losses, increased care activities and competing expenses. If the mother is dying or has died, children, particularly girls, are needed for household duties. If the father dies, children may be less likely to stop their schooling. In three South African provinces, a survey of 771 AIDS-affected households reported that more than 40% of primary caregivers took time off work or school to care for an ill HIV-infected family member. Almost 10% of households removed a girl from school (compared with 5% for boys) (Steinberg et al., 2002). In these ways, AIDS reinforces gender inequities, deepens household poverty and threatens future generations.

Student enrolment

The epidemic may negatively affect student enrolment in other ways. Some of this is caused by reduced fertility and young adults dying from AIDS, meaning there are fewer school-

The negative impact of school fees

School fees also pose significant problems for AIDS-affected households; families simply cannot afford them. It is the primary reason children are withdrawn from school (Mutangadura, 2000; Badcock-Walters, 2001). At a societal level, these fees also negatively affect development and poverty alleviation. Yet, low- and middle-income countries' school systems often rely on these fees to cover teacher salaries and other critical expenses. Some countries are now acting to reduce the negative effect. For example, Uganda and Kenya have removed education user fees. Another approach provides families with subsidies for travel to and from school, school meals and learning materials. Several studies point to a need for assistance with secondary school fees (Mutangadura, 2000).

age children, thus decreasing social demand for education in some hard-hit areas.

Children orphaned or otherwise made vulnerable by AIDS may not attend school because they have to look after the household, care for younger siblings, or simply because they cannot afford the fees. In high-prevalence countries, the number of these children is still growing. It is crucial they have locally appropriate, affordable, non-stigmatizing, innovative educational options, such as home-based learning and distance education.

To date, in high-prevalence countries, too few governments have created policies or funding to enable children from AIDS-affected households and communities to go to school. However, Zambia's Ministry of Education has completed extensive policy and planning to meet these children's educational needs. It now actively works with the Ministry of Community Development to identify children who need subsidies to gain and keep access to education. Countries such as Kenya, which have adopted free and compulsory primary education, provide children—who would not otherwise be able to attend school—with an invaluable opportunity.

However, these children need more than short-term solutions. The impact of AIDS on education needs to be tackled in a social and economic development context (Gould and Huber, 2002). Poverty reduction efforts are critical because macroeconomic factors (e.g., the impact of structural adjustment programmes) are as likely as the AIDS epidemic to reduce a family's ability to keep children in school.

Impact on quality

Education quality may also suffer as more teachers succumb to the disease. This is because more inexperienced and under-qualified teachers and increased class sizes reduce quality student-teacher contact. In rural areas, where schools are dependent on only one or two teachers, a teacher's illness or death is especially devastating. However, there are subtler reasons why education may suffer, including the lack of motivation or ability to teach and learn because of 'AIDS in the family' or among colleagues (Harris and Schubert, 2001).

Moreover, skilled teachers are not easily replaced. In hard-hit countries, more teachers need to be trained, but this is currently beyond the capacity of many countries' university or college systems. Other possible strategies include reducing the teacher training period, enticing former teachers to return to the education system, and allowing teachers to work after retirement age.

Extraordinary actions are required to prevent the epidemic from doing permanent damage to education systems and students. However, in sub-Saharan Africa, little is being done to deal with current or future teacher shortages.

Taking action

The Fast Track Initiative on Education for All grew out of the Monterrey consensus in 2002 (see 'Finance' chapter). This initiative seeks to ensure that no country with a credible education-sector plan embedded within a poverty reduction strategy fails to achieve the Millennium Development Goal of Universal Primary Completion by 2015 due to unpredictable long-term finance.

The Fast Track Initiative partners—which comprise all the major bilateral donors, the World Bank, UNICEF, UNESCO, UNAIDS, NGOs and recipient countries—seek to catalyse sound education-sector policies that include HIV and gender strategies, encourage appropriate domestic financing, improve aid effectiveness, and mobilize increased aid for primary education.

Impact on the health sector

Effective strategies to address AIDS need robust, flexible health systems. However, the epidemic hit just when many countries were reducing public-service spending to repay debt and conform to international finance institutions' requirements. On top of this, the epidemic itself has contributed to rapid health-sector deterioration by increasing burdens on already-strapped systems and steadily depriving countries of essential health-care workers. Staff losses and absenteeism caused by sickness and death mean health-care sectors must recruit and train more staff. At the same time, large numbers of uninfected workers are suffering from burnout and emotional exhaustion.

In African countries, studies estimate AIDS causes between 19% and 53% of all government health employee deaths (Tawfik and Kinoti, 2001). For example, Malawi and Zambia have experienced five- to sixfold increases in health-worker illness and death rates (UNDP, 2001). In fact, the epidemic is quickly outstripping growth in the supply of health-sector workers (Liese et al., 2003). This comes when the need for health-care services is increasing rapidly in heavily-affected countries.

Health-care workers need to be sensitized to the effects of AIDS, so they can provide non-stigmatizing care. But AIDS also adversely affects uninfected patients' quality of care, as overburdened health-care sectors adopt a triage approach that de-emphasizes patient care for conditions less severe than AIDS (USAID, 2002).

Taking action

In most low- and middle-income countries, action is urgently required to strengthen chronically weak health systems and protect the health and safety of personnel. Opinions remain varied on possible strategies, but consensus emerged at a high-level forum on the health Millenium Development Goals on the following key actions:

- Policy initiatives to address push-pull factors that encourage health-sector personnel to migrate to other regions or countries, which leads to chronic understaffing. Other widely promoted actions include: targeting HIV-positive health workers for antiretroviral treatment; improving salaries and benefits to retain and attract back highly trained staff; and reducing rigid application of professional rules so health and non-health professionals can take on additional functions.
- A 'system-wide approach' that harmonizes multiple-donor support, as well as giving low-and middle-income countries a greater role in setting priorities and deploying resources.
- Strengthening countries' health-management information systems and establishing structures to monitor progress towards the health-related Millennium Development Goals.
- Expanding pre-service and in-service training.
- Ensuring workers' occupational safety and health by providing information, protective clothing, and adequate equipment.
- Expanding the service-provision roles of NGOs and private providers.

Impact on public-sector capacity

An effective and functioning public sector is vital for delivering essential goods and services, and developing successful national AIDS responses. Before the epidemic, several worst-affected countries were already struggling with daunting development challenges, excessive debt burdens, and declining trade. In many low- and middle-income countries, adjustment programmes involved deep public-spending cuts, and governments currently struggle to provide basic social services, support and infrastructure. In the worst-affected countries, AIDS has additionally undermined the public sector's functional effectiveness (Cohen, 2002). When essential services falter, the poor and most vulnerable endure the worst consequences.

UNDP's comprehensive study, *The impact of HIV/AIDS on human resources in the Malawi public sector* showed the country's annual loss of governmental staff rose almost sixfold between 1990 and 2000, primarily due to premature AIDS deaths (UNDP, 2002). During the study period, public-service mortality increased by a factor of 10. Deaths were disproportionately high among young adults of both sexes—a strong indication AIDS was primarily responsible. In 2000, more than half of the country's established posts in the education and water departments stood vacant (Malawi Institute of Management/UNDP, 2002). Furthermore, other Southern African countries' key ministries report half or more of their posts are unfilled (Cohen, 2002).

Few studies have comprehensively analysed the epidemic's impact on public-sector productivity. However, it is reasonable to conclude that such high vacancy rates inevitably lead to poorer coverage and quality of government services.

Impact on workers and the workplace

AIDS threatens economic security and development because it primarily strikes the working-age population. This has implications for survival of communities and enterprises, as well as long-term maintenance of productive capacity. The epidemic erodes economic growth through its impact on labour supply and productivity, savings rates, and the delivery of essential services. Individuals living with HIV lose jobs, incomes and savings. As a result, they consume and invest less. The workplace—farms, factories, market stalls or government offices—becomes less productive or sometimes fails, reducing output, profits, tax revenue and investment.

In hard-hit countries, AIDS is likely to reduce the labour force's growth rate. The International Labour Organization (ILO) projects that the labour force in 38 countries (all but four in Africa) will be between 5% and

Ministries of agriculture staff and HIV

In Eastern and Southern Africa, a recent report examining AIDS and agriculture concluded illness and death among government agricultural employees undermined governmental capacity to respond adequately to the epidemic. In Kenya's Ministry of Agriculture, AIDS caused 58% of all staff deaths in the past five years. Meanwhile, some 16% of staff in Malawi's Ministry of Agriculture and Irrigation are HIV-positive (Topouzis, 2003).

35% smaller by 2020 because of AIDS. The epidemic also affects workforce quality, since AIDS-affected workers are replaced by younger, less-experienced men and women. At the same time, the loss of teachers and trainers results in future generations with lower skill levels (Lisk, 2002). South Africa's Labour Department says an estimated 3% of the country's workforce (or roughly 500 000 workers) could be in the terminal stages of AIDS by 2010—a threefold increase over the 2001 estimate.

Increasing the cost of doing business

AIDS reduces output by squeezing productivity, adding costs, diverting productive resources, depleting skills and distorting the labour market. For employers, employee health expenses and funeral costs are rising as productivity and profits decline. The epidemic increases absenteeism, organizational disruption, and the loss of skills and 'organizational memory'. The loss of supervisory workers can have an especially harsh impact, since their acquired knowledge and skills are seldom replaced simply by hiring others. In hard-hit areas, the general shortage of skilled workers and management-level staff can mean positions stay vacant for months or even years—at a significant cost to productivity.

The effects can be even harsher for small businesses and the informal economy—both sources of work for most women and men in low- and middle-income countries. Almost invariably, workers in the informal economy lack health insurance or access to medical facilities at their workplaces, and their livelihoods are heavily reliant on their labour and skills. Workers in the informal economy also have little access to AIDS workplace programmes.

Reducing workplace impact

Supporting workplace prevention programmes for employees and management makes good economic and developmental sense. So, too, does providing health care in workplace settings, and endorsing policies of non-discrimination against employees living with HIV. A major South African insurance company's 2003 health-care survey found more than two-thirds of 26 major companies questioned said they had developed an AIDS strategy. Thailand's American International Insurance has an evaluation and accreditation programme to test and acknowledge when companies have appropriate AIDS-prevention policies. Companies that secure accreditation and continue to pass prevention policy audits are given discounted group-life insurance premiums.

A Pan-African Employers' Confederation survey found all national employers' organizations had an AIDS policy and had encouraged their members to implement workplace programmes and collaborate with National AIDS Councils. Increasingly, companies advocate voluntary, confidential counselling and testing, and provide antiretroviral treatment to workers. At the same time, they assure them that testing HIV-positive will not cause them to lose their employment.

The ILO encourages a comprehensive approach to workplace polices and programmes, based on protecting infected and affected workers' rights, and offering prevention and care services. Its Code of Practice on HIV/AIDS and the world of work is a framework for action that establishes policy development principles, and provides practical programming guidance on prevention and behaviour change; protecting workers' rights and benefits; and treatment, care and support needs.

In partnership with the Global Fund to Fight AIDS, Tuberculosis and Malaria, and the Global Business Coalition on HIV/AIDS, the ILO works to extend care and treatment access through occupational health services, and supports community outreach. But many HIV-positive workers are reluctant to participate in such programmes because they fear losing their jobs or being ostracized. Developing a climate that encourages workers' participation can be facilitated by involving trade unions or workers' representatives in planning and implementing workplace programmes.

Trade unions, and confederations of trade unions, are playing an increasingly important role in strengthening national AIDS responses. For example, the South African Clothing and Textile Workers' Union provided HIV and AIDS training to 1100 shop stewards between 2002 and 2004. The union also actively supports voluntary, confidential counselling and testing, and develops union-based support groups for HIV-positive workers. Furthermore, the South African Clothing and Textile Workers' Union and other unions are dynamic participants in the Treatment Action Campaign, which helped persuade the South African Government to provide antiretroviral therapy through the public sector (see 'Treatment' chapter and 'People living with AIDS' focus).

Macroeconomic impact

In high-prevalence countries, the combined negative effects of AIDS on finances—of households, employers and key sectors—are likely to have tangible macroeconomic impact; however, most estimates of this impact appear to be relatively modest (see Figure 14). These estimates apply to the highest prevalence countries. Lower prevalence countries, such as those in Latin America and the Caribbean, Eastern Europe, and South and South-East Asia, are likely to have smaller macroeconomic impacts. For the most part, available estimates apply to short- or medium-term projections (10–25 years). Over this period, the models estimate that the effect of AIDS on Gross Domestic Product growth is approximately matched by the impact on total population over the same period. That is, negative effects on production are counterbalanced by similar reductions in resource consumption. As a result, the epidemic's impact on per-capita Gross Domestic Product is relatively small—and even positive in some of the scenarios considered.

This results from the implicit assumption that most low- and middle-income countries have a surplus of unskilled labour in the formal sector, so that the short-term effect of excess mortality will include a reduction in the unemployment rate and a rise in skilled wages. In addition, lower population growth reduces the pressure on land and physical capital, so that production becomes more capital-intensive, and labour productivity increases. Available models used assume that the economies of affected countries have sufficient flexibility for these adjustments to occur.

These modelling exercises may underestimate the longer-term impact on economic growth in heavily affected countries, should the number of people affected and infected continue to grow rapidly. Few models can capture the economic costs of institutional dysfunction, for example, or the costs of a severe distortion in the supply and distribution of labour power, intergenerational transmission of knowledge and skills, or of the disruption of lifetime capital acquisition and inheritance.

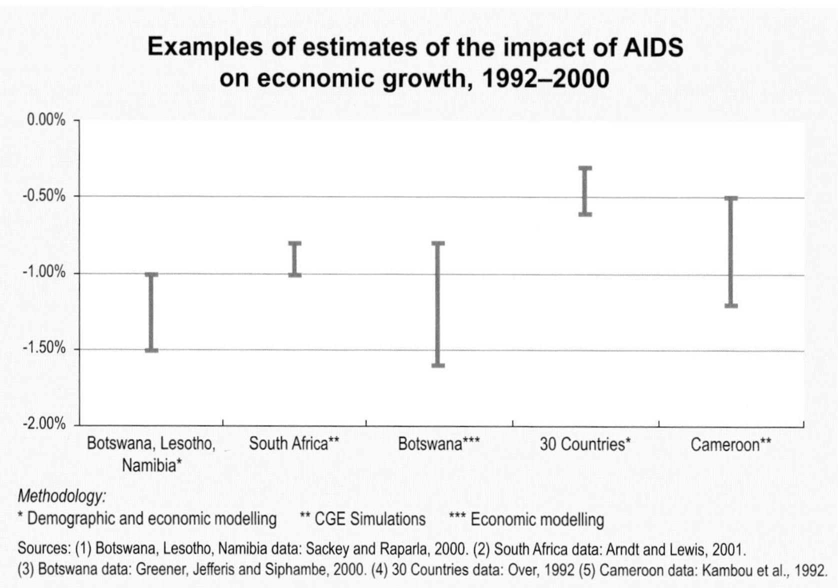

Figure 14

Pessimistic estimates of macroeconomic impact in the long run were reported in a recent joint study by Heidelberg University and the World Bank (Bell et al., 2003), using South Africa as a test case. The long-term economic costs of AIDS could be 'devastating' because of the cumulative weakening from generation to generation of human capital. To avoid such an outcome, the study advised greater spending to contain the epidemic, more funds to provide treatment and care for those infected, increased aid for orphans via income support or subsidies that are linked to school attendance, and taxes to finance these expenditures.

Perhaps the most significant impact of the epidemic will be on government budgets. Governments will witness reduced growth in tax revenues as economic growth slows, while budgetary demands for health care and social welfare will increase. Governments will face the same increased AIDS-related employment costs as those faced by the private sector, including increased training and recruitment costs and changes to the structure of health insurance and pensions. These combined effects are likely to complicate efforts to balance government budgets for many years to come, and will significantly inhibit the capacity of governments in high-prevalence countries to mount an adequate response without external assistance.

Challenges of the 'Next Agenda'

The impacts of AIDS on the development capacity of poor countries will significantly undermine their ability to make substantive progress towards the Millennium Development Goals, particularly in regard to poverty reduction, education and health targets and the care of orphans. The epidemic has placed multiple challenges before the international community, cutting across every sector. These challenges include:

- Embedding the message that AIDS is both a global emergency and a long-term development crisis that requires an exceptional and sustained response, far beyond the scale of what we have seen to date.
- Ensuring there is universal recognition that AIDS is reversing decades of development progress in the most-affected countries. Therefore, strengthening the response to

AIDS must be a central part of development programming and practice.

- Reorienting situation assessment and early warning systems to a 'people focus' with greater attention to household impacts.
- Developing new strategies to deal with the disproportionate impact of the epidemic on women, girls and orphans, including microcredit, school support and food assistance programmes.
- Developing strategies for radical and innovative approaches to restoring human capacity in the worst-affected countries; for example, massive antiretroviral therapy programmes, a complete re-thinking of how skills will be built, retained and sustained, salary support, stopping the drain of health and administrative workers, etc.
- Developing long-term strategies to replace the short-term 'Band-Aid' approaches which have dominated the response up until now. The epidemic is not going to be resolved in the short-term; strategists need to be looking 10–20, even 30, years ahead.

Focus

AIDS and orphans: a tragedy unfolding

"We wanted to stay together after our parents and grandparents died of AIDS. I want to go back to school, but there is no money… I must work hard to get a good life and look after myself not to get the disease my mother and father had." – *Felix, 15 years old, the sole income earner in a household that includes his five younger siblings and an 80-year-old great uncle*

Children orphaned by AIDS are found in almost every country of the world. In some countries, there are only a few hundred or a few thousand. In Africa, there are millions. All have suffered the tragedy of losing one or both parents to AIDS, and many are growing up in deprived and traumatic circumstances without the support and care of their immediate family (see Figure 15).

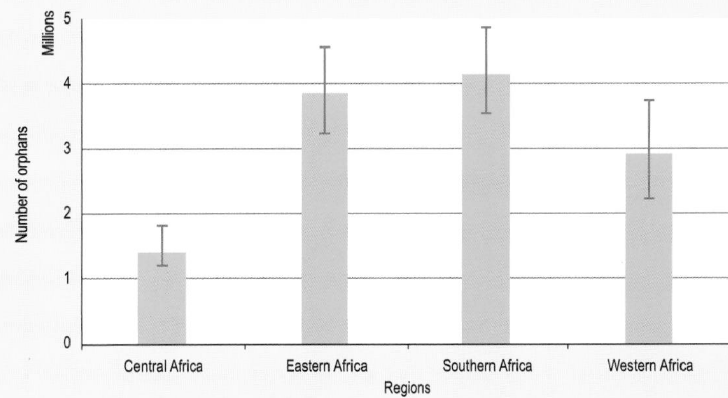

Figure 15

Children orphaned by AIDS range in age from a few days or months old to 18 years of age. In countries with low-level and concentrated epidemics, it is impossible to reliably estimate the number of children orphaned by AIDS, or to determine what percentage they represent of all orphans.

The worst orphan crisis is in sub-Saharan Africa, where 12 million children have lost one or both parents to AIDS. By 2010, this number is expected to climb to more than 18 million. As staggering as these numbers are, the crisis will worsen if parents struck by HIV do not get access to life-prolonging treatment and effective prevention services.

Some countries have yet to experience the full impact of parental deaths. For example, in South Africa, the number of orphans is expected to increase from 2.2 million (12% of all children) in 2003 to 3.1 million (18% of all children) by 2010. Even in countries where HIV prevalence has stabilized or declined, the number of orphans continues to rise due to the time lag between when parents become infected and when they die.

Despite the daunting numbers, children orphaned by the epidemic can still have safe, healthy and productive childhoods, but only if all sectors of society respond with immediate, sustained and coordinated efforts that give high priority to protecting children and preserving the family unit.

Who is an 'orphan'?

An orphan is defined as a child under the age of 18 who has had at least one parent die. A child whose mother has died is known as a maternal orphan; a child whose father has died is a paternal orphan. A child who has lost both parents is a double orphan.

Many agencies now avoid using the term 'AIDS orphan' as it is stigmatizing. Extensive research shows that stigma prevents governments and communities from effectively responding to the orphan problem, as well as hindering the emotional recovery of affected children themselves (Stein, 2003). Stigma and discrimination also intensify violations of these children's rights—in particular, their access to education, social services, and community and familial support (see 'Human Rights' focus).

The impact on children

Even people who work with orphaned children struggle to understand the emotional anguish a child experiences as he or she watches one or both of his or her parents die. When one parent is HIV-infected, the probability is high that the other parent is as well. Therefore, children often lose both parents in quick succession. An orphan's caregivers may also succumb to AIDS, with the result that children may suffer multiple bereavements. The child's suffering is often compounded by being separated from his or her siblings.

For example, in a report from Zambia, separated siblings said they see each other less than once a month (Family Health International, 2002). Many experience depression, anger, guilt and fear for their futures. This experience can lead to serious psychological problems such as post-traumatic stress syndrome,

Figure 15a

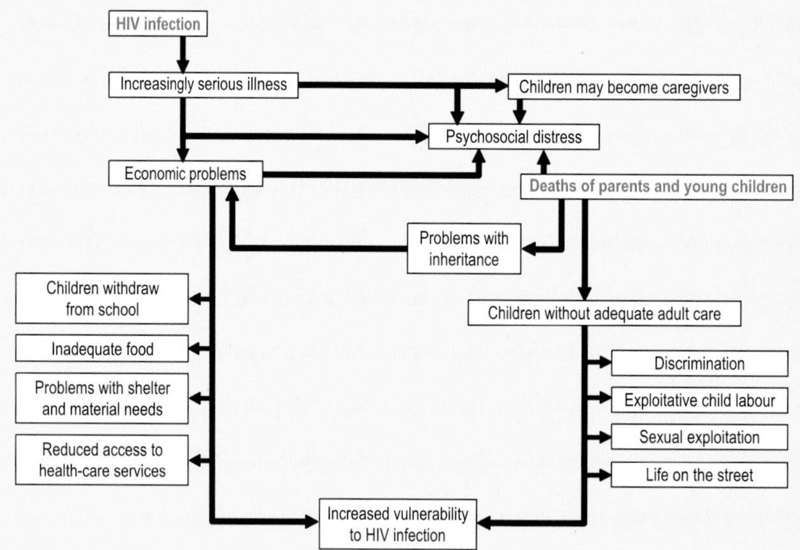

Source: Williamson, J. (2004) *A Family is for Life* (draft), USAID and the Synergy Project. Washington.

alcohol and drug abuse, aggression, and even suicide (Foster, 2002).

Poverty and social dislocation also add to an orphaned child's emotional distress. Factors such as loss of household incomes, the cost of treating HIV-related illnesses, and funeral expenses frequently leave orphaned children destitute. A parent's death also deprives them of the learning and values they need to become socially knowledgeable and economically productive adults. Recent research suggests that this breakdown in intergenerational knowledge may play a part in a country's economic decline (Bell et al., 2003).

Orphans at risk

Without the protective environment of their homes, orphaned children face increased risk of violence, exploitation and abuse. They may be ill-treated by their guardians, and dispossessed of their inheritance and property. Those living with foster families are more likely to be malnourished, underweight, or short for their age in comparison to non-orphans (Monasch and Snoad, 2003). In worst-case scenarios, orphaned children may be abducted and enrolled as child soldiers or driven to hard labour, sex work, or life on the streets.

In Cambodia, a recent study by the Khmer HIV/AIDS NGO Alliance and Family Health International found that about one in five children in AIDS-affected families reported that they had to start working in the previous six months to support their family. One in three had to provide care and take on major household work. Many had to leave school, forego necessities such as food and clothes, or be sent away from their home. All of the children surveyed had been exposed to high levels of stigma and psychosocial stress, with girls more vulnerable than boys.

However, there are many examples of successful help for orphans in these situations. In Zimbabwe, since 1998, the Salvation Army's Mayise Camp has provided psychosocial support to orphaned children. It recently expanded its care services to tackle violence, exploitation and abuse. Since children often have trouble obtaining medical, psychological and legal services, the Camp started a Mobile Law Clinic that brings essential services to the children. In Cambodia, the nongovernmental organization *Mith Samlanh* ('friends') runs 12 interlinked programmes for 1500 street children, ranging from HIV prevention and care, to reproductive health education and income-generating activities.

Ensuring access to education is critical in responding to the orphan crisis. Orphans often fall behind or drop out of school, compromising their psychosocial development and future prospects. This also affects a country's long-term recovery from the epidemic. For instance, research in the United Republic of Tanzania revealed that the school-attendance rate among orphans who had lost one parent was only 71%. Among double orphans it was even lower at 52% (Monasch and Snoad, 2003).

Staying in school offers orphaned children the best chance of escaping extreme poverty and its associated risks. Thus, everything possible needs to be done to keep them in school. For example, China's Henan Province recently announced that orphans living with their extended family would receive free primary and secondary schooling, and financial support for further studies. Similarly, Jamaica's National AIDS Committee helps some of the country's orphaned children with school-related expenses, including school fees, uniforms and books.

Grandmothers to the rescue: the 'Go-Go Grannies'

The Go-Go Grannies are a group of grandmothers in South Africa's Alexandra Township who help and encourage each other as they raise their orphaned grandchildren. They have lost their own children to AIDS and are now finding it difficult to cope, both emotionally and physically. The Grannies are part of the Alexandra AIDS Orphans Project, which runs support-group programmes for children and caregivers living with, and affected by, the epidemic. The project currently provides psychosocial, financial and material support to 30 grandmothers. This includes one-time building grants to ensure adequate shelter for their growing families, as well as seeds and fertilizers so the women can start their own gardens to bring in food and income for their families.

Strengthening the capacity of families to protect and care for children

Preserving some sort of family life is extremely important for children who have lost one or both parents to AIDS, whether the family is headed by the lone remaining parent, a grandparent, or another relative. Women and girls of all ages are shouldering much of the burden of the orphan crisis. Young girls may drop out of school to tend to ailing parents, look after household duties, or care for younger siblings. Mothers are more likely than fathers to continue to care for their children after the death of the spouse, and women are more willing to take in other orphans.

Then there are the grandmothers—older women who care for their own children when the latter fall ill, and eventually become surrogate parents to their bereaved grandchildren, often with few resources (see Figure 16). For example, studies in Thailand show that almost half of the country's orphaned children live with their grandparents. Projects to support these elderly caregivers have been developed in response. In Chiang Mai, the Mother Child Concern Foundation helps to strengthen older people's associations, develops volunteer schemes to assist older caregivers, and provides low-interest loans to set up small businesses.

Formal institutions, such as orphanages, may provide a last resort for a limited number of orphaned or sick children. In the early days of the orphan crisis, countries such as Zimbabwe built a number of orphanages. But it quickly became apparent that the orphanage solution was unsustainable and conflicted with a child's fundamental right to grow up in a family environment.

If preserving the family is the best option for orphaned children, then the family's capacity to care for, and protect, these children must be urgently strengthened. This means adopting programmes that keep parents living with AIDS alive and healthy as long as possible, improve a household's money-earning capacity, and provide children and their caregivers with psychosocial and other support.

Thailand is one country in which family capacity has been strengthened. There, the MTCT-Plus Programme (mother-to-child transmission plus antiretroviral treatment) provides antiretroviral treatment for HIV-positive mothers, their infected partners, and children (Beckerman, 2002). The programme was launched by UNICEF and Columbia University's Mailman School of Public Health, and links preventing mother-to-child transmission with treatment and care options in antenatal-care clinics. The programme also operates in Côte d'Ivoire, Kenya, Mozambique, Rwanda, South Africa, Uganda and Zambia (UNICEF, 2003).

Growing role of grandparents

Relationships of double orphans and single orphans (not living with surviving parent) to head of household, Namibia, 1992 and 2000

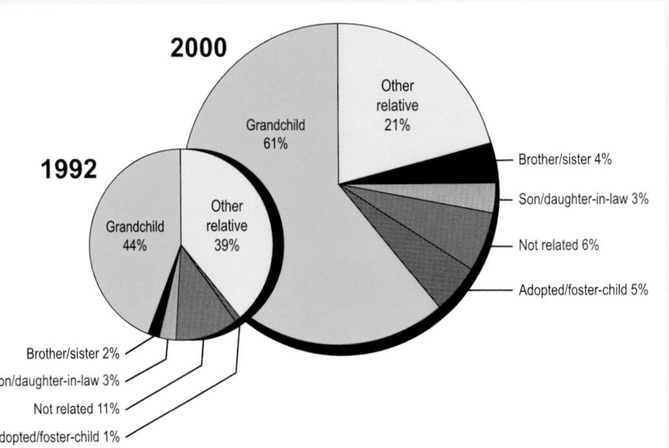

Sources: UNICEF-MICS, Measure DHS, 1992 and 2000

Figure 16

Better nutrition and food security will improve a family's overall health and increase the time parents and children have together. For instance, in Haiti, the international NGO, Hunger Grow Away, is promoting a new micro-intensive gardening system that uses limited viable soil, water resources, tools and labour to offer orphaned children and their caregivers food security and incomes.

Mobilizing community-based responses

Communities are capable of responding effectively to the plight of orphans and children whose parents are dying of AIDS. A wide variety of relatively formal projects has sprung up from the concern of families, neighbours and religious groups. A case in point is Cambodia. The monks at Wat Kien Kes Temple provide some of the country's orphans and vulnerable children with vocational training and income-generating skills to improve their standard of living. They also mobilize local communities to donate food, land and material goods to affected families. The monks have also stimulated HIV-oriented dialogue within the community, which raises AIDS awareness, engenders compassion and reduces discrimination (USAID, 2004). If properly recognized and supported, these initiatives can provide the backbone of national strategies (Foster, 2002).

National action plans needed

Until now, most orphan-support interventions have been piecemeal and have not matched the scale of the problem. In Uganda, officials recognized the orphan crisis early on. Yet government assistance fell short of the need, with only an estimated 5% of orphans receiving some sort of help between 1998 and 2000 (Deininger, et al., 2003). Clearly, urgent steps to scale up and replicate successful interventions are required and should include the following 'country commitments' to:

- conducting participatory situation analyses;
- implementing a national policy and legislation review to better protect children;
- establishing national coordination mechanisms for responding to the orphan challenge;
- developing and implementing national action plans addressing both orphan prevention and the needs of orphans; and
- implementing monitoring and evaluation activities based on indicators that specifically measure effects on the well-being of orphans and children made vulnerable by HIV and AIDS (UNICEF et al., 2004).

The 2003 report on progress in meeting the 2001 UN Declaration of Commitment on HIV/AIDS goals notes that 39% of countries with 'generalized epidemics' have no national policies to provide orphaned and vulnerable children with essential support (UNAIDS,

2003). Some 14% of these countries are developing policies, but 25% have no plans to do so.

The orphan challenge needs to be met through resolute political will before it reaches crisis proportions. In countries, a wide range of government and civil society stakeholders need to provide financial help to children, families and communities, along with HIV prevention, care and support.

National policies, such as those developed by Honduras, Jamaica, Malawi, Rwanda, Swaziland, Thailand and Uganda, are a good starting point. But policies are meaningless if there is no commitment to translate them into practical action. Families and communities often demonstrate strong commitments and resiliency, and are leading the responses to protect children affected by AIDS. Policy frameworks and national plans need to provide environments that foster these efforts so that orphans can survive and thrive in the future.

4

Bringing comprehensive HIV prevention to scale

4

Prevention needs of girls and women

Despite women's higher biological vulnerability, it is the legal, social and economic disadvantages faced by women and girls in most societies that greatly increase their HIV vulnerability. Therefore, gender-sensitive approaches are key when designing prevention programmes.

Not as easy as ABC

For years, prevention programmes for the general population have focused on the 'ABC' strategy—abstain and delay sexual initiation; be safer by being faithful or reducing the number of sexual partners; and use condoms correctly and consistently. For many women and girls, this approach is of limited value. They lack social and economic power, and live in fear of male violence. They cannot negotiate abstinence from sex, nor can they insist their partners remain faithful or use condoms.

Ironically, trust and affection within marriage and other long-term relationships are sometimes part of the problem. Studies from various parts of the world suggest married couples have sex more frequently than unmarried individuals, but use condoms less often. Global studies of relationships between sex workers and their clients show a similar pattern: condom use was less consistent if sex workers felt a level of intimacy with their regular clients. For example, in Kenya's Nyanza Province, surveyed clients of sex workers reported using condoms less consistently if they were with their usual sex worker (Helene et al., 2002).

A range of approaches needed

Many women are denied the knowledge and tools to protect themselves from HIV. Surveys in 38 countries found extremely low HIV-transmission knowledge among 15–24-year-old women (UNFPA, 2002). It is vital to implement comprehensive strategies, including gender-specific and culturally specific services that help women counteract discriminatory social and economic factors. Key components include: access to education (particularly secondary education); strengthening legal protection for women's property and inheritance rights; eradicating violence against women and girls; and ensuring equitable access to HIV care and prevention services. Men are often regarded as a major part of the problem. However, they need to be a substantial part of the solution by: taking responsibility for fidelity and safer sex; committing themselves to their daughters' education; alleviating women's burden of care; and embracing a zero-tolerance attitude towards violence against women.

In June 2002, the World Health Organization (WHO) and the International Center for Research on Women led a consultation of experts to rethink classic HIV prevention based on women's and girls' distinct needs. They also aimed to improve HIV interventions that target men (WHO, 2003). The experts described a continuum of approaches to integrate gender into prevention programmes:

- *Gender-sensitive approaches*, at a minimum, recognize that women and men have different prevention, care and support needs. For example, diagnosing and treating sexually transmitted infections need to be integrated into family planning/reproductive health clinics. Then women will be able to gain access to these services without fear of social censure. Another example is promoting female-controlled prevention tools, such as female condoms or microbicides.
- *Approaches that transform gender roles*. These work with men and women to overturn gender norms that create HIV vulnerability. Involving men in these approaches is critical to fostering constructive roles for men in sexual and reproductive health. One of the best-known examples is the 'Stepping Stones' participatory approach to HIV, sexual health and gender. It was first developed in Uganda in the mid-1990s, and is now used in more than 100 countries. Peer groups of 10 to 20 people of the same sex and similar age are formed to discuss gender roles, money, attitudes to sex and sexuality and attitudes to death. These peer environments encourage women and men of all ages to explore their social, sexual and psychological needs, analyse the communication blocks they face and make changes in their relationships.
- *Interventions that empower women and girls* attempt to equalize the power balance between women and men. Examples include increasing women's access to assets and resources, such as land and inheritance rights, and facilitating women's networks and strengthening grassroots community organizations. Other projects go beyond immediate gender-specific needs. They are based on the belief that empowerment can only be achieved when women take control of all aspects of their lives. For instance, India's Sonagachi Project involving sex workers has a self-governing structure and uses peer educators, making it an international empowerment model for HIV prevention among sex workers and their clients.

Gender-sensitive programming can often be achieved in the short term since national policy-makers and international donors understand and accept it. Developing more discrete, female-controlled prevention tools, such as microbicides, will greatly enhance these approaches. In the longer term, modifying the gender-based realities that drive the epidemic will require wide-scale transformative and empowering approaches. The effects of doing this will take longer to become evident, but are essential to halting the epidemic.

Bringing comprehensive HIV prevention to scale

Prevention is the mainstay of the response to AIDS, but is seldom implemented at a scale that would turn the tide of the epidemic. Effective, inexpensive and relatively simple HIV prevention interventions do exist, but the pace of the epidemic is clearly outstripping most country efforts towards effective prevention programming. Globally, less than one-fifth of people who need it have any access to prevention services (Policy Project, 2004).

Today, expanded access to antiretroviral therapy is bringing hope to millions of people living with HIV; it is vital that this be matched by expanded prevention programming. Dramatically expanding prevention programmes would have a profound impact on HIV infection levels. Comprehensive prevention could avert 29 million of the 45 million new infections projected to occur this decade (Stover et al., 2002) (see Figure 17). Moreover, without sharply reducing HIV incidence, expanded access to treatment becomes unsustainable. Antiretroviral therapy providers will be swamped by demand.

Figure 17

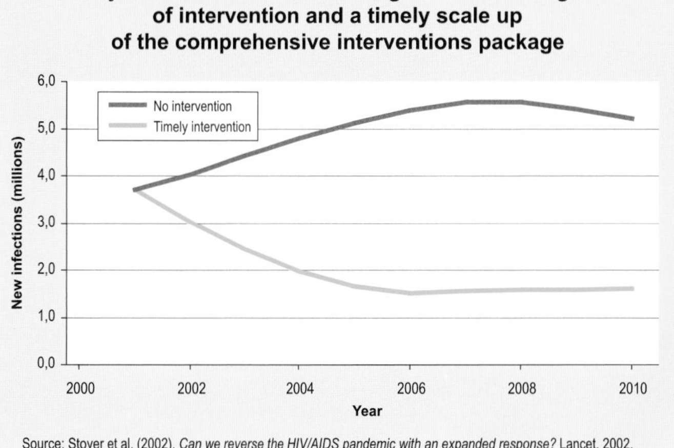

Source: Stover et al. (2002). *Can we reverse the HIV/AIDS pandemic with an expanded response?* Lancet, 2002.

In the 2001 UN Declaration of Commitment on HIV/AIDS, countries around the world committed themselves to massively scaling up prevention programmes. The Declaration's goal is to reduce HIV prevalence among young people (15–24 years old) by 25% in the most affected countries, and to reduce the proportion of infants infected with HIV by 20%, both by 2005.

If current trends continue, many countries will fall short of these targets. In the hardest-hit countries of sub-Saharan Africa, few people have access to prevention programmes despite extraordinarily high infection rates. In other regions where the epidemic is rapidly emerging, opportunities to stop its expansion still exist—but only if prevention efforts are accelerated.

Meeting new prevention challenges

Fortunately, a number of countries are demonstrating results in reducing HIV infection rates. Senegal, Thailand and Uganda pioneered early HIV prevention successes. In recent years, similar progress has been recorded in countries as diverse as Brazil, Cambodia and the Dominican Republic. The global community can learn from these prevention successes and adapt them. An overall lesson is that an effective

Progress update on the global response to the AIDS epidemic, 2004

Prevention programmes reach fewer than one in five people who need them

- According to estimates from 70 countries responding to a 2003 coverage survey, the proportion of pregnant women covered by services to prevent mother-to-child HIV transmission ranges from 2% in the Western Pacific, to 5% in sub-Saharan Africa, and 34% in the Americas.
- The proportion of adults needing voluntary counselling and testing who received it ranged from almost none in South-East Asia, to 7% in sub-Saharan Africa, and 1.5% in Eastern Europe.
- Condom use in sex acts with a non-cohabiting partner ranged from 13% in South-East Asia, to 19% in sub-Saharan Africa.
- Fewer than 10% of surveyed countries with significant HIV transmission among injecting drug users have access to harm-reduction programmes.
- In the Americas, nearly 30% of men who have sex with men have access to prevention services, compared with 6% in sub-Saharan Africa. In South-East Asia, 16% of the estimated 2.2 million sex workers benefit from basic prevention services, compared with around 32% of the estimated 2.5 million sex workers in sub-Saharan Africa.
- In sub-Saharan Africa, nearly 60% of primary school students receive basic AIDS education, compared with 13% in the Western Pacific region.

Source: *Progress report on the global response to the HIV/AIDS epidemic,* UNAIDS, 2003; *Coverage of selected services for HIV/AIDS prevention and care in low- and middle-income countries in 2003,* Policy Project, 2004.

Reinforcing strategies of risk, vulnerability and impact reduction

Figure 18

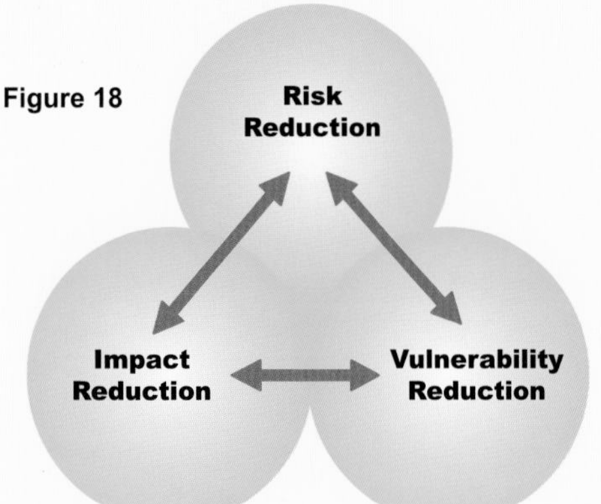

Source: UNAIDS, The Global Strategy Framework on HIV/AIDS (Reinforcing strategies of risk, vulnerability and impact reduction: The expanded response to the epidemic), 2001

response is anchored in three strategies, which are highly inter-related (UNAIDS, 2002):

- decreasing the risk of infection to slow down the epidemic;
- decreasing vulnerability to reduce both risk and impact; and
- reducing impact in order to decrease vulnerability.

At the same time, HIV prevention needs to evolve and be more innovative in addressing changes in the epidemic. For example, in several industrialized countries, risk behaviours and new infections are rising again among populations in which prevalence had stabilized or declined—particularly among young men who have sex with men. This has been linked to the promise of antiretroviral therapies (Ostrow et al., 2002; Suarez et al., 2001) as well as 'prevention fatigue' and the fact that many young people are now coming of age without having experienced the epidemic's devastations.

New or greatly increased efforts are needed to prevent HIV in women and girls, as even the best-designed interventions will have limited success unless supported by sustained efforts to attack the root causes of their vulnerability (see box on page 68). Equally, the challenge of 'keeping the next generation HIV-free' means that far more resources must be invested in prevention among young people of both sexes.

Expanded access to antiretroviral therapy and other treatment offers a critical opportunity to

Reducing vulnerability among mine workers

Most of South Africa's 300 000 gold and platinum miners work far from home and see their families only once a year—a system that originated under colonialism and flourished under apartheid. This system is one of the factors driving the country's HIV epidemic, exposing miners to a host of risk situations. Today, that is changing for many men as companies work to replace crowded, all-male hostels with low-cost, family housing, often working with local governments to build houses and convert old hostels.

Lonmin Platinum is one of the leaders in these efforts. It is the world's third-biggest platinum group metals producer and employs 16 000 regular mine workers. It has built more than 1000 dwellings to date and aims to build an additional 2000 in short order. And the company has gone even further. On World AIDS Day 2003, it started providing HIV-positive employees with antiretroviral treatment, and is considering the possibility of extending the programme to their families.

strengthen prevention efforts, by encouraging vastly more people to learn their HIV status. This is likely to occur both because the promise of treatment should stimulate greater use of voluntary counselling and testing, and because health-care providers will increasingly make the offer of diagnostic testing a routine practice in clinical settings. This, combined with visible treatment successes, should encourage more open dialogue about HIV. Messages of care and compassion from political, religious and community leaders will also help reduce stigma towards people living with HIV.

Reducing vulnerability

Effective prevention requires policies that help reduce the vulnerability of large numbers of people—in effect, creating a social, legal and economic environment in which prevention is possible. An effective response to AIDS goes hand in hand with basic socioeconomic development. Studies in sub-Saharan Africa show that men and women living in areas with higher indicators of development such as life expectancy and literacy are significantly more likely to use condoms (Ukwuani et al., 2003). Boys in Zimbabwe who remain in school and have intact families are more likely to practise safer sex (Betts et al., 2003). Studies in sub-Saharan Africa and the Caribbean indicate that women are less likely to use condoms than men due to gender-related power dynamics, which make it more difficult for women to request the use of condoms (Norman, 2003).

Initiatives that enhance economic and social development and empower women and girls also contribute to effective AIDS responses. Such prevention-friendly efforts take many forms and can often be implemented by both public and private sectors. For example, in South Africa, mining companies are building migrant mine workers family housing to replace the overcrowded, single-sex hostels that have been an important contributor to HIV transmission in the region (see box above). Eliminating school fees in Uganda and Kenya helps get new poor pupils into school and keep young people, notably girls, in school. Legislation legalizing the purchase and possession of sterile injecting equipment can reduce HIV transmission among injecting drug users without contributing to increased drug use. Similarly, international cooperation to prevent human trafficking for sexual exploitation reduces the number of young people exposed to an extremely high risk of HIV, violence and other human rights abuses.

Comprehensive prevention

Comprehensive prevention addresses all modes of HIV transmission. Since HIV epidemics

4

are extremely diverse across regions, within countries and over time, programme planners need to place different emphases on the mix of strategies:

- in **low-prevalence settings**, prevention among key population groups (e.g., sex workers and their clients, injecting drug users, men who have sex with men) can be effective in keeping HIV at low levels in the general population;
- in **high-prevalence settings**, prevention among key populations continues to be important, but broad strategies reaching all segments of society are needed to turn the epidemic around; and
- in **all countries**, prevention is impeded if universal access to treatment, as well as impact and vulnerability-reduction measures, are not clearly parts of the response.

Vulnerability to HIV exposure—an individual or community's inability to control their risk of infection—is multifaceted, so no single prevention intervention will be effective on its own. Key elements in comprehensive HIV prevention include:

- AIDS education and awareness;
- behaviour change programmes, especially for young people and populations at higher risk of HIV exposure, as well as for people living with HIV;
- promoting male and female condoms as a protective option, along with abstinence, fidelity and reducing the number of sexual partners;
- voluntary counselling and testing;
- preventing and treating sexually transmitted infections;
- primary prevention among pregnant women and prevention of mother-to-child transmission;
- harm reduction programmes for injecting drug users;
- measures to protect blood supply safety;
- infection control in health-care settings (universal precautions, safe medical injections, post-exposure prophylaxis);
- community education and changes in laws and policies to counter stigma and discrimination; and
- vulnerability reduction through social, legal and economic change.

Preventing sexual transmission through 'combination prevention'

The term 'combination prevention' is sometimes used to mean comprehensive prevention. However, more frequently it refers to the combination of strategies required to prevent sexual transmission. Combination prevention includes various strategies that individuals can choose at different times in their lives to reduce their risks of sexual exposure to the virus.

Countries that have achieved sustained progress against HIV transmission have pursued an array of complementary prevention approaches, from the 'ABC' options for preventing sexual transmission at the individual level (see box on page 73) to the integration of prevention and care efforts. Brazil, Thailand and Uganda exemplify very different but effective responses: they emphasized getting the right combination of interventions to fit the specific risk factors and vulnerabilities that characterized the epidemic in each country.

Uganda is one of most inspiring examples of an effective national response, having successfully reduced overall prevalence of HIV since its peak in 1992. This was done through a variety of prevention approaches including community mobilization, pioneering nongovernmental

The ABCs of combination prevention

Just as combination treatment attacks HIV at different phases of virus replication, combination prevention includes various safer sex behaviour strategies that informed individuals who are in a position to decide for themselves can choose at different times in their lives to reduce their risk of exposing themselves or others to HIV (Global HIV Prevention Working Group, 2003). These are often referred to as the ABCs of combination prevention.

- **A means abstinence**—not engaging in sexual intercourse or delaying sexual initiation. Whether abstinence occurs by delaying sexual debut or by adopting a period of abstinence at a later stage, access to information and education about alternative safer sexual practices is critical to avoid HIV infection when sexual activity begins or is resumed.
- **B means being safer**—by being faithful to one's partner or reducing the number of sexual partners. The lifetime number of sexual partners is a very important predictor of HIV infection. Thus, having fewer sexual partners reduces the risk of HIV exposure. However, strategies to promote faithfulness among couples do not necessarily lead to lower incidence of HIV unless neither partner has HIV infection and both are consistently faithful.
- **C means correct and consistent condom use**—condoms reduce the risk of HIV transmission for sexually active young people, couples in which one person is HIV-positive, sex workers and their clients, and anyone engaging in sexual activity with partners who may have been at risk of HIV exposure. Research has found that if people do not have access to condoms, other prevention strategies lose much of their potential effectiveness.

A, B, and C interventions can be adapted and combined in a balanced approach that will vary by cultural context, the population addressed and the stage of the epidemic.

organization (NGO) projects and public education campaigns emphasizing delayed sexual initiation, partner reduction and condom use. Strong political leadership, destigmatization and open communication were key aspects of the Ugandan response to AIDS. Behavioural changes in the early 1990s—in particular, delayed sexual debut and reduced numbers of casual partners—were pivotal in reducing new infections. Following these initial changes, increased condom use appears to have played an important role in stabilizing the epidemic, which preserved and accelerated the response's momentum over the past decade (Singh et al., 2003; Shelton et al., 2004).

Thailand also applied a variety of approaches, with high-profile critical leadership beginning in the early 1990s. As well as mass media campaigns, Thailand pioneered a '100% Condom Use' policy for sex workers and their clients. This led to an increase in condom use, particularly in sex work, and a decrease in the number of sexual partners (UNAIDS, 2000).

Brazil reduced national infection rates by investing in mass media campaigns on AIDS awareness, harm reduction programmes for injecting drug users, behaviour change programmes for sex workers and men who have sex with men, and by promoting voluntary counselling and testing (Levi and Vitória, 2002). Strong civil society advocacy was an essential element, including by organizations of HIV-positive people. This advocacy effort supported and strengthened government-administered prevention activities and encouraged integrating care and treatment in the National AIDS Programme, including universal access to antiretroviral therapy.

The responses of these three countries were based on correct assessment of the unique mix of factors driving their respective epidemics. For example, Thailand's primary emphasis on condom use in sex work settings would have been less successful in Uganda since sex work was not the main factor driving its epidemic.

AIDS education and awareness

Although the epidemic is well into its third decade, basic AIDS education remains fundamental to the response. For instance, in India, behavioural survey data showed that 30% of women had not heard of HIV or AIDS (NACO, 2003). Rural women were the least informed: less than 25% of rural women in the states of Bihar (18.7%), Gujarat (22.7%) and Uttar Pradesh (24.3%) were aware that HIV could be transmitted sexually. Figure 19 indicates the difference in knowledge about transmission of HIV between men and women, and between urban and rural respondents.

Most studies of prevention programmes in low- and middle-income countries indicate that effective behaviour-change projects include educational and communications components, using a range of media, from traditional theatre and music, to global television and radio networks (Merson et al., 2000). Countries that have significantly reduced rates of new infections have typically invested heavily in AIDS education and awareness initiatives.

Media campaigns have become increasingly involved in HIV and AIDS programming. National broadcasters such as China's CCTV and the South African Broadcasting Corporation have made strong efforts, as have global media organizations such as the British Broadcasting Corporation, France's TV5 and the international music broadcaster Music Television (see 'Young People' focus).

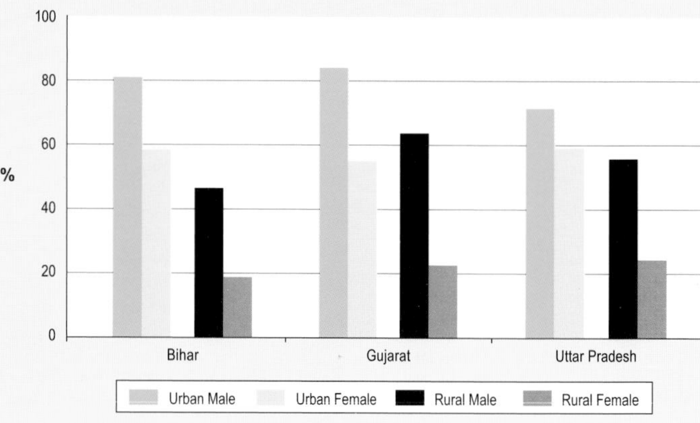

Source: National AIDS Control Organization, *National Baseline General Population Behavioural Surveillance Survey 2001*

Figure 19

However, information alone is not enough to produce sustained behaviour change. A recent study in Zimbabwe found that many young people who were educated about AIDS and sexually transmitted infections still did not use a condom during sexual intercourse (Betts et al., 2003). Clearly, as a prevention tool, HIV education alone has its limits. Nevertheless, information is critical to helping people gain an accurate understanding of how HIV is transmitted and how it can be prevented—the first step towards reducing risk.

National youth councils, health-care provider networks, religious networks and other structures can provide established communication channels for conveying facts. In China, Anhui province launched a 'train the trainers' approach to diffusing HIV-related information among health-care workers. Fifty-five staff were initially trained at various health institutions, and follow-up workshops were conducted in local provincial health-care settings. Eighteen months after the training, surveys found that basic HIV-related knowledge was up to 100% higher in counties where the training occurred,

China moves ahead with prevention among populations

China has 840 000 people living with HIV, with over 50% of infections acquired through contaminated drug injecting equipment. More recently, there has been a large increase in the number of people infected through commercial sex, especially in coastal areas in east and south China, and in big cities. In response, the government has declared a policy of vigorous behavioural intervention among groups at higher risk of HIV exposure. Although some of the measures—which include condom promotion, needle exchange and methadone maintenance therapy—have proved controversial with some government departments and the public, the new policy actually supports activities already under way in various parts of the country. For example, in 2001, the cities of Wuhan in Hubei Province and Jingjiang in Jiangsu Province began a pilot study with World Health Organization (WHO) support to promote 100% condom use in entertainment establishments. In 2002, a pilot project for marketing syringes and needles was conducted in Guangxi Zhuang Autonomous Region and Guangdong Province, using staff of local centres for disease control (Ministry of Health/UN Theme Group, 2003).

compared with counties where staff received no training (Wu et al., 2002).

Programmes to change HIV risk behaviour and sustain healthy behaviour

Dozens of studies have demonstrated that a variety of strategies can help individuals initiate behaviour change and sustain healthy behaviour to reduce risk. Evaluations of programmes have documented sexual behaviour change among adolescents and adults, men and women, people in low-, middle- and higher-income countries, and among groups that are especially vulnerable to infection (Global HIV Prevention Working Group, 2003).

Behaviour change and maintenance programmes provide essential health information, motivate people to reduce risk and increase individuals' skills in using condoms and negotiating safer sex. Effective approaches for young people and children involve life-skills-based education that promotes the adoption of healthy behaviours. These include taking greater responsibility for their own lives, making healthy choices, gaining strength to resist negative pressures and minimizing harmful behaviours.

Successful behaviour change programmes are usually accompanied by the other components of comprehensive prevention mentioned earlier. They are also supported by collecting solid information on the behaviours, attitudes, and social networks of the target population. A variety of techniques can be used, from surveys to sophisticated geographic information systems. For example, a recent South African study in three townships and a business district demonstrates how formative research plays a potentially useful role in developing prevention strategies. Researchers found that social networks in these areas were relatively diffuse, but that respondents were broadly able to identify public sites where people meet new sexual partners. The study showed that most of these sites lacked condoms, and helped identify potentially important venues for interventions (Weir et al., 2003).

Promoting male condom use

HIV prevention efforts have long focused on encouraging correct and consistent condom use as part of a combination prevention strategy. Scientific data overwhelmingly confirm that male latex condoms are highly effective in preventing sexual HIV transmission (CDC, 2002). Evidence also indicates that the poly-

Nepal's unique prevention efforts

In Nepal, Population Services International has implemented an awareness campaign that takes advantage of the reach of the national postal service. The campaign places a sticker saying 'Protect yourself and others from HIV/AIDS' on every letter or package entering and leaving the country. The stickers have the logo of the Number One brand of condoms which Population Services International has been distributing in Nepal since 2003. Other promotion efforts have focused on non-traditional outlets serving populations at higher risk, including people in entertainment establishments such as various types of restaurants and massage parlours. In the first year of operation, this resulted in almost four million condoms being distributed, far exceeding the first-year target of one million.

urethane female condom is comparably effective in protecting against sexual transmission (WHO/UNAIDS, 1997). In addition, condoms prevent other sexually transmitted infections associated with increased risk of acquiring and transmitting HIV.

Condoms have always played a key role in successful national prevention programmes. Yet despite clear public health benefits, condom use is still low in many countries. Studies of nearly 4300 adults in Kenya, Tanzania and Trinidad found that only 19% had used a condom with their most recent sex partner (Norman, 2003). The United Nations Population Fund (UNFPA) has identified more than 200 myths, misperceptions and fears that hinder access to and use of condoms (UNFPA/UNAIDS, 2004).

Effectively promoting condom use requires clear messages that dispel myths and misperceptions, such as the idea that only promiscuous people use them or the fallacy that HIV is small enough to pass through latex. However, it requires more than just education. Individuals—particularly women and girls—who wish to use condoms often experience difficulty in negotiating their use with sex partners (Norman, 2003). These findings underscore the need to address gender issues within condom promotion efforts (see Figure 20).

Globally, condom distribution has increased substantially in recent years, but a large supply gap remains. In South Africa, between 2000 and 2002, condom distribution rose by almost 70%. In Brazil, between 1996 and 2000, total condom sales increased by about 62% (Levi and Vitória, 2002). In India, condom sales increased by 13% during 2003–2004. Meanwhile, the Chinese government currently purchases 1.2 billion condoms a year from domestic sources, primarily for free distribution as contraceptives.

Despite the clear need, there are still not enough condoms available in many regions where HIV is rampant. UNFPA estimates that the current supply of condoms in low- and middle-

Figure 20

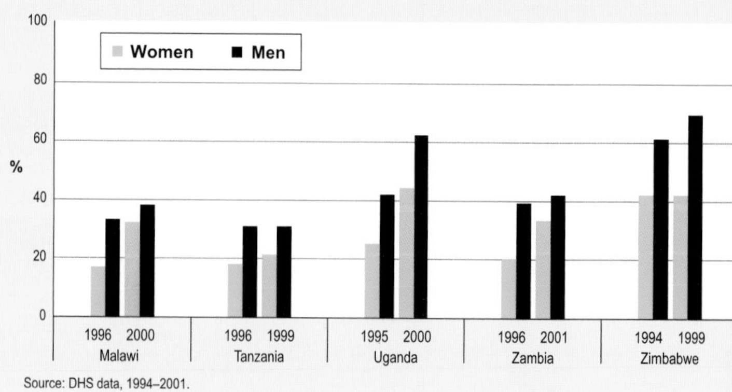

income countries falls 40% short of the number required. Unfortunately, international funding for procuring condoms has declined in recent years. The World Bank's Multicountry AIDS Programme and the Global Fund to Fight AIDS, Tuberculosis and Malaria are serving as important new channels of financial assistance for condom promotion. Despite this, a substantial condom gap remains and could grow much worse in coming years, unless all relevant stakeholders act to increase condom supply.

Female condoms

The female condom was launched in the early 1990s. Since 1997, more than 90 countries have introduced it. Promotion efforts have occasionally been resisted at the local level for a variety of reasons related both to providers and to users. But ministries of health in Brazil, Ghana, Zimbabwe and South Africa have been able to significantly increase the numbers of women using female condoms. The key ingredients of successful female condom introduction include training for providers and peer educators, one-to-one communication with potential users, a consistent supply, and combining private- and public-sector distribution. Other critical factors for scaling up female condom use include involving a broad range of decision-makers and influential people (programme managers, service providers, community leaders and women's group members), as well as political leadership and funding by governments and donors.

Market factors also often prevent the effective promotion of female condoms. For one thing, they cost more than male condoms, which makes them inaccessible in many resource-limited countries. In response to these challenges, donor countries are working to obtain preferential prices, and increase financial assistance for promoting female condoms. A second-generation female condom that will cost one-third less than the current version has entered Phase II and III trials in South Africa.

Young people

Young people are a critical focus for behaviour-change programmes, since people 15–24 years old make up an estimated one-half of all new infections. However, young people in different parts of the world face different kinds of risks, and prevention programming must be designed accordingly. For example, interventions aimed at children who do not attend school are very different from those in school. In countries where injecting drug use poses a higher risk of HIV infection than sexual transmission, the curricula for life skills training have to be adjusted accordingly. Fortunately, a great deal of experience on prevention among young people has been built up in the past two decades and this is being applied in various parts of the world (see 'Young People' focus).

Women and girls

The special vulnerability of women and girls is well documented. For example, in sub-Saharan Africa overall, women are 30% more likely to be infected with HIV than men (see 'Global Overview' chapter). Among young people, the gender disparity in infection rates is particularly pronounced. In household surveys in seven countries in sub-Saharan Africa, 15–24-year-old women were found to be 2.7 times more likely to be HIV-infected than their male counterparts (WHO, 2002a) despite the fact that they were far less likely to report having non-marital, non-cohabiting partners in the previous 12 months (see Figure 21).

Starting young is central to most prevention strategies, and one of the best means of protecting girls from HIV exposure is to keep them in school (see 'Impact' chapter). In line with

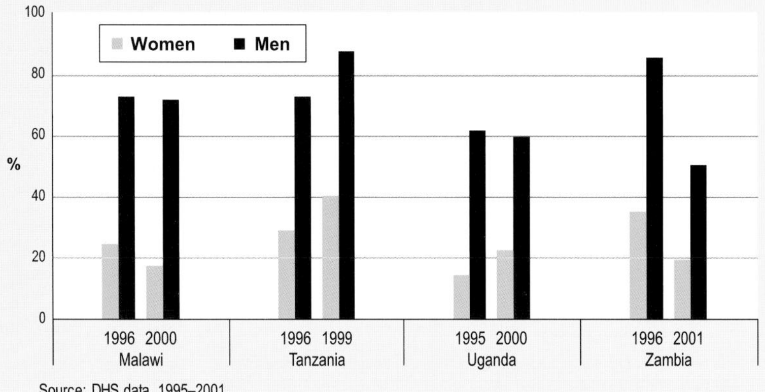

Figure 21

the international initiative 'Education for All', three key action lines have been identified as being central to the education sector response to HIV and girls:

1. Get girls into school, and ensure a safe environment that can keep them at school and learning.
2. Ensure HIV prevention education is provided as part of the overall quality education that all children and young people deserve.
3. Ensure special measures for those not in schools to extend the definition of education well beyond schools alone, and to consider the needs of working children, street children, and those who are exploited or made vulnerable by poverty and poor living conditions.

As girls grow older, other prevention activities become increasingly important. Reducing women's vulnerability to HIV must address a variety of gender-related legal, social and economic disadvantages.

Married and cohabiting couples

Married and cohabiting couples have sex more frequently than people who are not living together, but they use condoms less often (Population Report, 1999). Some of this low condom use is certainly due to trust, but it also reflects women's lack of power to negotiate safer sex, even when a woman suspects her husband has engaged in high-risk sex either before or during the marriage.

Being safer by being faithful to one's partner is integral to ABC, but the idea that no protection is ever needed with regular partners can be dangerous. Faithfulness is only protective when neither partner is infected with HIV and both are consistently faithful. For example, a 1999 study in Thailand found that although three-quarters of HIV-infected women were most probably infected by their husbands, nearly half thought they were at no or low risk for HIV infection. Sex with their husband was the only HIV risk factor reported by these women (Xu et al., 2000).

This highlights the value of voluntary counselling and testing services for couples, which can increase knowledge of HIV status and assist partners to talk about sex and plan to reduce their risk. Studies have found that after voluntary testing and counselling, HIV sero-discordant couples (couples where only one partner is infected) and HIV-positive participants reduced unprotected intercourse and increased condom use at a greater rate than HIV-negative and untested participants (Weinhardt et al., 1999).

India: Condom use among men who have sex with men

The Humsafar Trust in Mumbai, which works with the Lokmanya Tilak municipal hospital, is one of India's two HIV surveillance sites for men who have sex with men. In a survey among the Trust's clients, 82% of men and 75% of transgendered people reported that their sex partners would be angry if they insisted on condom use. About half of both groups said that condoms were costly, difficult to find and embarrassing to purchase, and reported harassment by police for carrying them. Equally alarming, 85% of both groups believed condoms were unnecessary with someone who appears healthy (Mathur et al., 2002.)

Men who have sex with men

This population accounts for 5–10% of all HIV cases worldwide, including the largest share of infections in most industrialized countries and in Latin America. In Central and Eastern Europe, HIV prevalence among men who have sex with men is much higher than that of the general population (Hamers and Downs, 2003). In Indonesia, men who have sex with men represent 15% of reported AIDS cases; 29% in Singapore; 32% in Hong Kong; and 33% in the Philippines (Colby, 2003). Less is known about HIV prevalence in this population in sub-Saharan Africa.

In many parts of the world, men who have sex with men typically do not self-identify as gay, homosexual or bisexual. Incarceration or military service may also create contexts where there is sexual expression among men who are not gay-identified. Men who have unprotected sex with men may also have unprotected sex with women and thus serve as an epidemiological bridge to the broader population. In China, a survey of over 800 men who have sex with men found that 59% reported having had unprotected sex with women in the previous year (Ministry of Health/UN Theme Group, 2003).

Prevention programmes must take into account the fact that this group is highly stigmatized throughout much of the world. As of 2002, 84 countries had legal prohibitions against sex between men (International Lesbian and Gay Association World Legal Survey, 2002). In 13 Latin American countries, they receive a substantially smaller allocation of funds from national prevention programmes than their representation among all those infected would merit (see 'National Responses' chapter).

In the 1980s, men who had sex with men in North America, Western Europe and Australia were early HIV-prevention pioneers. They developed community-based programmes that forged safer sex norms and contributed to substantially reducing new HIV-infections. Such leadership is also apparent in low- and middle-income countries, through groups such as Malaysia's Pink Triangle, Gays and Lesbians of Zimbabwe, and the Dominican Republic's *Amigos Siempre Amigos* ('friends always'), to name only a few.

In many countries, NGOs play a critical role in delivering HIV-prevention services to men who have sex with men. For example, the Indonesian government and Family Health International have implemented specially designed peer education among *waria* (transvestite sex workers), more than one in five of whom tested HIV-positive in 2002 in Jakarta (Ministry of Health, 2003).

Peer-based interventions that target social networks of men who have sex with men can be highly effective in promoting risk reduction. Recently, prevention workers recruited and trained young men in St Petersburg, Russia, and Sofia, Bulgaria, to deliver HIV prevention interventions to 14 social networks of men who have sex with men in these cities. An evaluation found that the programme promoted discussion of HIV and AIDS within the networks, and increased both knowledge levels and condom use (Amirkhanian et al., 2003).

Sex workers

HIV prevalence is generally higher among sex workers than in the general population. Surveys of sex workers in some urban areas between 1998 and 2002 detected extraordinarily high rates of infection: 74% in Ethiopia, 50% in South Africa, 45% in Guyana and 36% in Nepal (UNAIDS, 2002). Rising levels of HIV among sex workers can provide early warning of increasing probability that the epidemic will expand into the general population.

At the same time, there is substantial evidence that prevention programmes for sex workers are highly cost-effective, and that sex workers can be strong partners in prevention if programmes are based on recognizing their human rights. Acknowledging the broad diversity of sex workers is important in creating prevention programmes. In addition to women, sex workers can be male or transgender, young or old, and work in a range of settings from highly organized brothels to roadside bars and the street.

The most effective prevention programmes for sex workers include condom distribution, access to diagnosis and treatment of sexually transmitted infections and HIV, counselling and other services. Several such projects have had some success in increasing safer sex practices and reducing new cases of infection, as shown in studies in Benin and Côte d'Ivoire (Alary et al., 2002; Ghys et al., 2003). For example, the Clinique de Confiance in Abidjan has seen a marked reduction in prevalence of HIV and other sexually transmitted diseases among its clients since 1992 (see Figure 22), much of it attributable to prevention programming.

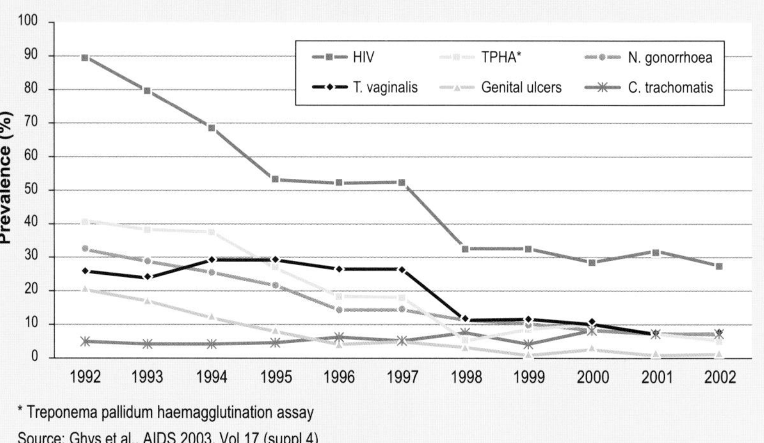

Figure 22

Trafficking of women and girls

Trafficking for the sex trade is a growing threat to women and girls. The International Labour Organization's 2002 report, *Unbearable to the human heart: child trafficking and action to eliminate it*, states that an estimated 28 000 to 30 000 children are in prostitution in South Africa, with half between the ages of 10 and 14. In Europe, the International Organization for Migration estimates that between 2000 and 6000 women and girls are trafficked each year into Italy, while France, the Netherlands, Switzerland and the United Kingdom are also destination countries. Viet Nam faces widespread trafficking of rural children into prostitution in large cities. In the Americas, Mexico has considerable internal trafficking of girls for sex at Mexican tourist resorts (ILO/IPEC, 2002).

The '100% Condom Use' programme, first implemented in Thailand, is one of the best known sex-work-related interventions and has been replicated in other countries such as the Dominican Republic and Cambodia. Following implementation of the programme in Cambodia, adult prevalence, which had reached 3% in 1997, remained stable at that level through 2002. Meanwhile, HIV prevalence among sex workers who work in brothels declined from 43% in 1997 to 29% in 2002 (Cohen, 2003).

Recently, some sex worker organizations have criticized the way this programme has been applied in some countries (Wolffers and van Beelen, 2003). One study found that certain features of the Cambodian programme, such as lack of consultation with sex workers, reduced programme effectiveness, while its mandatory testing provisions raised significant human rights concerns (Lowe, 2002). A subsequent programme evaluation in 2003 led to the programme addressing some of these concerns. In contrast, the voluntary approach used in the Dominican Republic encourages condom use by mobilizing and educating sex workers, managers and other establishment staff (Kerrigan et al., 2003).

In many countries, a high percentage of sex workers are foreigners. An estimated 30% to 40% of sex workers in European Union countries are from Eastern Europe (Brussa, 2002). In Abidjan, Côte d'Ivoire, most sex workers come from neighbouring Ghana, Liberia and Nigeria (Ghys et al., 2002). In these circumstances, prevention programmes need to be carefully tailored to address the heightened vulnerability of foreign workers—particularly those who have been trafficked against their will (see box on page 80). One example is the European Network for HIV/STD Prevention in Prostitution. It operates in 24 European countries, including nine in Central and Eastern Europe. Its 'cultural mediators' work to contact sex workers from low- and middle-income countries and link them with health providers and other services (Brussa, 2002).

Human rights violations against sex workers (including high levels of violence) by police and by criminals are as pervasive as the sex trade itself, and seriously undermine prevention efforts (Human Rights Watch, 2003). Strategies to address this include education and awareness training for police officers, protective regulations, and enforcement of existing laws and workplace sanctions that prohibit discrimination and punish violence.

Prisoners

At any given time, there are approximately 10 million people imprisoned worldwide. This has serious implications for the global epidemic, since prisons and other custodial settings are breeding grounds for infectious diseases such as HIV, tuberculosis and hepatitis. Prison populations come largely from the most marginalized groups in society—people in poor health and with chronic untreated conditions, the vulnerable and those who have engaged in activities with high risk of HIV exposure such as injecting drugs and sex work. The vast majority are released into the wider community at some point.

Evidence of high HIV prevalence in prison is widely available. In South Africa, where prevalence of HIV infection for adults is more than 20%, the level in prisons is double (Goyer, 2003). In the United States, the proportion of confirmed cases of AIDS in prison is estimated to be four times higher than that in the general population (Braithwaite and Arriola, 2003). In Europe, reported HIV infection levels are as high as 26% in Spain; 17% in Italy; 13%

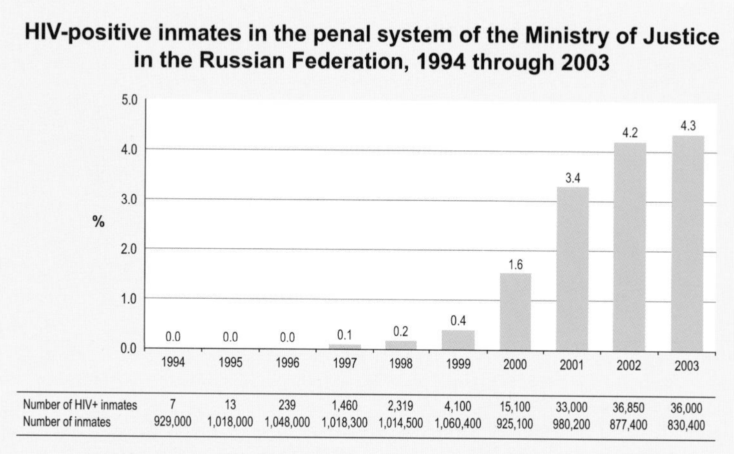

	1994	1995	1996	1997	1998	1999	2000	2001	2002	2003
Number of HIV+ inmates	7	13	239	1,460	2,319	4,100	15,100	33,000	36,850	36,000
Number of inmates	929,000	1,018,000	1,048,000	1,018,300	1,014,500	1,060,400	925,100	980,200	877,400	830,400

Source: Based on GUIN (Department of Penalty Execution) data - Main Directorate of Corrections of the Ministry of Justice

Figure 23

in France; and 11% in both Switzerland and the Netherlands. Many HIV infections have also been reported from prisons in countries in Eastern Europe, such as Ukraine and, more recently, Lithuania, while prisons in Brazil have infection levels varying from 11% to 22% (Jürgens, 2003).

Globally, most prisoners are men, but women prisoners are also at risk of HIV. In Brazil, Canada and the United States, women prisoners are more likely to be HIV-positive than their male counterparts, largely because a high proportion are incarcerated for drug use and sex work (De Groot et al., 1999; Human Rights Watch, 1998).

In the Russian Federation, as injecting drug use has increased in society, the proportion of prisoners who are injecting drug users has increased and the number of HIV-positive prisoners has grown, as Figure 23 demonstrates. HIV-positive inmates are now about 4.3% of the total prison population.

Prison authorities sometimes deny it, but behaviours which carry high risk of HIV transmission are common in prisons, including injecting drug use, tattooing, male-male sexual relations and violence (including rape). In South Africa, up to 65% of male prisoners have sex with other prisoners, and an estimated 80% of prisoners awaiting trial are robbed and raped by convicted prisoners with whom they share a cell (Goyer, 2003; International Centre for Prison Studies, 2003).

Fortunately, a growing number of prison systems are working to protect prisoners from HIV. Many EU countries now provide free access to condoms, substitution treatment, and needle and syringe programmes in prison. In Spain, for example, an estimated 60% of incarcerated drug users receive methadone (Stover and Ossietzky, 2001). The Russian Federation is working with the AIDS Foundation East-West to develop a model programme which includes prevention education for prisoners and staff, access to condoms and providing bleach to sterilize injecting equipment (AFEW, 2003). Among low- and middle-income countries, Uganda is a leader in providing HIV prevention training for prisoners and staff, and has shared this expertise with South Africa's prison system.

Antiretroviral treatment and drug substitution therapy are now available in some European prisons. This reflects the principle that treatment and care for prisoners should be equivalent to that available outside the prison setting, as most recently stated in the February 2004 Dublin Declaration on HIV/AIDS in Prisons in Europe and Central Asia. Ultimately, however, some of the most effective interventions for this group will be those aimed at breaking the vicious circle of drug use, crime and imprisonment. These include expanded substitution treatment for drug users in general, and increased use of non-custodial sentences.

Migrant workers and mobile populations

In recent years, increasing numbers of people have been on the move—from place to place within their own country, or to different countries altogether. The International Organization for Migration estimates that the number of international migrants (those who crossed national borders) increased from 105 million in 1985 to 175 million in 2000 (IOM, 2003), while a similar number of people may move within national borders.

There is a strong link between various kinds of mobility and heightened risk of HIV (see 'Global Overview' chapter). However, while there is a widespread prejudice that migrants 'bring AIDS with them,' the fact is that many migrants move from low HIV prevalence areas to those with higher prevalence, increasing their own risk of being exposed to the virus.

HIV-related risk often depends on the reason for mobility. A recent study in India found that 16% of truck drivers working a route in the south were HIV-positive, compared to adult national HIV prevalence of below 1% (Manjunath et al., 2002). In South Africa, HIV prevalence is twice as high among migrant workers (26%) than among non-migrant workers (Lurie et al., 2003). In Sri Lanka, housemaids who have returned from working in the Middle East account for about half of reported HIV cases (UNDP, 2001a). Armed conflicts can increase HIV risk in a very short time as thousands are forced to flee their homes and communities (see 'Conflict' focus).

The wide variety of conditions facing migrants requires that HIV prevention be carefully tailored to the specific circumstances of different groups. On a global level, there is increasing attention on prevention among mobile popula-

Rights to entry, treatment and care

A growing number of HIV-positive people are migrating to countries in Europe. Recent studies show that these individuals are typically diagnosed late in the course of infection and consequently miss the benefits of early care and treatment (Haour-Knipe, 2002). Some countries have prioritized voluntary counselling and testing, care and treatment for HIV-infected migrants and asylum seekers. But other countries have opted for mandatory testing and exclusion. This is particularly the case for migrants planning to remain in the host country for longer than six to twelve months. Some countries exclude HIV-positive immigrants altogether, while others insist on evidence that the individual has the means to finance his or her own treatment and care while in the country.

In the United Kingdom, this debate came to a head in 2003 when it was revealed that an estimated 80% of new heterosexual HIV infections had been acquired in sub-Saharan Africa. Intense media coverage suggested that asylum seekers were absorbing too many public services, which led to calls for mandatory HIV testing for immigrants.

In response, the All-Party Parliamentary Group on AIDS and its counterpart group on refugees held a series of hearings to investigate the matter. The resulting report concluded that testing and exclusion were both impractical and undesirable on human rights and public health grounds. It recommended that the government adhere to recognized guidelines against mandatory testing, while encouraging voluntary testing to ensure improved access to treatment and care. The group also called for national guidelines on providing care to HIV-positive asylum seekers living in the United Kingdom (All-Party Parliamentary Group on AIDS, 2003.)

Matching the intervention with local conditions

Governments often fear that providing access to clean needles and syringes might result in more injecting drug use. But there is no evidence to support this view. Studies in Australia, Canada, Sweden, the United Kingdom and the United States have all shown that such programmes (particularly in concert with other interventions) help reduce the use of non-sterile injecting equipment and the transmission of HIV. There was no evidence that they increased either the number of injectors or the frequency of injecting drug use (Riehman, 1996). However, programmes must fit local conditions. For example, research in Canada has shown that cocaine injectors tend to inject much more frequently than heroin injectors, and therefore require much greater quantities of needles and syringes than usually provided by needle-syringe programmes (Strathdee and Vlahov, 2001).

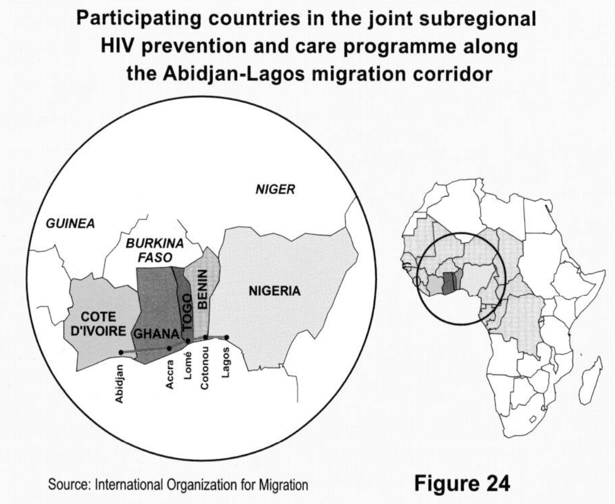

Participating countries in the joint subregional HIV prevention and care programme along the Abidjan-Lagos migration corridor

Source: International Organization for Migration

Figure 24

tions that regularly cross international borders such as truck drivers, traders and sex workers. A recent review found that as many as 56 programmes are operating in Africa and 27 different organizations are working in this field in South and South-East Asia (IOM/UNAIDS/UNDP, 2002; UNDP, 2001). Five countries are participants in a recently launched joint subregional HIV prevention and AIDS care programme along the Abidjan-Lagos Migration Corridor (see Figure 24).

Cooperation across borders is increasing in various parts of the world. For example, in October 2003, ASEAN countries took a major step forward when they agreed to incorporate HIV prevention programmes within large construction projects. As a pre-condition to bidding on these projects, contractors' bids must include HIV prevention for construction workers and surrounding communities.

Injecting drug users and their sex partners

Using contaminated injecting equipment to inject drugs is a highly efficient mode of HIV transmission and continues to play a major role in HIV epidemics in several regions of the world (see Figure 25). Worldwide there are more than 13 million injecting drug users, and in some regions more than 50% of them are infected with HIV. Today, drug injecting with contaminated equipment is the major HIV transmission mode in many countries in Europe, Asia and Latin America, and is also driving HIV transmission in North Africa and the Middle East. In recent years, transmission among injecting drug users has been responsible for the world's fastest spread of HIV infection, which has occurred in Eastern Europe and Central Asia (see 'Global Overview' chapter).

However, experience shows that it is possible to prevent and even reverse major epidemics among injecting drug users through a mixture of interventions. Cities such as London, United Kingdom, and Dhaka, Bangladesh, have managed to keep HIV prevalence among injecting drug users to less than 5%. In New York City

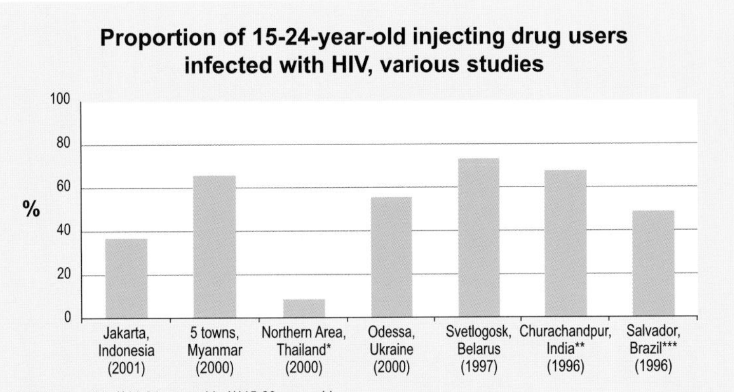

Figure 25

in the United States, Edinburgh, Scotland, and several Brazilian cities, prevalence among injecting drug users has actually fallen (Burrows, 2003).

The best responses are built on the three pillars of supply reduction, demand reduction and harm reduction. A range of programming options should be used: discouraging people from using drugs, making treatment available to users, providing appropriate substitution therapies and making sure that clean needles and condoms are available. A review comparing HIV prevalence in cities across the globe with and without needle and syringe programmes found that cities which introduced such programmes showed a mean annual 19% decrease in HIV prevalence. This compares with an 8% increase in cities that failed to implement prevention measures. In Australia alone, these programmes prevented an estimated 25 000 HIV infections, and saved hundreds of millions of dollars in HIV treatment costs (Drummond, 2002).

Currently, the proportion of injecting drug users reached by prevention interventions is extremely low—less than 5% of the total in countries where this is a significant mode of transmission (UNAIDS, 2003). In many countries, there are still policy and legal barriers to using proven approaches such as access to clean needles and substitution therapy. This is despite statements by international bodies such as the International Narcotics Control Board confirming that these measures do not contravene international drug control conventions (INCB, 2003). Moreover, few interventions take into account the sex partners of injecting drug users, a key consideration in avoiding further expansion of the epidemic.

Prevention efforts are also hampered by the stigma associated with drug use. In some countries, health-care providers actively avoid serving injecting drug users. In the Russian Federation, more than 90% of the estimated one million people living with HIV were infected through injecting drug use. Yet injecting drug users make up only 13% of people receiving antiretroviral therapy (Malinowska-Sempruch et al., 2003).

HIV testing

Knowledge of HIV status is the gateway to AIDS treatment and has documented prevention benefits; however, the current reach of HIV testing services is poor and uptake is often low, largely because of fear of stigma and discrimination.

The cornerstones of HIV testing scale up include strengthened protection from stigma and discrimination as well as assured access to integrated prevention, treatment and care services. Public health strategies to increase knowledge of HIV status and human rights protection are mutually reinforcing and should be integrated for greatest effect in reducing HIV transmission and improving the quality of life of people living with HIV. The testing

HIV testing

UNAIDS promotes expanded access to both client-initiated and provider-initiated voluntary, confidential HIV testing, conducted with informed consent and accompanied by counselling for both HIV-positive and HIV-negative individuals. With respect to provider-initiated testing, in all settings, individuals retain the right to refuse testing, i.e. to 'opt out' of a routine offer of testing. All testing needs to be accompanied by referral to medical and psychosocial services for those who receive a positive test result, and by community education and legal and policy reform to counter stigma and discrimination.

process, regardless of context, must remain voluntary, with the confidential nature of the test result preserved. The '3 Cs' are the underpinning principles advocated since HIV testing of individuals began in 1985. They are:

- confidentiality
- testing accompanied by counselling
- testing only with informed consent, meaning that it is voluntary.

HIV testing options for individuals urgently need to be greatly expanded to enhance access to treatment and prevention. *Client-initiated* voluntary counselling and testing services which focus on increasing knowledge of HIV status, particularly of sexually active people, are run by NGOs or public services at freestanding or designated facilities. Rapid scale up requires:

- effective marketing of knowledge of HIV status for people who may have been exposed to HIV through any mode of transmission;
- pre-test counselling provided either on an individual basis or in group settings with individual follow-up;
- the use of rapid tests that provide results in a timely fashion to permit immediate post-test counselling follow-up for both HIV-negative and HIV-positive individuals.

New strategies to enhance the effectiveness of both treatment and prevention programmes require a *provider-initiated* routine offer of HIV testing with assured referral to effective prevention and treatment services. *Diagnostic HIV testing* is indicated whenever a person shows signs or symptoms that are consistent with HIV-related disease, including tuberculosis, to aid clinical diagnosis and management. A routine offer of HIV testing by health-care providers should be made to all patients in:

- sexually transmitted infection clinics—to facilitate tailored counselling based on knowledge of HIV status;
- maternal and child health clinics—to permit antiretroviral prevention of mother-to-child transmission;
- health-care settings where HIV is prevalent and antiretroviral treatment is available (injecting drug use treatment services, hospital emergencies, internal medicine hospital wards, etc.)

Figure 26

Changes in voluntary counselling and testing in South Africa: more sites = more tested

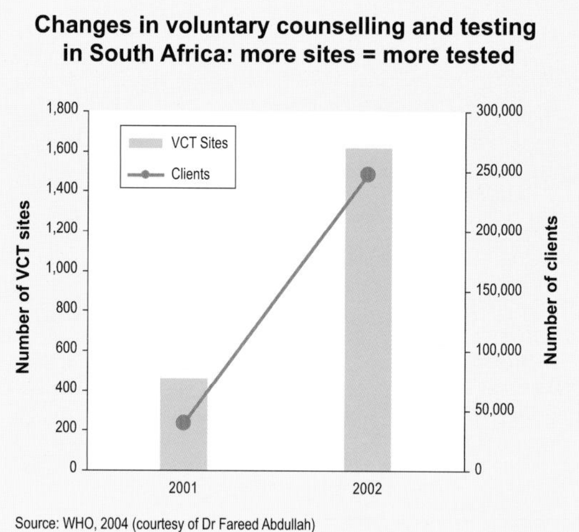

Source: WHO, 2004 (courtesy of Dr Fareed Abdullah)

Referral to post-test counselling services emphasizing prevention, for all those being tested, and to medical and psychosocial support, for those testing positive, must be assured—whether diagnostic testing is being performed or testing is being offered routinely (see Figure 27). The basic conditions of confidentiality, consent and counselling apply but the standard pre-test counselling used for client-initiated testing is adapted simply to ensure informed consent, without a full pre-test education and counselling session.

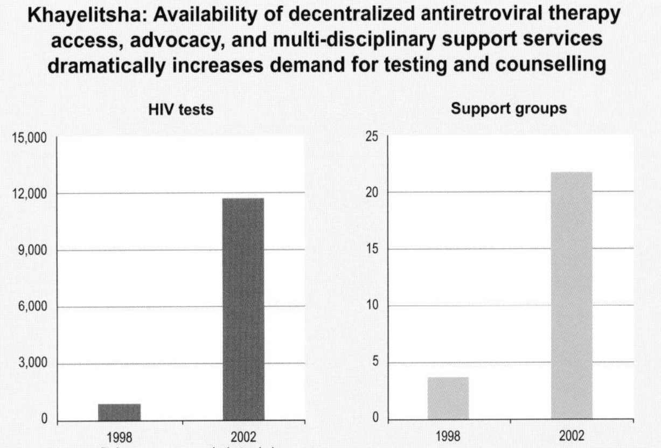

Figure 27

To provide *informed consent* to a provider-initiated offer of HIV testing, patients need to be informed of the following:

- the clinical and prevention benefits of testing;
- the right to refuse;
- the follow-up services that will be offered; and
- the importance of informing others, if the result is positive, who are at ongoing risk and would not suspect they were being exposed otherwise.

For provider-initiated testing, whether for purposes of diagnosis, offer of antiretroviral prevention of mother-to-child transmission or encouragement to learn HIV status, patients retain the right to refuse testing, i.e. to 'opt out' of a systematic offer of testing. HIV testing without consent may be justified in the rare circumstance in which a patient is unconscious, his or her parent or guardian is absent, and knowledge of HIV status is necessary for purposes of optimal treatment. All blood donors should be advised that their blood will be tested confidentially for HIV, and HIV-infected blood donations should be removed from the blood supply.

Preventing and treating sexually transmitted infections

Preventing, diagnosing and treating sexually transmitted infections are essential components of an effective HIV prevention strategy. Untreated sexually transmitted infections dramatically increase the risk of HIV transmission through unprotected sex. Most of these sexually transmitted infections can be prevented by using condoms and seeking treatment early. Moreover, many bacterial sexually transmitted infections (e.g., syphilis, gonorrhoea and *Chlamydia*) and parasitic infections (e.g., *Trichomonas* infection) can be treated easily and inexpensively with antibiotics.

Unfortunately, in many countries, poor sexually transmitted infection diagnosis and treatment is hampering HIV prevention efforts. In 2003 in Viet Nam, only 38% of sexually transmitted infection cases were properly diagnosed, counselled and treated. Comparable figures for Botswana and Kenya were 30% and 50% respectively (UNAIDS, 2003). However, in Cotonou, Benin, pharmacists trained to diagnose and recommend treatment for sexually transmitted urethritis in men were far more likely to identify cases and recommend effective treatment than other pharmacists.

While there is general agreement that sexually transmitted infection control efforts need to be significantly scaled up—in a variety of ways—there is debate among researchers about the relative impact of large-scale sexually transmitted infection treatment programmes on HIV incidence. In Mwanza, Tanzania, a large-scale community-based sexually transmitted infection treatment trial reduced HIV incidence at the community level. However, two other trials in Uganda (in Masaka and Rakai) showed no effect (Kamali et al., 2003). This is likely due to the relatively advanced stage of the epidemic when these latter trials were undertaken. Control of sexually transmitted infections may be more effective in reducing HIV incidence in low and slowly rising epidemics (Hitchcock and Fransen, 1999).

Preventing mother-to-child transmission

In 2003, an estimated 630 000 children worldwide became infected with HIV—the vast majority of them during their mother's pregnancy, labour and delivery, or as a result of breastfeeding. Meanwhile, some 490 000 children died of AIDS-related causes in 2003.

At least a quarter of newborns infected with HIV die before the age of one. Up to 60% die before reaching their second birthday. Overall, most die before they are five years old (Dabis and Ekpini, 2002; Elizabeth Glaser Pediatric AIDS Foundation, 2003). In 1999, in Botswana, 40% of all children who died before their fifth birthday were killed by AIDS. In Zimbabwe, AIDS killed more than 35% in the same age group compared to 25% in Namibia and Swaziland, and over 20% in Kenya, South Africa and Zambia (Walker et al., 2002).

Many of these children acquire HIV through mother-to-child transmission, starkly illustrating current global health inequities. In low- and middle-income countries, there is at least a 30% likelihood that an HIV-positive breastfeeding mother will pass the virus to her newborn child (UNAIDS, 2003). By contrast, in industrialized countries, HIV transmission to infants is rare due to antiretroviral prophylaxis, Caesarean delivery and alternatives to breastfeeding (Dabis and Ekpini, 2002; WHO, 2003b). Transmission rates below 2% can be achieved in non-breastfeeding populations in resource-constrained settings with a combination of zidovudine from 28 weeks of pregnancy, supplemented by a single dose of nevirapine at the onset of labour for the mother and a single dose of nevirapine and a week of zidovudine for the newborn.

In the 2001 UN Declaration of Commitment on HIV/AIDS, the world pledged to reduce the proportion of infants infected with HIV by 20% by 2005; and by 50% by 2010. Achieving

Reducing mother-to-child transmission… and beyond

MTCT-Plus is a multi-partner initiative funded by several private foundations and, more recently, the United States Agency for International Development. Launched in 2001, the initiative seeks to accelerate prevention programme scale up by providing long-term antiretroviral treatment to women participating in programmes to prevent mother-to-child transmission who need it themselves (WHO, 2003a). By November 2003, MTCT-Plus had enrolled more than 900 mothers, children and partners who needed antiretroviral therapy. The goal is to recruit 10 000 patients at 11 demonstration sites in Côte d'Ivoire, Kenya, Mozambique, Rwanda, South Africa, Uganda and Zambia. Another 12 planning grants have been awarded to projects in these countries and others.

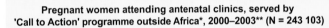

these targets will require immediate and dramatic scale up of activities, such as expanding primary HIV prevention services for women of childbearing age, access to voluntary counselling and testing for pregnant women, comprehensive reproductive health services, and antiretroviral prophylaxis to prevent mother-to-child transmission.

Since July 2000, Boehringer Ingelheim has offered nevirapine to low-income countries for mother-to-child transmission prevention programmes. Since July 2002, Abbott Laboratories announced a donation programme of its HIV rapid tests for the same purpose. Through these donation programmes, HIV rapid tests have been donated free of charge to test more than 450 000 pregnant women and donations of both products have been made to 48 programmes in 24 countries. In many participating countries, however, infrastructures to deliver these interventions remain a challenge.

Progress in expanding access to antiretroviral prevention regimens has so far been slow with only 10% of pregnant women offered this service (Policy Project, 2004). In Burkina Faso, Ethiopia, Malawi, Nigeria and South Africa, less than 1% of HIV-infected women who gave birth in 2003 had access to a regimen to prevent mother-to-child transmission. In Cambodia, Myanmar and Viet Nam, coverage is less than 3% (UNAIDS, 2003). Many barriers hinder scaling up these prevention programmes, including inadequate prenatal care service coverage, lack of financial and human resources, low knowledge of serostatus among childbearing women, fear of stigma and discrimination and the tendency of many women in some low- and middle-income countries to give birth at home instead of in health-care settings.

Figure 28

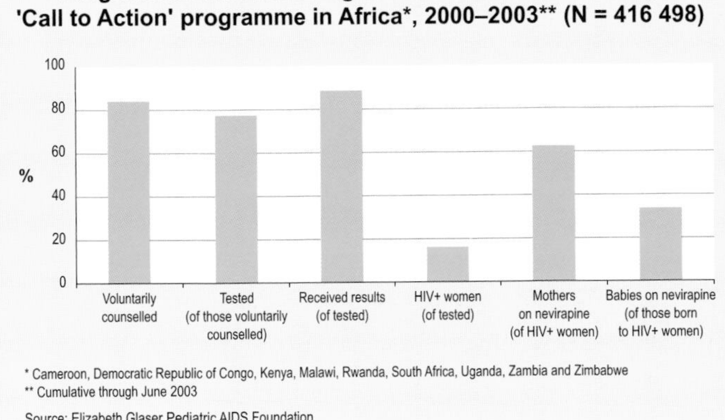

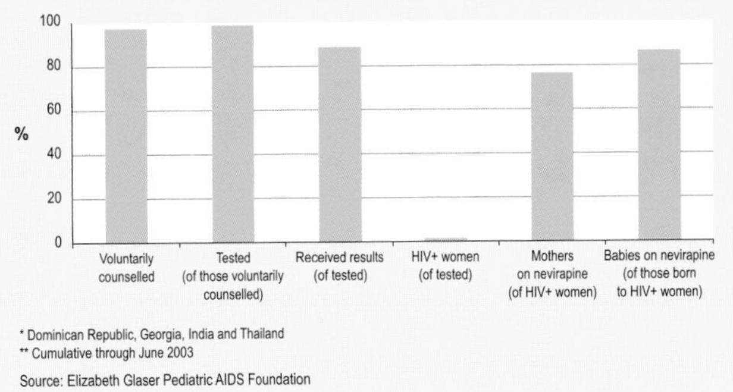

Figure 29

Since 1999, UNICEF has been an international leader in establishing projects to reduce mother-to-child transmission in low- and middle-income countries. Between April 1999 and July 2002, projects supported by UNICEF and partner agencies in 16 countries reached almost 600 000 pregnant women in antenatal care centres, and provided antiretroviral treatment to more than 12 000 HIV-positive women following counselling and testing. The Elizabeth Glaser Paediatric AIDS Foundation has made a key contribution through its Call to Action Initiative in 17 countries. Figure 28 shows the cascade of services and their uptake in nine African countries. At African sites, 63% of HIV-positive pregnant women received prophylaxis compared with 77% in sites outside Africa (see Figure 29).

More comprehensive approaches linking prevention and care show great promise in increasing the number of women who enrol in mother-to-child transmission prevention programmes and in reducing mortality in children under five years of age who would otherwise lose their mothers. This includes offering additional care services for HIV-positive mothers and their families—notably treating opportunistic infections and providing antiretroviral therapy, nutritional support, and reproductive health care including family planning services. This approach may also be a gateway to changing the attitudes of male partners if they are offered access to health services through their partners' pre- and postnatal care (UNFPA, 2003).

HIV transmission in health-care settings

Transfusion with contaminated blood, unfortunately, is an extremely efficient form of HIV transmission. According to the WHO, blood transfusions may account for 5–10% of all cumulative infections worldwide (WHO, 2002). However, the incidence of this type of transmission has significantly declined due to practices such as mandatory screening of donated blood, relying on low-risk donors, and promoting appropriate clinical use of transfused blood. For example, in the United States this combination has reduced the risk of HIV transmission to approximately one in every 500 000 transfusions.

Substantial progress has also been made in promoting blood safety in low- and middle-income countries (WHO, 2003). But some countries still have not fully implemented proven blood safety policies. They risk HIV transmission due to inconsistent blood screening and using paid donors. Prevalence in these groups is higher than in groups which volunteer to give blood and are not paid for doing so (WHO, 2003).

An estimated 5% of new infections worldwide and 2.5% of HIV infections in sub-Saharan Africa (Hauri et al., 2004) stem from using unsterilized needles or syringes in settings such as hospitals and clinics.

UNICEF, WHO and UNFPA recommend that all countries should use only auto-disable syringes for immunizations. These are syringes which become unusable after one injection. The Global Alliance for Vaccines and Immunizations partnership supports the widespread introduction of auto-disable syringes with immunizations, requires that auto-disable syringes be used with all vaccinations procured through UNICEF, and distributes safety boxes for safe disposal of injection equipment.

To prevent transmission of HIV or other blood-borne diseases, health-care workers should adhere to 'universal precautions', an approach that assumes all individuals are potentially infectious. This requires wearing gloves when exposure to any body fluid is possible, and using gowns, masks and goggles if splattering is likely.

Taking comprehensive prevention to scale

Comprehensive prevention programming can become a reality if concerted action is taken on several fronts. These include:

- Financing. Global spending on HIV prevention in 2003 was estimated to be only one-third of the figure needed by 2005 for a comprehensive response (Global HIV Prevention Working Group, 2003).

- Multisectoral action. There is still room for involving many more political, social and economic partners in prevention. Key collaborators include faith-based organizations, NGOs, organizations of people living with HIV and private industry and workers' organizations.
- Responding to changes in the epidemic. As epidemics evolve, HIV prevention strategies must also evolve to meet new challenges. This imperative is particularly relevant in industrialized countries where risk behaviours are rising and new HIV transmission is occurring, coinciding with the availability of antiretroviral treatment and rising 'prevention fatigue' (CDC, 2003; Valdisseri, 2003). Thailand had early success in reducing sexual HIV transmission but did not effectively address transmission among injecting drug users. Addressing this route of transmission has become more important, as has addressing HIV transmission within married and cohabiting couples.
- Prevention opportunities in the treatment era. Expanding treatment access in low- and middle-income countries (see 'Treatment' chapter) will increase incentives for individuals to be voluntarily tested. It also holds the promise of reducing HIV-related stigma, and can potentially bring millions into health-care settings to receive prevention interventions designed to assist people living with HIV in enacting a policy of 'HIV?—It stops with me'.
- Research on vaccines and microbicides. The first Phase III trial of a preventive HIV vaccine did not prove effective, but several potentially promising vaccine candidates continue to progress through the clinical trial process. These include a combination vaccine that will be tested on 16 000 volunteers being enrolled in a Phase III trial in Thailand. The pace of research on microbicides is also accelerating with more than 50 microbicidal products being developed; four are anticipated for Phase III testing in 2004 (Foss et al., 2003). If these trials are successful, effective microbicides could be on the market in five years.

Challenges of the 'Next Agenda'

If the spread of HIV is sustained at its current pace, hard-hit countries strain even more under the impact of the epidemic and have increasing difficulty keeping up with the demand for treatment and support for children orphaned by AIDS. Furthermore, countries will fail to reach their Millennium Development Goals and the 2001 UN Declaration of Commitment on HIV/AIDS targets.

It would be a grave mistake, with severe consequences for future generations, if prevention efforts flagged. We have both scientific knowledge and empirical evidence to address the prevention challenge. Expanding treatment access is also providing new opportunities now to integrate prevention and treatment.

The goal of an AIDS-free generation within the next 15–20 years is attainable if political and social leadership is shown in all sectors and at all levels of society, right down to individuals and families. Each new infection prevented today cuts off a potential chain of HIV transmission tomorrow.

Future challenges include:

- Closing the prevention gap—in 2004, less than 20% of those in need have access to HIV prevention services. Without effective comprehensive prevention for all, the numbers of people living with HIV will continue to escalate, with disastrous short- and long-term effects.

- Ensuring that prevention is comprehensive and involves a variety of effective interventions, since no single element is enough. Achieving the most successful strategies and activities will depend on the stage and nature of each country's epidemic, the needs of different populations at risk, and the participation of people living with HIV.
- Fully integrating comprehensive prevention activities into '3 by 5' and other antiretroviral scale up programmes by using clinical settings to encourage both HIV-positive people and those who test negative to adopt safer behaviour.
- Effectively addressing all vulnerability factors driving the epidemic, including societal injustices, gender inequality, human rights deprivation, social exclusion of marginalized groups and the lack of youth involvement in AIDS-related decision-making.
- Eliminating AIDS-related stigma and discrimination through effective legal frameworks and by protecting the rights of all individuals.
- Speeding up development, financing and accessibility for effective HIV vaccines and microbicides.
- Reinvigorating prevention programmes in high-income countries to reduce prevailing prevention 'fatigue' and to avoid the epidemic's resurgence.

Focus

HIV and young people: the threat for today's youth

Today's youth generation is the largest in history: nearly half of the global population is less than 25 years old (UNFPA, 2003). They have not known a world without AIDS.

Young people between the ages of 15 and 24 are both the most threatened—globally accounting for half of all new cases of HIV—and the greatest hope for turning the tide against AIDS. The future of the epidemic will be shaped by their actions. Experience proves this. The few countries that have successfully decreased national HIV prevalence have achieved these gains mostly by encouraging safer behaviour choices among young people.

Young people are exposed to HIV in different ways. In high-prevalence, sub-Saharan Africa, the main mode of transmission is heterosexual intercourse. This region contains almost two-thirds of all young people living with HIV—approximately 6.2 million people, 75% of whom are female (UNAIDS, 2003.) In Eastern Europe and Central Asia, HIV prevalence among young people is rising rapidly due to drug injecting with contaminated equipment and, to a lesser extent, unsafe sex (see Figure 30 and 'Prevention' chapter).

High risk, high vulnerability

A variety of factors place young people at the centre of HIV vulnerability. These include lack of HIV information, education and services; the gambles many must take in order to survive; and the risks that accompany adolescent experimentation and curiosity.

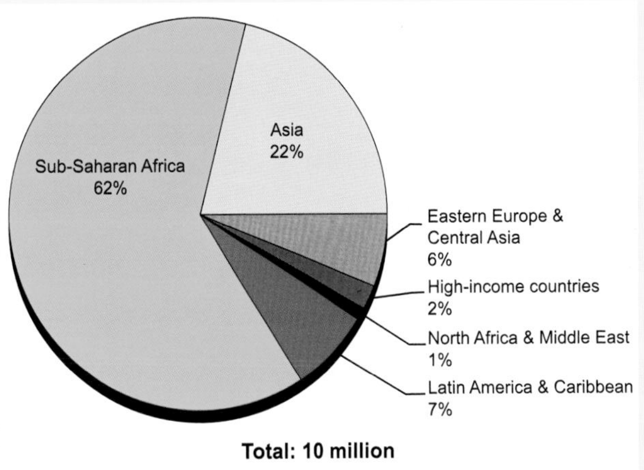

Figure 30

Early sexual debut

Most young people become sexually active in their teens, and many before their 15th birthday. Factors such as increasing urbanization, poverty, exposure to conflicting ideas about sexual values and behaviour, and the breakdown of traditional sexuality and reproduction information channels are encouraging premarital sexual activity among adolescents.

Studies show that adolescents who begin sexual activity early are likely to have sex with more partners and with partners who have been at risk of HIV exposure. They are not likely to use condoms (WHO, 2000). In Kisumu, Kenya, 25% of sexually active young boys and 33% of young girls said they had not used a condom during their first and subsequent sexual encounters (Glynn et al., 2001). Erratic

Barriers to prevention information in India

In India, premarital sex and pregnancy are more common than generally acknowledged. The country's capacity to provide sexual and reproductive health services to young people faces the twin constraints of cultural resistance to open discussion of sexuality and an overall lack of basic information about it. Although sex education is part of school AIDS education, some state officials dilute messages they disagree with, and teachers often avoid topics that make them uncomfortable. When they seek information or services, young people may be scolded or face judgemental health providers. Moreover, since sexual health services frequently offer little privacy or confidentiality, girls often seek substandard or illegal services (Greene et al., 2002).

Sexual and reproductive health status of 15–19-year-old girls in 2000 and 2001

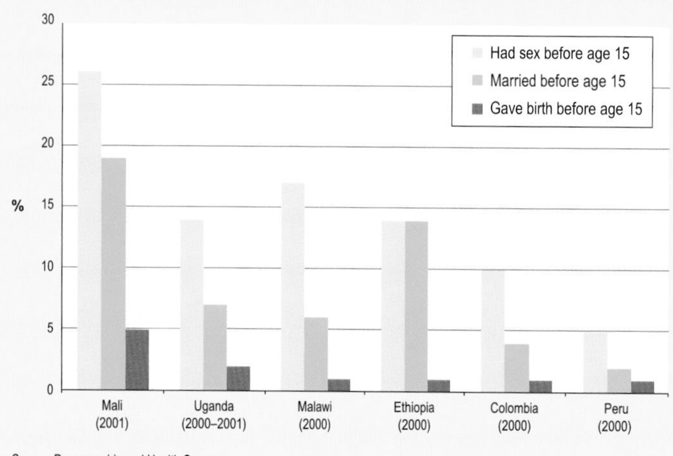

Source: Demographic and Health Surveys

Figure 31

condom use with regular and non-regular sexual partners was also reported in studies in Argentina, Korea and Peru (WHO, 2000).

Gender disparities

When the primary mode of HIV transmission is heterosexual, young women are the worst affected. The proportion of women living with HIV who are over 15 years old is 1.7 times higher in sub-Saharan Africa than in other regions (Population Reference Bureau, 2003). In Trinidad and Tobago, the number of women between 15 and 19 years old with HIV is five times higher than among adolescent males (Pisani, 2003) (see 'Global Overview' chapter).

The higher biological vulnerability of girls and women to HIV infection is one explanation for the growing numbers of young women infected with HIV. However, gender power imbalances, patterns of sexual networking, and age-mixing are important factors that tip the balance further against them. In sub-Saharan Africa, girls are having sex at an earlier age than boys (see Figure 31), and their sexual partners tend to be older.

Over 45 quantitative studies in sub-Saharan Africa on age differences between girls 15 to 19 years old and their sexual partners show that many male partners are six or more years older (see box on page 95). Typically, girls in cross-generational relationships have limited power to resist pressures to agree to unsafe sexual practices (Luke and Kurz, 2002). Abstinence before marriage may not be a successful strategy for these girls, because they marry early and their older husbands may already carry the virus.

Economics, sexuality and HIV in Africa

Why do girls in sub-Saharan Africa often have much older sexual partners? The most common explanation is that poverty and hardship drive girls into transactional sex with older men. However, a regional survey found that economic necessity is one of several factors. Many girls also sought out older men because they were viewed as good marriage partners or providers of a better life who could help the girls with education or work opportunities. Many reported that gifts of clothes, jewellery and perfume enhanced their self-esteem and their status among their peers (Luke and Kurz, 2002).

Whatever the reasons, the UN Secretary-General's Task Force on Women, Girls and HIV/AIDS in Southern Africa has found that both transactional sex and intergenerational sex have become the norm in many countries. For example, a study in Zimbabwe found that nearly 25% of women in their 20s are in relationships with men at least 10 years older (United Nations, 2003). It is also clear that these relationships are a major factor in the 'feminization' of AIDS in Africa. African men are expected to have many sex partners, and on average, those living with HIV became infected in their mid-to-late 20s.

In comparison, girls generally form long-term sexual relationships with one partner. Despite this relative fidelity, many living with HIV were infected soon after they started having sex. A Zambian study showed that 18% of women who said they became sexually active within the last year were HIV-positive. In South Africa, 20% of sexually active girls between the ages of 16 and 18 were infected (Pisani, 2003). Intergenerational sex appears to be a driving factor in the epidemic in Southern Africa. These relationships are based on equations of power and economics that leave girls vulnerable to abuse, exploitation, violence and HIV.

Coerced sexual relationships

From a very early age, many young women experience rape and forced sex. For example, 20% of all young girls interviewed in Kisumu, Kenya, and Ndola, Zambia, said their first sexual encounter involved physical force (Glynn et al., 2001). Similarly, around 25% of 15–24-year-old girls in KwaZulu-Natal, South Africa said they had been 'tricked' or 'persuaded' into their first sexual experience (Manzini, 2001). Violent or forced sex can increase the risk of transmitting HIV because forced vaginal penetration commonly causes abrasions and cuts that allow the virus to cross the vaginal wall more easily.

Injecting drug use: emerging threat

In Central Asia and Eastern Europe, there is evidence that the age of initiation of injecting drug use is falling (Rhodes et al., 2002). Furthermore, overall drug use appears to be increasing, due to rapid social and political change, sharp declines in living standards, and an increase in regional heroin availability (UNDP, 2003). Young injecting drug users are particularly at risk, since they may not have the knowledge or skills to protect themselves from infection via contaminated injecting equipment (UNAIDS, 2003).

Linking increased knowledge to behaviour change

Knowledge and information are the first lines of defence for young people. Some countries have taken bold steps to address the AIDS information needs of young people, but this education is still far from universal. For instance, in sub-Saharan Africa, only 8% of out-of-school youth and slightly more in-school youth have access to prevention education. The equivalent figures for Eastern Europe and Central Asia are 3% of out-of-school youth and 40% of in-school youth; and for the Caribbean and Latin America, 4% and 38% respectively (Global HIV Prevention Working Group, 2003). One global study showed that 44 out of 107 countries did not include AIDS in their school curricula (Lopez, 2002).

It is not surprising that data from 20 high-prevalence countries reveal that although most young people have heard of HIV and AIDS, they are mostly unable to recognize three misconceptions about HIV and to identify two prevention methods (see Figure 32). A recent survey in Egypt had similar findings. Most respondents had heard of AIDS and believed it to be a dangerous disease, but many had little additional knowledge.

Access to AIDS information alone is no guarantee of behaviour change, but education does have an impact. An analysis of 250 North American programmes found that among sexually active young people, AIDS education programmes were effective in decreasing the number of sexual partners and increasing condom use (Kirby, 2002). In Tanzania, the

Percentage of young women (15–24 years old) with comprehensive HIV and AIDS knowledge, by region, by 2003

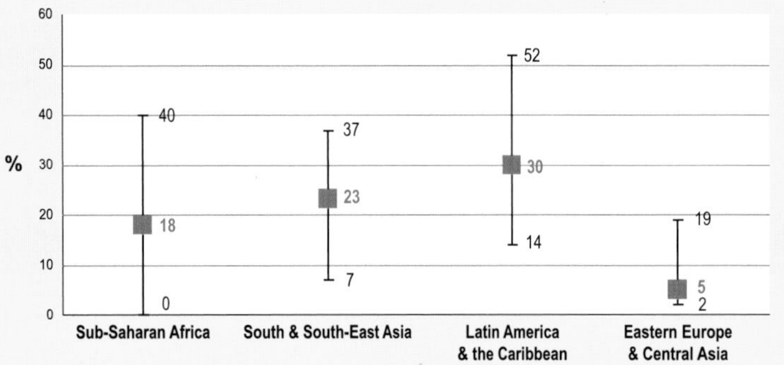

Note: For each region, the percentage is shown for countries with low, median and high values

Sources: United Nations Development Programme (2002), *Botswana AIDS Impact Survey (BAIS 2001): Survey Results and Indicators Summary Report. Gaborone*; UNICEF, *Multiple Indicator Survey (2000)*; FHI, *Behavioural Surveillance Survey (2001)* and; Measure DHS+, *Demographic and Health Surveys (1998–2002).*

Figure 32

MEMA kwa Vijana ('good things for young people' in Swahili) AIDS education project targeted 15–19-year-olds in 20 rural communities (Obasi et al., 2003). The three-year effort substantially improved both knowledge and reported condom use among young people and will now be rolled out to 600 communities.

Supportive environments

A vital lesson learned by the *MEMA kwa Vijana* project was that changing the norms and beliefs of adults in the community, particularly among men, increased the effectiveness of youth-targeted, behaviour-change interventions. Programme and policy directions in several countries have been hampered by adult beliefs of what young people should be permitted to know. Many adults, including political leaders, still find it difficult to acknowledge the sexuality of young people, and they fear that sexual education will lead to promiscuity.

However, various global studies have consistently found little evidence that sex education encourages sexual experimentation or increased sexual activity (Cowan, 2002). Successful young people's AIDS and sexual health education initiatives have worked to allay the fears of adults by taking into account social norms, cultural practices, gender roles and expectations.

In Haiti, the *Fondation pour la santé reproductive et l'education familiale* ('Foundation for reproductive health and family education') has dramatically increased the use of AIDS reproductive health services for young people through a multifaceted approach that builds

Mass media, HIV prevention and youth

Mass media are increasingly important in most young people's lives, and in many countries they represent excellent channels through which to reach youth with HIV prevention messages. Research has shown that media campaigns are most effective when combined with local education efforts.

To encourage delays in sexual initiation, a mass media campaign in Jamaica uses a targeted, age-based approach to encourage young people. For 10–12-year-olds, abstinence messages are the focus. Children between 13 and 15 years of age are targeted with self-awareness and abstinence messages; older youth are targeted with information on protection from pregnancy, HIV and sexually transmitted infections.

In South Africa, a survey found that the innovative media approaches and messages of 'loveLife', the national young people's HIV prevention programme, have been helpful in breaking down social taboos regarding adolescent sexuality, promoting responsible sexual behaviour and increasing use of comprehensive health services. Working through 900 government-run clinics to promote youth-friendly health services, 'loveLife' has 'Y-Centres' or youth centres that provide HIV education and sexual health services in a recreational environment.

MTV Networks International's 2003 version of the Staying Alive campaign, conducted in partnership with UNAIDS, the World Bank and many others, reached 942 million households in some 171 countries. The television programmes and concerts promoted favourable HIV-prevention attitudes, knowledge and skills among young people. These programmes further formed the basis of in-depth campaigns launched in local areas across the globe. For example, Family Health International used the same television campaign to help build a national media campaign in Senegal (Family Health International, 2003).

a support network among peers, parents and educators. Support from these 'gatekeepers' is a vital strategy that has also succeeded in breaking down social resistance in Cameroon, Madagascar and Rwanda.

Agenda for action

Young people are especially vulnerable to HIV, but they are also our greatest hope for changing the course of the AIDS epidemic. When young people are given appropriate tools and support, they can become powerful agents for change. Nothing short of a comprehensive HIV prevention strategy for young people is required. Early sexual debut, transgenerational sex and gender disparities highlight the fact that education alone will not protect the world's youth from infection. Access to confidential health services and condoms, and protecting the rights of young girls, are also required to lower HIV prevalence among young people.

For example, in Uganda, political commitment and active community mobilization led to a dynamic youth movement concerned with AIDS. Between 1990 and 2000, HIV prevalence among pregnant teenagers (15–19 years) in Kampala fell from 22% to 7%. Delayed sexual debut, reducing the number of partners and increased condom use were all significant factors in this success (Cohen, 2003; UNICEF/UNAIDS/WHO, 2002).

In a world with AIDS, many young people's life choices easily vanish. The AIDS agenda for young people needs to translate the 2001 UN

Declaration of Commitment on HIV/AIDS into concrete actions. These include:

- **Creating a supportive environment** so young people can obtain HIV and reproductive health information, education and services. Policies and laws need to ensure that available resources focus on advancing young people's rights to health care and on reducing all discriminatory structures and practices.
- **Reaching those who influence young people.** Parents, extended families, teachers, political and community leaders and celebrities are strong influences on young people. When their mentors act as positive role models and provide safe environments, meaningful relationships and space for self-expression, young people take the initiative for responsible behaviour.
- **Placing young people at the centre of the response.** There is no age restriction for leadership. Young people are assets, not liabilities; their voices need to be heard and their talents cultivated so they can be instruments for change.
- **Mobilizing the educational system** to become a vehicle for a comprehensive prevention and care programme for school-age youth.
- **Mainstreaming HIV prevention and AIDS care for young people into other sectors.** Young people are often interested in religion, workplaces, sports and the media. These sectors can be used to provide information and services.
- **Addressing gender inequalities** by improving young girls' opportunities to obtain education and skills training, by protecting their rights, and by boosting their income-earning prospects. There is also a need to change the damaging concepts of masculinity that define boys' lives—and negatively affect those of girls and women. Authorities need to clearly transmit the message that sexual exploitation of and violence against young girls and boys are unacceptable.
- **Opening dialogue on sensitive issues.** Adults and young people need to work together on adolescent sexuality, sexual health education, sexual violence and abuse, gender roles and traditional practices.

Treatment, care and support for people living with HIV

5

5

Treatment and care for women and girls

Biology matters

HIV affects men and women in different ways, and women's immune systems may respond differently to the virus (Farzadegan et al., 1998). On top of the many HIV-related diseases and ailments suffered by both sexes, HIV-positive women have a higher incidence of cervical cancer than women without the virus. When women are on antiretroviral treatment, they may experience stronger side effects. Studies suggest female hormones may play a role, as may the fact that both sexes take the same size dose of drugs, even though the average woman weighs less than a man (Project Inform, 2001).

Despite these differences, when treated equally, the differences between men and women's survival rates disappear. Unfortunately, in most parts of the world, the social and economic power imbalances between men and women raise fears that women are being denied equitable and timely access to treatment options.

Targets and obstacles

In many countries, prevailing gender attitudes mean women and girls are the last priority for health care. Husbands and elders often decide whether to spend family resources on health care, or whether a woman can take time away from her household duties to visit a health centre. AIDS has further complicated this situation. When male and female family members are HIV-infected, and resources are limited, addressing male treatment needs often comes first.

To reflect the global distribution of HIV by sex, which is nearly 50–50, women should constitute at least half of the millions of people in low- and middle-income countries expected to gain access to antiretrovirals in coming years. To account for regional differences (such as in sub-Saharan Africa, where women account for 57% of HIV infections), countries need to set national treatment targets based on the epidemic's sexual distribution. Furthermore, communities need to overcome barriers to women being tested for HIV, including the risk of violence they may face if they are found to be HIV-positive.

Adolescent girls face strong obstacles to gaining access to treatment. In many countries, they are at the highest risk of HIV due to gender power imbalances, early marriages, sexual violence, and intergenerational sex. Yet, they have the least power to demand treatment. They also often face legal barriers such as age-of-consent laws. These laws are meant to protect young people, but they may also deny them the ability to make important life decisions (Center for Health and Gender Equity, 2004).

Ensuring gender-sensitive access to treatment

Recently, the Center for Health and Gender Equality proposed essential elements for gender-sensitive access to AIDS treatment (Center for Health and Gender Equality, 2004). These include ensuring that:

- **eligibility criteria reflect both biomedical and socioeconomic vulnerabilities**—Treatment eligibility should consider factors such as the inequality in social status of many women and girls, as well as CD4 cell counts.
- **eligibility criteria do not discriminate against women depending on their pregnancy status, nor focus on women only in relation to their pregnancy**—Non-pregnant women and adolescent girls should not be neglected during efforts to expand access to services that prevent mother-to-child transmission.
- **criteria and processes for expanding access to treatment are transparent and accountable to communities in question.**
- **drug adherence programmes are gender-sensitive**—A service's hours of operation and staffing need to consider a woman's work and domestic schedules or responsibilities, as well as her need for privacy and dignity when accessing care.
- **sound efforts are made to achieve quality of care and an end to bias within health-care systems**—In many places, health-care infrastructure and procedures need to be improved to provide safe, comprehensive and sustained treatment. At the same time, health-care providers must model gender-sensitive behaviour and not perpetuate gender bias, even if it is rampant in the wider community.

In Botswana and South Africa, treatment programmes raise hopes that gender equity can be achieved. Both have observed that women outnumber men in gaining access to scaled-up treatment services. Various reasons may exist for this. Both programmes have strong roots in efforts to prevent mother-to-child transmission of HIV that do not target men. Also, it may be that general experiences with antenatal, maternity and child-related public health care make women more comfortable with accessing AIDS-related health services. It is still unclear whether the experiences of these programmes can be replicated in other acutely affected countries, especially those where public-health infrastructure is less developed and where women face greater obstacles in gaining access to general health care (Fleischman, 2004).

Treatment, care and support for people living with HIV

The global community is at a crossroads in expanding access to HIV treatment and care. Never before have the opportunities been so great: unprecedented political will in countries; unprecedented financial resources to fund treatment, care and support; and unprecedented affordability of medicines and diagnostics.

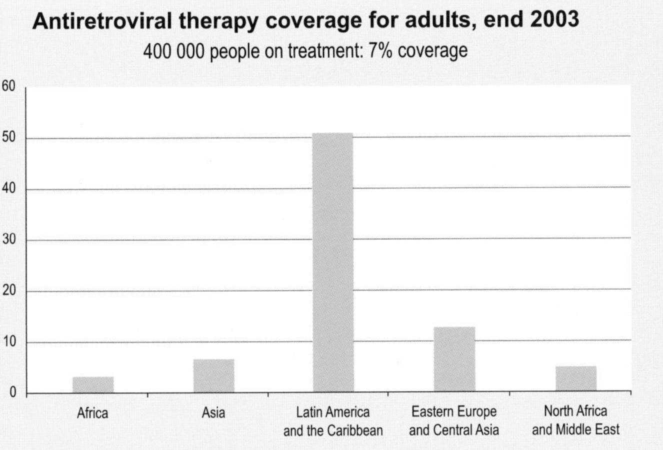

Figure 33

Despite these extraordinarily positive conditions, access to antiretroviral treatment and other HIV-related disease care remains abysmally low. Five to six million people in low- and middle-income countries need antiretroviral treatment immediately. However, the World Health Organization (WHO) estimated that only 400 000 people at the end of 2003 had access to it. This means that nine out of ten people who urgently need HIV treatment are not being reached.

Scaling up treatment and care

Nevertheless, the global movement to scale up access to HIV treatment has made critical gains during the past several years. In endorsing the 2001 Declaration of Commitment on HIV/AIDS, all UN member states pledged to progressively provide the highest attainable standard of treatment for HIV-related disease, including antiretroviral therapy. Most countries with national AIDS plans have incorporated antiretroviral treatment into them and have set specific antiretroviral treatment coverage targets. Meanwhile, UNAIDS and other partners have developed tools to measure progress and promote accountability in achieving this goal, and are actively monitoring and evaluating the situation in countries.

Globally, governments, the UN system, bilateral donors, the Global Fund to Fight AIDS, Tuberculosis and Malaria and civil society are increasingly focusing on treatment and care as part of their commitment to scaling up the global HIV response. For example, the World Bank's Multi-country AIDS Programme, which amounts to US$ 1 billion for Africa and US$ 155 million for the Caribbean, is allowing governments and other beneficiaries to use World Bank funds flexibly for HIV treatment, including for procuring medicines, strengthening health system infrastructures and training.

In May 2004, the Bank agreed to allocate US$ 60 million through a new Treatment Acceleration Programme to scale up treatment in three pilot countries: Burkina Faso, Ghana

Progress update on the global response to the AIDS epidemic, 2004

Less than one in ten people who need antiretroviral therapy receive it

- An estimated five to six million people in low- and middle-income countries will die in the next two years if they do not receive antiretroviral treatment. As of December 2003, only an estimated 400 000 people in these regions were obtaining it.
- On average, 80% of responding countries reported having a policy in place to ensure or improve access to HIV-related drugs. However, in reality, it is estimated that access to antiretroviral treatment is below 10% in every region except the Americas.
- Several South American countries have universal coverage for antiretroviral therapy, including Argentina, Brazil, Chile, Cuba, Mexico and Uruguay. Several others cover about two-thirds of people in need, including Barbados, Colombia, Costa Rica and Paraguay.
- In sub-Saharan Africa, an estimated 4.3 million people need AIDS home-based care, but only about 12% receive it. In South-East Asia, coverage drops to 2%.
- In South America and Eastern Europe, most patients receive at least the essential package of care services recommended by WHO and UNAIDS. In Africa and Asia, only one-third of people receive at least the essential package.

Source: *Progress Report on the Global Response to the HIV/AIDS Epidemic,* UNAIDS, 2003; *Coverage of selected services for HIV/AIDS prevention and care in low- and middle-income countries in 2003,* UNAIDS/USAID/WHO/CDC and the Policy Project, 2004.

and Mozambique. Meanwhile, the Global Fund to Fight AIDS, Tuberculosis and Malaria's HIV-related grant monies mean that 700 000 people will be able to gain access to antiretroviral treatment (Global Fund to Fight AIDS, Tuberculosis and Malaria, 2003). About 80% of the Fund's HIV/AIDS and integrated HIV/Tuberculosis approved proposals include provisions for strengthening antiretroviral programmes and procuring HIV medicines.

Bilateral donors are increasingly open to supporting care and treatment if they are part of comprehensive AIDS plans linked to broader national development plans. The United States of America has launched the *President's Emergency Plan for AIDS Relief* which includes the goal of reaching two million people with HIV treatment in priority countries in Africa and the Caribbean. France and seven other countries have initiated a 'twinning' project called Ensemble pour une solidarité thérapeutique hospitalière en réseau to help support antiretroviral programmes in several low- and middle-income countries.

Low- and middle-income countries are also increasingly allocating funds from national budgets and debt relief to support treatment services. For example, in 2003–2004 Cameroon allocated over US$ 30 million in debt relief under the Highly Indebted Poor Countries Initiative to support AIDS programmes—most of the money went to care activities. Meanwhile, South Africa's national AIDS care plan is based largely on domestic financing.

The private sector

Private sector efforts are also increasing. Advocacy to set up prevention and treatment programmes in the workplace has been mainly led by businesses themselves. Under the leadership of Ambassador Richard Holbrooke, the Global Business Coalition on HIV/AIDS has grown to include 145 major business corporations. Many of these companies and other large and small enterprises are establishing HIV treatment programming for their employees as called for by the International Labour Organization (ILO). These companies include Anglo American (see box on page 103),

Anglo American and AngloGold—providing antiretroviral treatment to miners in Southern Africa

Over the past 16 years Anglo American has implemented a comprehensive response to HIV and AIDS including non-discrimination, prevention, testing and care. From mid-2002 through 2003, the company initiated an antiretroviral treatment programme, one of the largest global employer-based HIV treatment initiatives, with over 1100 employees receiving treatment by January 2004. To accelerate providing comprehensive HIV services in government primary care clinics located in their communities, Anglo American is extending HIV services beyond the workplace through partnerships with 'loveLife' and other community-based organizations.

In November 2002, AngloGold, a large gold mining company, also recognized that human and economic factors justify investing in HIV workplace programmes, and extended its programme for HIV-positive employees to include antiretroviral treatment. Treatment activists and commentators in South Africa have applauded these initiatives. However, they stress it is also important to provide treatment to other HIV-positive family members in order to avoid inequity in treatment access within families and to ensure women and children can obtain treatment for HIV-related disease.

DaimlerChrysler (automobiles), Eskom (utilities), Lafarge (cement), Royal Dutch/Shell (petroleum) and Heineken (beer). Tata Steel in India and ChevronTexaco in Nigeria are also expanding treatment services within their companies and wider communities.

In March 2004, the Accelerating Access Initiative (a public-private partnership of six research-based pharmaceutical companies and the UN) reported that the quantities of antiretroviral medicines from these companies supplied to Africa doubled in the last six months of 2003.

Falling antiretroviral prices

In recent years, the prices of antiretroviral medicine have fallen dramatically; a major development that has helped to make wider treatment access possible. In 2000, the price of a first-line WHO-recommended combination antiretroviral regimen to treat one patient for one year was between US$ 10 000 and US$ 12 000 on world markets. Several factors converged to help bring down prices—including advocacy by people living with HIV and by world leaders. By early 2002, generic competition and the practice of differential pricing by pharmaceutical companies had contributed to dramatic price reductions, particularly for low-income countries. The price for certain generic combinations dropped to US$ 300 per person per year.

The William J Clinton Presidential Foundation has played a critical catalytic role in planning in individual countries and in engaging generic drug manufacturers from India and South Africa in moves to lower prices. By the end of 2003, it announced that it had negotiated antiretroviral prices as low as US$ 140 per

Equitable access to affordable medicines—the power of advocacy

"People no longer accept that the sick and dying, simply because they are poor, should be denied drugs which have transformed the lives of others who are better off."

—Kofi Annan, Secretary-General of the United Nations

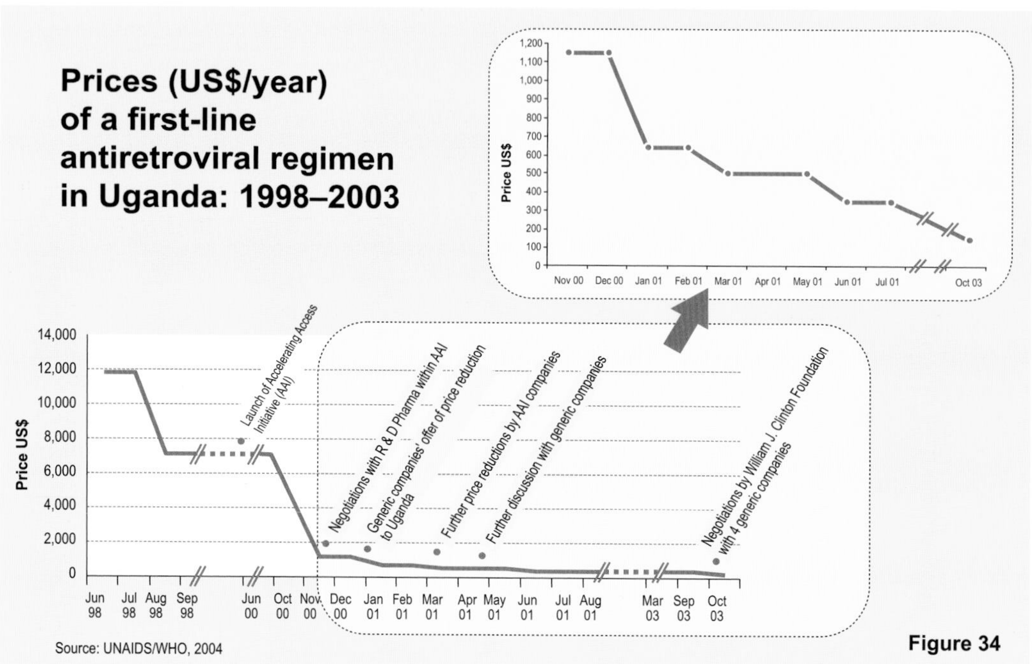

Source: UNAIDS/WHO, 2004

Figure 34

person per year (less than US$ 0.50 per day) under certain conditions. These preferential prices for generics are available for WHO-recommended, first-line regimens in countries in which the Foundation is working in Africa and the Caribbean.

Recently, the Clinton Foundation has offered the same prices for antiretroviral procurement to the United Nations Children's Fund (UNICEF) and to World Bank and Global Fund beneficiaries. These are important advances, but antiretroviral prices remain extremely high in a number of middle-income countries, including Russia, Serbia and other Central and Eastern European countries. The price offered by pharmaceutical companies for WHO-recommended, second-line regimens is also high, exceeding US$ 1000 per person per year—even in low-income countries.

Meanwhile, cooperation continues to increase between countries with antiretroviral medicine manufacturing capacity and countries wishing to set up local production facilities. Brazil, India, Thailand and several large African countries recently signed cooperation agreements. Then, at a January 2004 WHO meeting, they and other low- and middle-income countries agreed to cooperate with European and North American industrialized countries. Together, they will jointly promote and undertake antiretroviral production technology transfer to low- and middle-income countries interested and able to create local production capacity.

In sub-Saharan Africa, many more countries say they intend to set up their own production facilities. These include Ethiopia, Kenya, Mozambique, Nigeria, Tanzania, Uganda and Zambia. South Africa already launched its first antiretroviral drug in August 2003. All have plans to start manufacturing generics sometime during 2004–2005 (Dummett, 2003).

Treatment and prevention: mutually reinforcing

Some people oppose scaling up treatment with prevention-versus-treatment 'cost-effectiveness' arguments. But cost-effectiveness analyses comparing HIV prevention and treatment provide a simplistic and outdated view that prevention should be funded to the exclusion of treatment, merely because prevention programmes may be cheaper.

In July 2003, the World Bank concluded that most studies underestimate the long-term impact of the epidemic, and that AIDS can cause far greater long-term damage to national economies than previously assumed. The Government of Brazil has estimated that antiretroviral treatment has resulted in savings of about US$ 2.2 billion in hospital care that would have otherwise been required by people living with HIV. The government says antiretroviral treatment has contributed to a 50% fall in mortality rates, a 60–80% decrease in morbidity rates and a 70% reduction in hospitalizations among HIV-positive people.

Cost-effectiveness analyses pitting prevention against treatment ignore the mutually reinforcing synergy of integrating these interventions. Ultimately, there is no arbitrary threshold at which treatment can be valued. No nation hit by an expensive security breach would refrain from correcting it on the grounds that it would be cheaper to prevent future breaches. It would deal with the breach *and* take preventive measures. So it should be with AIDS.

Widespread access to antiretroviral treatment could bring millions of people into health-care settings, providing new opportunities for health-care workers to deliver and reinforce HIV prevention messages and interventions. Doctors, nurses and community health workers should be trained to integrate risk reduction promotion into antiretroviral adherence support. Simultaneous and aggressive expansion of both HIV prevention and AIDS treatment in a truly comprehensive approach can halt and begin to reverse the epidemic.

Antiretroviral medicines in resource-limited settings

With unprecedented opportunities now in place for scaling up treatment, it is almost universally agreed that antiretroviral medicines can

The link between prevention and care

The belated focus on AIDS treatment is highlighting the synergies between many aspects of prevention and treatment. For example, the fact that antiretroviral drugs are becoming more available means that more people are seeking voluntary counselling and testing and finding out their HIV status. Both treatment and prevention are needed simultaneously for a successful response.

- In South Africa, a health survey conducted after the start of Médecins Sans Frontières' antiretroviral programme in Khayelitsha found that, of eight sites reviewed, the Khayelitsha township had the highest level of condom use, willingness to join AIDS clubs, and willingness to be tested for HIV (WHO, 2003b).
- In Masaka, Uganda, a voluntary counselling and testing unit that had closed its doors for lack of clients was rehabilitated in 2002 at the same time an antiretroviral programme began on the same hospital premises. Attendance soared. By February 2003, a total of 5060 clients had received voluntary counselling and testing—a 17-fold increase on 2000 (Mpiima et al., 2003).
- In the first year of the HIV Equity Initiative, an antiretroviral programme run by Partners for Health in Cange, Haiti, demand for voluntary counselling and testing increased more than threefold (WHO, 2003a).
- A survey of 700 HIV positive people in Côte D'Ivoire in 2000 indicated that those with access to antiretroviral treatment were more likely to use condoms during sex than those without access (Moatti et al., 2003).

Providing antiretroviral treatment in Thailand

In Thailand, lower drug prices have contributed to a fivefold increase in the number of HIV-positive patients receiving antiretroviral treatment; from about 2500 cases in November 2002 to more than 15 000 cases by November 2003. The 2004 target is 50 000 people. The Thai government's antiretroviral treatment programme now offers free treatment to HIV-positive patients, and uses the locally produced combination drug GPOvir (d4T, 3TC and nevirapine) as the standard first-line treatment regimen. Using GPOvir has reduced the monthly cost for one patient's treatment from about US$ 300 to US$ 29. All 92 of the provincial hospitals under the Public Health Ministry are capable of providing antiretroviral treatment, and this capacity is to be rolled out to other hospitals in the near future.

be delivered safely and effectively in resource-limited settings. Beginning with the UNAIDS Drug Access Initiative in 1997 in Abidjan and Kampala, and then from Africa to Asia to the Caribbean, one after another, small-scale pilot projects have demonstrated programme effectiveness and safety.

Civil society has long been at the forefront of delivering HIV treatment. The Catholic Church reports that it delivers 26% of health care globally, and other faith-based groups are increasingly active in providing HIV care. Nongovernmental organizations (NGOs) have been treatment pioneers. They include Haiti's Zanmi Lasante (Partners in Health), San Eguidio in Mozambique, and international campaigners such as Médecins sans Frontières (see box on page 107). They have stimulated the energies and commitment of the international community, and have taught valuable lessons.

Many countries, including those with high HIV prevalence or with emerging epidemics in large populations, have already been mobilizing in response to the HIV treatment gap. Several countries in Latin America and the Caribbean now offer universal coverage for antiretroviral treatment, including Argentina, Barbados, Chile, Costa Rica, Cuba, Mexico and Uruguay. Bahamas and Guyana are advancing towards universal access. Brazil is engaged in a South-South cooperation programme with Bolivia and Paraguay to achieve universal access in those countries. Other countries that have made substantial progress include Botswana and Senegal. However, Brazil remains the only country with a large population to achieve universal access to AIDS treatment.

In Asia, as of November 2003, the national AIDS programmes in only two countries—India and Thailand—offered both first- and second-line treatment regimens. Only three others—Indonesia, Nepal and Sri Lanka—provided at least one first-line treatment regimen. The challenge now is to show that nationwide treatment programmes can be made available to millions of people in other low- and middle-income countries.

For development planners, the AIDS epidemic is a global public health emergency. Life expectancy of people with HIV is plummeting and the epidemic of infection is rapidly transforming into one of disease and death. Therefore, emergency approaches are needed to counteract the gradual approach to development that is often traditional to the health sector. At the same time, it is critical that expanded antiretroviral treatment coverage does not signal a return to disease-specific approaches to health care, but rather systematically builds and strengthens health systems across the board.

Médecins sans Frontières: pioneering HIV treatment in low- and middle-income countries

Since the early 1990s, Médecins sans Frontières has been caring for people living with HIV in low- and middle-income countries. Its first antiretroviral treatment programmes began in 2001. As of April 2004, approximately 13 000 people were on treatment in 42 of its projects in 19 countries in Africa, Asia and Latin America. The organization has been scaling up its programmes rapidly: from 1500 people in 10 countries in mid-2002, to a projected 25 000 in 25 countries by the end of 2004. At the same time, Médecins sans Frontières is sharing lessons learned through its diverse treatment experience. These lessons include:

- 'one pill twice a day'—adhering to treatment needs to be made as easy as possible; 80% of the organization's patients are on a WHO-recommended, triple fixed-dose combination.
- 'decentralize and adapt'—Médecins sans Frontières operates in areas with limited infrastructure and personnel. So, it uses mobile treatment clinics, delegates basic patient care to nurses and community health workers, and often begins treatment on the basis of a positive HIV test and clinical assessment by trained staff.
- 'available to the poorest'—cost should never be a barrier to treatment, and treatment will therefore have to be free for most people in the poorest countries.
- 'price matters'—the lower the price of medicines, the higher the number of patients who can be treated.
- 'involve the community'—community engagement helps to raise treatment and prevention adherence, and to break down the taboo surrounding HIV.

Voluntary counselling and testing, HIV prevention and treatment programmes, and sexual and reproductive health services need to be effectively integrated and form part and parcel of primary health services. An excellent example of prevention-treatment integration is provided by mother-to-child transmission prevention programmes that also include antiretroviral treatment for mothers who need it, both during and after pregnancy.

At the XIVth International Conference on HIV/AIDS in Barcelona, Spain in 2002, key participants set a global target of expanding antiretroviral treatment to three million people in low- and middle-income countries by the end of 2005. UNAIDS Secretariat, WHO and other partners concluded that this target was feasible if sufficient funds were raised and other measures taken. These 3 million people are among those who will die within two years if they do not receive antiretroviral treatment now.

Shortly after the Barcelona conference, additional steps were taken by the international community to mobilize around this target. This included establishing a global partnership of organizations working for expanded treatment access: the International HIV Treatment Access Coalition. The coalition grew to more than 120 members, but proved to be unsustainable as a vehicle for coordinating international community support.

The '3 by 5' Initiative

In September 2003, a crucial development occurred at the second UN General Assembly Special Session on HIV/AIDS. The Director-General of the World Health Organization and the Executive Director of UNAIDS declared the lack of treatment in low- and middle-income countries a global public health emergency and launched the '3 by 5' Initiative. They appealed to the global community to bridge the treatment gap, calling it one of the greatest human rights and public health crises of our times.

On World AIDS Day 2003, WHO took another important step, the announcement of its '3 by 5' Initiative. In the '3 by 5' context, WHO and UNAIDS have urged partners, including NGOs and the private sector, to join in mobilizing support to governments for scaling up treatment programmes in countries.

This '3 by 5' Initiative is an interim target, part of a global movement to mobilize support for vastly expanded—and ultimately universal—treatment access. Since its launch, many countries have announced, reconfirmed, or stepped up their commitments to bringing HIV treatment to their people who need it. To date, some 40 countries have formally said they wish to participate in the Initiative. With support from UNAIDS, WHO is seeking resources to expand the technical support that it can offer to countries in scaling up treatment programmes. As of June 2004, the governments of Canada, Sweden and the United Kingdom together with allocations from the UNAIDS Unified Budget and Workplan had provided important financial support for WHO to carry out its '3 by 5' strategy.

The strategy

The WHO strategy, *Treating 3 million by 2005—Making it happen*, includes a clear commitment by WHO to act in an urgent manner; involve people living with HIV in a central role; work in partnerships; safeguard equity and human rights; ensure sustainability for lifelong care; and make certain the Initiative is complementary with existing services. '3 by 5' will enshrine country ownership—the overriding feature of the 'Three Ones' approach initiated by UNAIDS (see 'National Responses' chapter). WHO's strategic framework contains 14 key elements which fall into five 'pillars': global leadership, strong partnership and advocacy; urgent, sustained country support; simplified, standardized tools for delivering antiretroviral therapy; effective, reliable supply of medicines and diagnostics; and rapidly identifying and reapplying new knowledge and successes.

Global leadership, strong partnership and advocacy

The most vital work of '3 by 5' is happening in countries and communities. But global leadership and alliances among international participants help create the conditions for success. Partnership is essential to making the Initiative work. The target of '3 by 5' and the longer-term goal of universal access far outstretch the capacities of any single organization. Innovative collaborative mechanisms are now being built that link national governments, international organizations, the private sector, civil society groups and communities.

A fundamental principle of '3 by 5' is that people living with HIV need to play a central role in designing, implementing and monitoring antiretroviral treatment programmes. Involving infected people in treatment-related activities contributes to reducing stigma and to making programmes more effective (Farmer et al., 2001). But stigma continues to be an obstacle to recruiting people living with HIV to work in antiretroviral programmes. Therefore, massive and creative efforts to combat stigma are required to create the supportive environment necessary for people living with HIV to play their full role in treatment scale up.

At the global and multilateral level, key partners supporting action in countries include international associations of treatment activists and treatment providers; WHO and other UNAIDS Cosponsors including the World Bank's Multi-country AIDS Programme; and the Global Fund to Fight AIDS, Tuberculosis and Malaria. To scale up country antiretroviral

Lack of health workers: a key impediment to antiretroviral programme success

The number of health workers available, including health administrators and training staff, is critical to country capacity to deliver services. Often health personnel have received no in-service training or even basic information about HIV and AIDS. According to a recent report, China has fewer than 200 doctors with any specialist skills in diagnosing and treating AIDS opportunistic infections.

In countries hard-hit by AIDS, research suggests that lack of health-worker capacity is a serious problem for all programmes, but particularly for those that plan to distribute antiretrovirals widely. For example, in Tanzania, the size of the health workforce must triple in order to deliver priority interventions to most of the population by 2015. In Chad, it must quadruple. In Botswana, health officials say that achieving universal coverage of antiretroviral treatment alone would require doubling the current nurse workforce, tripling the number of physicians and quintupling the number of pharmacists.

Unfortunately, in countries most affected by AIDS, health staff vacancy rates are extremely high. In 1998, Ghana had a vacancy rate of 43% for physicians in public facilities; in Malawi it was 36%. In 1998, Lesotho reported its public sector nurse vacancy rate was 48%, Malawi's was 50% in 2001. Another problem is that health workers are not evenly distributed in a country. In Tanzania, the nurse-per-100 000 population ratio in urbanized Dar es Salaam is 160, but in the rest of Tanzania there are districts with a ratio of fewer than 6 nurses per 100 000. Of course, this problem is not confined to countries with high HIV prevalence. In Nicaragua, approximately 50% of the country's health workers are concentrated in the capital city, Managua, where only 20% of the population lives.

Migration is a key reason that health workforces are shrinking in low-income countries. Better wages and benefits, career opportunities and active recruitment attract health workers with internationally-accepted degrees to industrialized countries. In Zambia, more than 600 doctors have been trained since independence, but only 50 remain in the country. More than 50% of physicians trained in Ghana during the 1980s practise abroad. The UN has estimated that 56% of all migrating physicians flow from low- and middle-income to industrialized countries, while only 11% flow in the opposite direction. The imbalance is even greater for nurses. Finally, far greater efforts must be made to improve working conditions and incentives for health and social service workers in rural areas.

treatment access, these partners are linking with key bilateral initiatives, including the United States *President's Emergency Plan for AIDS Relief*, the European Union and the United Kingdom's Call to Action on AIDS led by its Department for International Development, as well as efforts by other donors and the private sector.

Strengthening country capacity

When countries align their national AIDS treatment goals to the '3 by 5' Initiative, many request collaboration with WHO and its partners. During early 2004, special WHO missions worked with countries, international partners, health authorities and stakeholders to support national plan development and funding request preparation, and other activities to scale up antiretroviral treatment implementation.

For example, in conjunction with '3 by 5', Zambia raised its 2005 treatment target from 10 000 to 100 000. Kenya announced a similar increase. But achieving these ambitious targets requires overcoming major implementation obstacles. The challenges are enormous: the health services of many countries have been badly undermined by inadequate investment over decades, and by the burden of AIDS itself (UNAIDS, 2003a). Virtually everywhere, the number of available health sector personnel is too low to meet the needs (see 'National Responses' chapter).

If obstacles are not addressed systematically, expanding antiretroviral treatment on a massive scale will remain merely an aspiration; it could also drain staff away from elsewhere in the health-care system. On the other hand, '3 by 5' can play a catalytic role in drawing new personnel into health work. Key actions to increase staff include: intensified recruitment and training of new and existing staff; improving conditions of employment in the public sector; reassessing job specifications and tasks; and addressing 'brain drain' from poor countries, including providing incentives for attracting nationals home from abroad. Another possible solution is recruiting national and international volunteers to address urgent service delivery gaps.

One way to bridge the health staff gap is to actively train and involve community members. Successful pioneering antiretroviral programmes based in communities in Haiti, South Africa, Uganda and elsewhere have shown that community health workers can take on significant responsibilities in counselling, psychosocial support to patients and their families, adherence support, nutritional support, home care and palliative care and monitoring patients for drug toxicity and clinical failure. To be successful, community members require good training and ongoing support, as well as clear mechanisms for communicating and collaborating with other members of the health-care team.

Simplified, standardized tools

Reducing complexity is a major factor in accelerating the roll-out of treatment in areas with weak health-care systems and severe shortages of trained health professionals. The streamlined guidelines of '3 by 5' have cut the number of recommended first-line treatment regimens from 35 to four. Regimens are simple and pills are fewer, and the four combinations cover a variety of circumstances including co-infection with tuberculosis, and pregnancy.

Twice-a-day regimens also help patients adhere to treatment, resulting in more people remaining healthier, regimens working longer, and opportunities for drug-resistant viruses to be reduced. Just as rapid HIV tests need to be a key feature of voluntary counselling and testing roll-out (see 'Prevention' chapter), so must laboratory testing and diagnostic tools to monitor the health of people on treatment be simplified and made more readily available to the poorest populations. In the interim, the fact that sophisticated monitoring tests such as viral load tests are not currently available in resource-poor settings is not cause to delay scaling up.

Effective, reliable supply of medicines and diagnostics

Maintaining a reliable, affordable supply of quality medicines and diagnostics is one of the greatest challenges countries face in scaling up. UNICEF, the Dutch NGO International Dispensary Association and others are already experienced in procuring antiretrovirals for low-income countries. To provide expanded country support, WHO is creating the AIDS Medicines and Diagnostics Service to be undertaken jointly with UNAIDS, UNICEF, the World Bank and other UN partners. It will serve as an information clearinghouse to help countries gain access to quality antiretroviral medicines and diagnostic tools at the best prices, including through providing information on forecasting need and demand, prices, sources, patents, customs and regulatory matters. The Service will also provide information on quality through its links with WHO's quality assessment programme—the

The commitment to equity must be more than window-dressing

How can we ensure that we make fair decisions about where to locate services and which patients to serve first? In the face of limited resources, ensuring that access to antiretroviral treatment is truly fair and equitable involves making the right choices: how and where to spend the money to set up services, and who gets priority for treatment among those within reach of facilities. There is no single formula for making such choices, but selecting people fairly requires an equitable deliberative process involving various levels of decision-making in society. The *process* of decision-making should be guided by the following key principles and be:

- *inclusive*—to involve a wide range of participants representing all interest groups;
- *impartial*—to avoid conflicts of interest;
- *transparent*—to ensure that the criteria set and rationales for treatment eligibility are open to scrutiny;
- *public*—to satisfy people's basic need to know the grounds for decisions that fundamentally affect their well-being;
- *relevant*—to ensure stakeholders can agree that priorities are based on appropriate and pertinent situational factors;
- *revisable*—to allow for changing decisions in light of new evidence; and
- *accountable*—to maximize fairness, appropriate individuals or institutions need to be responsible to communities for the principles and procedures they implement.

Prequalification Project—in collaboration with UNICEF, the UNAIDS Secretariat and with support from the World Bank.

Providing antiretrovirals in an equitable manner: who gets what and when

In many resource-limited settings, universal access to HIV-related disease treatment cannot be achieved immediately. Indeed, the interim target of expanding antiretroviral treatment access to 3 million people by 2005 is an admission that all people in need today will not be reached. Until resources and programmes are available for all people who need them, ensuring equity of access to services—fair distribution of treatment—will be a key challenge for governments and health-care providers.

Some governmental authorities and health services managers may be reluctant to make decisions about who should be served first and may not foresee the ethical implications of where to site services. In the absence of an explicit structured approach to the ethical roll-out of HIV-related treatment, eligibility may be determined without reference to ethical standards and procedures. When not all people in need can be served, distributing HIV treatment services needs to be guided by principles of equity and human rights such as freedom from discrimination, as well as agreed-upon procedures.

Given the urgency of the situation, antiretroviral treatment will inevitably be delivered initially from those facilities that already have the basic requirements. To ensure this does not simply perpetuate and deepen existing inequalities in health-care delivery, substantial resources need to be directed simultaneously at building the infrastructure to serve people who are considered 'hard to reach' or whose needs have been neglected up to now, including women, young people and the poor.

In many countries, ensuring equitable access for women and girls will require changing attitudes, removing structural impediments to treatment such as discriminatory laws and regulations and monitoring practices for accountability. The same holds true for people whose behaviour is widely stigmatized—injecting drug users, sex workers and men who have sex with men. Specific proactive measures are needed to ensure that gender inequities and barriers to care for vulnerable groups are addressed, and ultimately eliminated. Treating children with antiretrovirals also requires special planning (see box on page 117).

Antiretroviral treatment: part of a comprehensive package

The effect of antiretrovirals on individual lives is often near-miraculous. They are not a permanent cure, but by reducing viral load, they can extend the lives of people living with HIV by years, hopefully until a cure for AIDS is found. But antiretroviral therapy must be part of an integrated package of interventions that includes prevention, care and support activities, all of which complement and reinforce each other (see 'Prevention' chapter).

People on these drugs may still need treatment for opportunistic infections from time to time and treatment for pain that may be a side effect of the drugs they are taking. Some will need substitution maintenance therapy for opiate dependency and many will continue to need psychosocial support in coping with an illness with serious implications for behaviour and lifestyle. They also need sexual and reproductive health services.

Antiretroviral prevention of mother-to-child transmission should avoid compromising future treatment options for women and use dual and triple combinations rather than single dose nevirapine wherever possible (WHO, 2004). Moreover, it must be remembered that even if '3 by 5' achieves all its targets, millions of HIV positive people with advanced immune deficiency will not have access to antiretrovirals for some time to come.

Services for people living with HIV-related disease need to be coordinated to create a 'continuum' of care—i.e. a system of care that meets the multiple and changing needs of infected individuals and their families, and that extends from the home and the community, to the clinic or hospital and back again. Services should be delivered at times and places that are convenient for HIV-positive people and their carers, and in a manner that is culturally sensitive. In addition, there should be efficient and effective referral mechanisms between the different services and levels of care.

Cuba: a comprehensive care success story

Cuba offers a rare example of comprehensive care across the continuum. In the early 1990s Cuba's HIV policies were the focus of controversy and criticism when HIV-positive people were quarantined. Now, people diagnosed with HIV are given a thorough clinical and psychological assessment and then offered the choice of outpatient care provided by a hospital and their family physician, or inpatient care at an AIDS sanatorium. They receive special high-calorie food rations and take part in an eight-week course on all aspects of living with HIV, including the progression of disease and safer sex. Their immune systems and general health are monitored regularly and entered on an electronic database, and health problems are treated promptly. Antiretrovirals are part of the package; about 1500 people currently have access to treatment (WHO, 2003e).

Public-private partnership with strong government leadership—the Botswana model

Botswana has one of the highest HIV prevalence rates in the world—nearly 40% of the adult population is living with HIV. It was the first country in Southern Africa to actively move towards scaling up antiretroviral treatment. President Festus Mogae's strong political leadership (he used the word 'extinction' to describe the threat of AIDS to the Tswana people) was instrumental in mobilizing domestic and international support for treatment programmes. Since 2000, the Botswana national treatment initiative—now called *Masa* (or 'new dawn')—has been supported by the African Comprehensive HIV/AIDS Partnership. This strong, unique public-private partnership involves the Government of Botswana, the Bill and Melinda Gates Foundation, and the Merck Company Foundation. The Botswana-Gates-Merck partnership supports the comprehensive national response and enhances local capacity through the strengthening of health-care infrastructure and the transfer of managerial and technical skills for sustainable health-service delivery.

By early 2004 *Masa* was the largest government HIV treatment programme in Africa, despite Botswana having a small population of 1.7 million and the fact that HIV stigma slowed initial uptake. As of April 2004, more than 24 000 people were enrolled in the programme, with more than 14 000 patients on antiretroviral therapy. However, inadequate capacity to rapidly increase people's awareness of their HIV status is considered the major barrier to expanding access. So Botswana is instituting a routine offer of HIV testing in clinical settings and engaging traditional healers as a potential source of referrals. In terms of equitable access for women and girls, so far more women are receiving treatment than men, by a 3 to 2 ratio.

Comprehensive care approaches are standard in Botswana (see box above), Brazil and other countries that have achieved universal access or are moving rapidly towards it. However, on the whole, comprehensive HIV care remains the exception.

In Africa, WHO estimates that less than 30% of HIV-infected people with tuberculosis—the most important opportunistic infection—are receiving anti-tuberculosis drugs (WHO, 2003c). In 2001, only about 1% of people in need in Zambia and Malawi, and 2% in Uganda, were receiving tuberculosis prophylaxis with isoniazid (Garbus and Marseille, 2003; Garbus, 2003a; Garbus, 2003b; Garbus, 2003c).

Food—an essential part of the response to AIDS

One of the key elements of comprehensive care is having enough to eat. This is the single most pressing preoccupation for many people with AIDS. Disease quickly impoverishes families and leaves many struggling to feed themselves adequately (see 'Impact' chapter). Therefore, relieving hunger is a high priority to help people cope with illness. But good nutrition

Essential medicines are hard to find in many poor countries

The majority of HIV-positive people in low- and middle-income countries do not have access even to relatively simple medications. Furthermore, some countries with high burdens of AIDS have poor and unequal access to essential drugs for *any* condition (World Bank, 2003). For example, in Haiti, Kenya, Malawi and India, coverage of essential medicines ranges from 0–49% across their populations. WHO reports that although access to essential medicines has doubled in the past 20 years, over one-third of the world's population still lacks such access and pays a heavy price in terms of poor health and high death rates. In the poorest parts of Africa and Asia, over 50% of the population lacks access to even the most basic essential medicines.

also has an important role to play in helping people with HIV stay healthy, in counteracting physical wasting due to HIV infection and in boosting energy levels. Moreover, many medicines, including some anti-tuberculosis drugs and antiretrovirals, cannot be taken on an empty stomach. Therefore, food support needs to be part of the comprehensive care package. This is important for the well-being of carers too: many say that one of the most stressful aspects of their job is visiting homes where there is no food and having nothing to offer (UNAIDS, 2000).

To help with food and nutrition issues, the World Food Programme (UNAIDS' ninth Cosponsor) is expanding its food assistance programmes to include HIV-positive people on treatment, as well as hard-hit communities. It is doing this in the context of AIDS treatment and HIV prevention programmes and is working with UNAIDS and other Cosponsors. The Programme has also helped to call attention to the problem of AIDS and food security in the most-affected countries.

Tuberculosis and HIV

In many countries where AIDS has hit hardest, tuberculosis is the leading cause of death in people living with HIV. The greatest impact of HIV on tuberculosis has been in sub-Saharan Africa, where up to 70% of tuberculosis patients are also infected with HIV. The virus is already increasing the incidence of tuberculosis in much of South-East Asia, Eastern Europe and Central Asia, especially where sub-groups of often marginalized people are at high risk of both diseases.

About one-third of the world's population carries latent tuberculosis infection (where *Mycobacterium tuberculosis* bacteria lie dormant in the body without causing disease). But, in the absence of HIV, only about 5% of them will *ever* progress to active disease. Infection with HIV dramatically increases the probability that someone already harbouring latent tuberculosis will develop the active disease to 5–10% *annually*.

It is not expensive to treat tuberculosis. If the medication is taken properly, most cases will be completely cured. In 1991, the World Health Assembly set targets to be reached by 2005 of 85% cure rates and 70% case detection among infectious cases. WHO's recommended DOTS (directly observed treatment, short course), is a highly cost-effective strategy to reach these targets. It has proven feasible for scale up both in a range of low- and middle-income countries and in a variety of formal, informal and private health provider settings (Raviglione, 2003). In 2001, the Stop TB Partnership was formed to expand, adapt and improve strategies to control and eliminate tuberculosis. It develops advocacy, coordinates resource mobilization and monitors progress towards the goals.

In sub-Saharan Africa, the advent of the HIV epidemic has severely compromised the promise of tuberculosis control, with tuberculosis notification rates increasing at 6% per year (De Cock and Chaisson, 1999). In countries of the former Soviet Union, a dramatic rise in tuberculosis has occurred since the mid 1990s. Tuberculosis now constitutes a serious danger for the growing numbers of HIV-positive people in the region.

Tuberculosis and HIV programmes complement each other

In 1998, WHO recognized the need for tuberculosis (TB) and HIV programmes to work together in sub-Saharan Africa. So it began ProTEST projects for joint tuberculosis and HIV programming in Malawi, Zambia and South Africa (WHO, 2004a). Similar joint intervention initiatives that build on collaboration between STOP TB and ProTEST have also been carried out in other parts of Africa and elsewhere (Family Health International, 2001; Piyaworawong et al., 2003). They show there are important benefits in coordinating key activities in tuberculosis and HIV programmes. For instance, in Malawi over a period of four years, an estimated 14 000 cases of HIV infection were avoided through ProTEST pilot projects.

WHO and the Stop TB Partnership's Global TB/HIV Working Group have members from both the HIV and tuberculosis communities. The Group has formulated an interim policy based on field experiences that provides guidance on which joint activities should be implemented (WHO, 2004b). The principle behind this policy of 'two diseases, one patient' encourages delivery of joint services at every tuberculosis or HIV and AIDS service outlet. First, collaboration between national tuberculosis and AIDS programmes needs to be established. Then, among people found to be HIV-positive, tuberculosis treatment or prevention can be provided at a relatively low cost and with high probability of success.

People with latent tuberculosis infection can be provided with isoniazid preventive therapy to prevent active tuberculosis disease, while those with active tuberculosis can be treated with six months of anti-tuberculosis medicines. Additionally, cotrimoxazole helps prevent HIV-related opportunistic infections, reducing the risk of death in people with both tuberculosis and HIV. In addition, intensifying tuberculosis case finding in HIV testing and counselling centres and in other HIV service outlets is essential. Currently, this is a huge missed opportunity to provide adequate care.

Effective HIV and tuberculosis collaboration needed

Antiretroviral treatment improves quality of life and survival among tuberculosis patients in the same way it does for other people living with HIV. In sub-Saharan Africa, tuberculosis patients with HIV infection form a large proportion of those eligible for antiretroviral treatment. The targets laid out in the 2001 UN Declaration of Commitment on HIV/AIDS, the '3 by 5' Initiative and the Millennium Development Goals for tuberculosis and HIV will be impossible to meet without effective collaboration between tuberculosis and HIV programmes in settings with high levels of both infections. Close collaboration is required to ensure community-level delivery of a comprehensive prevention, treatment, care and support package.

Tuberculosis control programmes face several challenges to achieving case finding and treatment goals; challenges that AIDS programmes have worked to overcome using innovative strategies. These include how to: address stigma, conduct outreach, engage with communities, involve patients and families in programme design and management, and undertake initiatives to deal with structural barriers to the prevention of tuberculosis such as poverty and social marginalization. Many of these challenges can be most effectively addressed if HIV and tuberculosis programmes work together in synergy.

AIDS medicines and the rules of global trade

The global trade in medicines is regulated by both national laws and regulations and international rules such as those in the World Trade Organization's Agreement on Trade-Related Aspects of Intellectual Property Rights—or

The Doha Declaration—the primacy of public health in international trade

The Doha Declaration on the TRIPS Agreement and Public Health was issued by the ministerial conference of the World Trade Organization in November 2001. It made it clear that public health and access to medicines for all are primary concerns in applying international trade rules. The Doha Declaration reaffirmed the flexibility that the TRIPS Agreement provides to countries in authorizing use of patented products—often called 'compulsory licensing'—in the interests of public health. The Declaration also extended the transition period to 2016 for least-developed countries to issue patents in the pharmaceutical sector.

The World Trade Organization Ministers at the Doha conference acknowledged (in paragraph 6 of the Declaration) that countries with insufficient pharmaceutical manufacturing capacities could face difficulties in effectively using compulsory licensing under the TRIPS Agreement because of the limitation on exports under compulsory licensing.

On the eve of its Ministerial meeting in Cancun in September 2003, the Organization agreed to a case-by-case system for waiving the export limitation in TRIPS so that countries without manufacturing capacity of their own could find sources of generic medicines. However, by mid-2004 the waiver system has not been used by any country. It is essential that governments, and partners in civil society and the private sector, actively evaluate the flexibility that the TRIPS Agreement affords to promote access to affordable HIV medicines in their countries. Countries may need to amend their patent legislation in order to take advantage of flexibilities such as the 2016 transition period, and the paragraph 6 waivers.

TRIPS. The Agreement protects intellectual property rights including patents, which provide important incentives for creating new and better HIV medicines and, hopefully one day, an HIV vaccine. At the same time, the exclusive control provided by patents can hinder access to affordable medicines, so the Agreement contains a number of 'safeguards' or flexibilities which national authorities can use to promote more affordable access. The World Trade Organization's Doha Declaration offered additional flexibility, as described in the box above.

In addition to offering lower prices to certain low- and middle-income country markets, some research-based companies have announced that they will not enforce patent rights for HIV medicines in some low- and middle-income countries. For instance, Roche, a major pharmaceutical company, produces saquinavir and nelfinavir used in WHO-recommended, second-line regimens. It has a written policy that it will not file or enforce existing patents on HIV-related medicines in sub-Saharan Africa or in any least-developed countries elsewhere. Bristol-Myers Squibb, which produces d4T used in WHO-recommended first-line regimens, had earlier announced a similar policy of not letting its patents prevent access to affordable HIV treatment in sub-Saharan Africa.

A few countries have begun to take measures to use the TRIPS Agreement more effectively. In May 2004, Canada reformed its patent legislation to allow Canadian generics producers to export to countries eligible under the WTO Doha paragraph 6 implementation arrangement. Meanwhile, Malaysia and Mozambique announced they were issuing compulsory licences for some HIV antiretrovirals. However, challenges continue as some regional and bilateral trade agreements—such as those between the United States and Colombia and the United States and Chile, as well as the Central American Free Trade Agreement—contain provisions that overly protect patent rights, which, in those countries, offsets much of the flexibility provided to governments under the TRIPS Agreement.

Developments in combination therapy: simplifying for better adherence

Triple combination antiretroviral therapy has long been the standard for treating HIV infection. The pharmaceutical industry is contributing to simplifying treatment regimens through developing and manufacturing fixed-dose combination formulations. Fixed-dose combinations permit all three individual molecules to be taken in one tablet, capsule or, in the future, a solution which is of special importance to children.

Three fixed-dose combinations, one each from Indian generics producers Cipla and Ranbaxy, and one from GlaxoSmithKline, have been approved by the WHO pre-qualification quality assessment programme. The generic fixed-dose combinations provide a WHO recommended, first-line regimen. Patents for individual components are often held by different originator companies, and the research-based industry is exploring multi-company arrangements to allow their products under patent to be combined or packaged together in blister packs.

Fixed-dose combination antiretrovirals offer a number of possible advantages. They can:

- increase patient adherence to treatment;
- delay the development of resistance;
- lower the total cost, including production, storage, transport, dispensing and other health system costs;
- reduce the risk of medication errors by prescribers, dispensers and patients themselves;
- simplify supply-system functioning and increase security; and
- facilitate patient counselling and education, and reduce waiting time for patients.

Based on its experience delivering antiretroviral treatment, Médecins sans Frontières strongly advocates fixed-dose combinations. Patients taking the most widely prescribed fixed-dose combination [d4T/3TC/Nevirapine(NVP)] are able to take one pill twice a day, in contrast with six pills a day if taken separately. Fixed-dose combinations can also be far

5

Romania's children with HIV—from tragedy to hope

Romania has the largest number of children living with HIV in Europe—more than 7500. It is believed that transfusion of unscreened blood and repeated contaminated medical injections between 1987 and 1991 led to more than 10 000 new born and young children becoming HIV-infected. In rising to meet this challenge, Romania was one of the first countries in Central and Eastern Europe to introduce antiretroviral treatment. The Romanian Government's strong commitment to improving access has included passing a special 2002 law guaranteeing HIV prevention and care, including publicly funded free treatment and a dietary supplement for all people who need it. Since 2001, a strong UN-facilitated public-private partnership has led to significant price reductions by six pharmaceutical companies involved in the Accelerating Access Initiative. Today, all those determined to be 'in need' according to international guidelines have access to HIV treatment in Romania. This covers some 5700 patients, including 4350 children. Romania is a special case; one in which treatment access for children sparked a campaign that led to achieving universal access to HIV treatment.

more affordable than the same combination procured as separate elements. Médecins sans Frontières says it pays US$ 270 per patient, per year for the d4T/3TC/NVP combination, compared with US$ 562 for separate products from originator companies (Médecins sans Frontières, 2004).

Antiretroviral treatment for children: a special challenge

Antiretroviral treatment for children presents special challenges. Few HIV medicines are produced in paediatric formulations, and those available as syrups have limitations. They have a short shelf-life, children sometimes object to the taste, carers may have difficulty measuring out the correct doses and they remain very expensive.

5

The indications that a child might benefit from antiretroviral treatment are different from those in adults, so different criteria for eligibility need to be set. However, the biggest challenges in treating children are not technical, but social and financial. Children are totally dependent on adults to identify their treatment needs, to take them to a clinic, and thereafter, to supervise them when they take their medicines and ensure they adhere to their regimens.

Children's treatment may be a low priority in a family with several HIV-positive members. Furthermore, many infected children have lost their mothers to AIDS, and it is often difficult to find a relative or guardian who will consistently supervise a child's treatment. A characteristic example, is the guardian of a small orphaned boy in Botswana who was supervising his treatment very reliably. Then the guardian died, leaving the child with other relatives who knew nothing of his treatment plan, and did not understand its requirements. When the boy seemed to get better, his relatives did not see the need to take him to the clinic, and he dropped out of treatment (UNAIDS, 2003).

A successful approach to counter this has been achieved at the Mildmay International Jajja's Home in Uganda. It is a small-scale pioneer in treating children with AIDS. Each of the 85 children in the project has a 'care plan' worked out with parents or guardians, and only those with a supportive home environment are offered antiretroviral treatment (UNAIDS, 2003).

Across the board, greater investment is required to address the special needs of children, including the technical challenges of developing fixed-dose combination antiretroviral formulations for them. National laws need to ensure that children have access to HIV treatment as a human right. National policy-makers and programme managers need to pay far more attention to the special requirements of children in designing and implementing treatment programmes. Knowing when to involve a child in his or her own treatment is another major challenge, since in most cases health workers have only their personal judgement to go on. Everywhere there is a pressing need for national health-care policies and guidelines on treating children with HIV.

Care in the community

Almost universally, relatives and friends provide up to 90% of care for people with AIDS within the home of the sick person. Many community-based programmes, often with few links to public health services, have sprung up around the world to support their efforts. In Uganda, The AIDS Service Organisation (TASO) is the biggest provider of treatment and care services, and offers an increasing number of its more than 60 000 members a full package of services from psychosocial support and counselling, to

Morphine—essential medicine for AIDS care

Unfortunately, initiatives to deliver palliative care cover only a minute proportion of people who require them. In addition, morphine is not yet widely provided in home-care kits. In many countries, a major stumbling block is that morphine and other strong painkillers are often forbidden by law. Yet morphine is recommended on the WHO Model List of Essential Medicines; WHO has produced guidelines indicating that opiates, including oral morphine, are necessary to relieve suffering.

Regulations stipulating that physicians alone can prescribe them need review so that opiates can be widely administered by nurses and others working at the community level. Uganda and Tanzania are the only African countries in which oral morphine is generally available, and only Uganda specifically provides for palliative care in its national health plan (Ramsay, 2003). A WHO joint project with African countries shows that strong partnerships are needed between regulating authorities and health workers to overcome this 'opiophobia' (WHO, 2002).

medication for opportunistic infections and palliative care.

The huge contribution of community-based initiatives is widely recognized: home-based care is a part of almost all countries' health plans. However, despite some notable examples of good practice, progress in drawing them into the wider public health system has been extremely limited.

As described above, the '3 by 5' Initiative recognizes community-based care as the building block of treatment programmes. Communities must play a key role in treatment advocacy, information and literacy, as well as in providing treatment, and monitoring and supporting patients on antiretrovirals (WHO, 2003d). However, most community-based programmes work in isolation with precarious funding. They require support to enable them to take on and maintain the extra burden of antiretroviral treatment over the long term.

Governments need to ensure that they provide a supportive environment for carers, which means reviewing and reforming existing laws, such as those relating to female property and inheritance rights, as well as other policies and guidelines that regulate their lives. It also means working on structural issues such as providing clean water and sanitation, shelter, education for girls, employment, old age pensions and other social security nets.

At the same time, individual carers need support so they will not succumb to fatigue and despair. They need information and training on what to expect of AIDS, how to care for a patient and access food support, and where to receive counselling for their own emotional needs. These 'informal' carers are a vital link in the chain. If they fail to cope, the whole system of community care begins to unravel. Systematic research needs to shed light on exactly who they are, what they do, and how they fit into the framework of community-based care. This information is a basic requirement for addressing their needs, strengthening their capacity and integrating them into the formal health-care system (Ogden and Esim, 2003).

Palliative care

One of the most neglected aspects of HIV care is palliative care, which is treatment to relieve pain and other distressing symptoms in people who are incurably and often terminally ill. It is estimated that at least half of all people with HIV will suffer from severe pain in the course of their disease (WHO, 2002). This is a source of intense distress to carers, relatives and friends who must stand by helplessly witnessing this suffering. It is vital that people who need palliative care receive it.

Pain relief is an essential part of this care, yet morphine (see box on page 119) and other effective pain medications often cannot be obtained. Even if a person is on antiretroviral treatment, palliative care is needed because HIV can still cause considerable illness and death. For instance, in the United States, around 14 000 people died of AIDS in 2003. Besides pain control, palliative care for people with AIDS encompasses:

- treating other symptoms such as diarrhoea, nausea and vomiting, coughing and shortness of breath, fatigue, fever, skin problems and mental impairment;
- psychosocial support, including relieving depression, anxiety and spiritual pain; and
- support for families and carers, including practical assistance with nursing, respite care and counselling to help them work through their emotions and grief.

In Zimbabwe and neighbouring countries, Island Hospice provides training in palliative care to communities and institutions. In Kenya, the Nairobi Hospice was founded in 1990 and offers a wide variety of training courses and practical experience in palliative care for health professionals, non-health professionals and volunteers.

In Botswana, a hospice at Bamalete Lutheran Hospital in Ramotswa village offers outpatient clinical services, as well as day care to terminally ill patients who are given transport to and from their homes. The hospice's respite care began in 2002, and is one of its most valued services (UNAIDS, 2003a). In addition, the Princess Diana Palliative Care Initiative, set up in 2000, is currently working in seven African countries. In 2001, WHO began a five-year joint initiative to set up national palliative care services for people with AIDS and cancer. It works through its Regional Office for Africa, health ministries and key partners in five African countries—Botswana, Ethiopia, Tanzania, Uganda and Zimbabwe.

Challenges of the 'Next Agenda'

Governments, civil society and their partners in countries face enormous challenges in bridging the treatment gap: the gap between aspiration and reality in scaling up antiretroviral treatment and comprehensive HIV care. Many questions still need to be answered. For example, how will it be decided who gets treated first when antiretroviral coverage is still limited? How can services best be provided to children? And how do governments strike a proper balance in service delivery for AIDS and other pressing health problems?

Final answers to most of these questions will be found at the national level, in accordance with local priorities and circumstances. These questions are difficult, controversial and often painful to resolve. But they must not be allowed to deplete global political will to dramatically expand HIV treatment throughout low- and middle-income countries.

The conditions for dramatically boosting access to HIV treatment have never before been so promising. There have been clear advances in high-level political commitment, international donor financing and affordability of medicines and other HIV-related commodities, as well as important progress in the work of civil society and the private sector in designing and implementing HIV treatment programmes in countries and communities. The '3 by 5' Initiative will succeed only if governments and partners in low- and middle-income countries lead the way. Future challenges include:

- Strengthening capacity in hard-hit countries facing the growing human resource crisis. Efforts need to quickly ensure that doctors, nurses and community health workers, along with others have access to HIV treatment. Public sector incentives and working conditions need to be improved, training and education programmes expanded and fast-tracked, and measures taken to allow strong reliance on nurses, paramedics and community workers in scaling up care.
- Ensuring widespread knowledge of HIV status, since it is the gateway to HIV treatment and prevention. Opportunities for voluntary testing and counselling need to be expanded, and a routine offer of HIV testing should be made to all patients with symptoms consistent with HIV-related disease and to those seen in sexually transmitted infection clinics, antenatal clinics and other sites (see 'Prevention' chapter).
- Rolling out antiretroviral treatment programmes in an integrated manner that strengthens, rather than depletes, the larger health system, and which is consistent with a country's overall development agenda.
- Providing greater support for technology transfer and exports—from countries with antiretroviral manufacturing capacity to countries without it. The tenfold increase in antiretroviral access currently being planned requires all partners within the pharmaceutical industry—originators and generic manufacturers—to be part of the AIDS response to ensure that sufficient quantities of HIV medicines, and the active ingredients for the finished formulations, are available.
- Ensuring countries can take advantage of their rights to use trade agreement provisions to widen access to HIV medicines and technologies. This also means resisting stricter-than-necessary patent provisions in regional trade agreements in order to avoid undermining much of the flexibility provided in global trade agreements and declarations for low- and middle-income countries.
- Reducing HIV-related stigma through action by social and community leaders, advocates, health-workers and the public at large so that treatment can reach people in need. International, regional and country-based treatment preparedness groups need sustained support to promote greater knowledge of and demand for HIV treatment.
- Placing equity at the forefront of policies and programmes to ensure fair access and open and transparent procedures within treatment services. Barriers to treatment access for women, children and other groups such as sex workers, injecting drug users and men who have sex with men, must be effectively addressed if '3 by 5', and ultimately universal HIV treatment access, are to become a reality.

Focus

AIDS and human rights: the need for protection

Safeguarding human rights is an essential part of responding effectively to the AIDS epidemic at individual, national and global levels. HIV strikes hardest where human rights are least protected, particularly among people and communities on the margins of society, including sex workers, injecting drug users and men who have sex with men. Conversely, safeguarding people's fundamental rights improves their ability to protect themselves and others at risk of HIV infection, helps reduce their vulnerability to HIV, and assists them in dealing with the epidemic's impacts.

In recent times, some have argued that human rights-based approaches to HIV prevention in efforts to scale up the AIDS response might have reduced the role of public health, which offers a more applied practical framework. However, experience has clearly shown that it is self-defeating to place public health and human rights in opposition. Public health strategies and human rights protection are mutually reinforcing. Their integration achieves the greatest effect in reducing HIV transmission and improving the quality of life of people living with HIV.

Rights-based achievements

Rights-based approaches to the AIDS epidemic have yielded results by:

- **Enhancing public health outcomes:** Protecting a person's right—particularly a person living with HIV—to achieve the highest attainable standard of physical and mental health has brought about increased confidence in health systems. In turn, this has led more people to seek and receive relevant information on HIV prevention, counselling and care.
- **Ensuring a participatory process** linking patients and care providers, which has improved the relevance and acceptability of public health strategies.
- **Fostering non-discriminatory programmes** that include marginalized groups more vulnerable to HIV infection. For example, the Stopping HIV/AIDS through Knowledge and Training Initiatives project in Bangladesh, and the Sonagachi project in Kolkata, India, have integrated the rights of people in sex work by ensuring that sex workers are part of planning, implementing and assessing all relevant AIDS programmes.
- **Scaling up the AIDS response** through empowering people to claim their rights to gain access to HIV prevention and care services. Several countries in Latin American, including Brazil, Costa Rica, El Salvador, Mexico, and Panama have entrenched this by providing free access to treatment and other related health services for many people living with HIV.
- **Enhancing the accountability of States** through people seeking redress for the negative consequences of health policies. Legal action based on human rights has been a vehicle to enforce people's right to gain access to health care, including antiretroviral treatment. For example, in South Africa, the Treatment Action Campaign won a court ruling that required the Government to supply the antiretroviral drug nevirapine to HIV-positive pregnant women at public health facilities, within a phased roll-out of a comprehensive national programme to prevent mother-to-child HIV transmission.

Progress at the national level

Despite challenges, there have recently been positive developments in addressing human rights issues at the national level. Through participatory processes, HIV-related human rights, particularly the principle of non-discrimination, have been integrated into programme tools such as national AIDS policies, strategies and legislative frameworks. For example, Cambodia adopted a law on HIV/AIDS in January 2003; the Parliament of Malawi adopted a rights-based policy on HIV/AIDS in January 2004; and similar policy and legal reforms have been announced in Belarus, India, Lesotho, Liberia, and the Russian Federation.

Meanwhile, supported by a Small Grants Facility established by the United Nations Educational, Scientific and Cultural Organization (UNESCO) and UNAIDS, young people in Malawi, Sri Lanka, Mozambique, Zambia and Bangladesh have developed and implemented programmes to address stigma and discrimination.

Rights and access to AIDS information and prevention

The right to seek, receive and impart information is a fundamental human right and is a *sine qua non* condition for ensuring effective HIV prevention and AIDS care. People have a right to know how to protect themselves from being infected with HIV. They also have the right to know their HIV status, and if they are infected, they have the right to know how to obtain treatment, care and support.

Adequate information, counselling and testing should be accessible to all those in need through rights-based, ethical and practical models of delivery. Globally, rights-based examples under way include: awareness campaigns targeting specific groups such as men who have sex with men, injecting drug users, medical professionals and prison populations (Guinea, Italy, Kuwait, Portugal); incorporating AIDS-related programmes into school curricula (Argentina, Cuba, Czech Republic, Mauritius, Saint Vincent); community development of education and prevention programmes (Lebanon, Thailand); and developing culturally specific education and prevention programmes for indigenous people, refugees, asylum-seekers and migrants (Canada, the Netherlands, Norway).

In March 2004, the UN Theme Groups on HIV/AIDS in Cambodia, Fiji, Nepal, and Thailand led national AIDS and Human Rights consultations. Furthermore, a meeting was held on AIDS and Human Rights in the Asia-Pacific region, sponsored by UNAIDS, the Office of the High Commissioner for Human Rights (OHCHR), the United Nations Children's Fund (UNICEF), the International Labour Organization (ILO), the United Nations Development Programme (UNDP), the United Nations Office on Drugs and Crime (UNODC) and the Policy Project. It was attended by representatives from 20 countries in the region, including government officials, national AIDS councils, lawyers, doctors, people living with HIV, injecting drug users, male and female sex workers, men who have sex with men, young people, mobile populations and ethnic minorities.

Recommendations from these consultations are contributing to advocacy activities, including the Asia-Pacific Leadership Forum. They are helping to improve training and guidance to increase the understanding of AIDS-related human rights issues in the region, and are assisting in identifying best practices.

In other regions, UNESCO and UNAIDS have provided support for young people's training sessions on human rights and AIDS. Sessions have been held in the Middle East and North

Africa (Beirut, Lebanon); in Francophone Africa (Yaoundé, Cameroon); and in Eastern Europe (Croatia). The training covered the knowledge, skills and attitudes needed to foster positive behaviour change. It also focused on the role of media and communications in rights-based messages, including how to dispel myths and fears that often create and reinforce AIDS-related stigma and discrimination. By the end of 2003, young people from over 60 countries had been trained.

AIDS mainstreamed into international human rights mechanisms

Increasingly, the UN and other organizations have focused on the principle that all people have the right to the highest attainable standard of physical and mental health. This has reinforced HIV-related human rights. In September 2002, the United Nations Commission on Human Rights appointed a Special Rapporteur on the Right to Health, who has paid close attention to AIDS-related issues. In June 2003, UNAIDS and the Office of the High Commissioner for Human Rights convened a meeting for Special Procedures on HIV/AIDS and Human Rights in order to develop a strategic approach to integrating AIDS-related issues into their respective mandates, and in so doing to strengthen AIDS-related human rights work at the country level.

AIDS issues have also been integrated into the work of other Special Rapporteurs, Independent Experts and Special Representatives on the situation of human rights in Cambodia, Haiti, Liberia, Myanmar, Somalia, Uganda and Yemen. In addition, Thematic Rapporteurs are monitoring AIDS-related rights. These include the Special Rapporteurs on violence against women, on housing and on the human rights of migrants.

The Special Rapporteur on the Sale of Children, Child Prostitution and Child Pornography has addressed the links between sexual exploitation of children and AIDS, and has identified practical steps governments can take to improve protection of children's rights in this regard. The Special Rapporteur Against Torture and Cruel, Inhuman or Degrading Treatment or Punishment has particularly focused on prisoners.

Resolutions on AIDS passed by the UN Commission on Human Rights, including the resolution relating to access to AIDS treatment, have catalysed political engagement and served to monitor AIDS-related rights.

In January 2003, the General Comment on HIV/AIDS and the Rights of the Child was issued by the UN Committee on the Rights of the Child, and was the first General Comment on the AIDS epidemic to be issued by a treaty-monitoring mechanism. The General Comment identifies good practices and specifically prohibits discrimination against children on the basis of real or perceived HIV status. It calls for countries to report on measures they have implemented to protect children from HIV.

The enduring challenge

Despite these gains, in various parts of the world grave AIDS-related human rights violations continue to occur with depressing regularity. Furthermore, serious gaps prevail between the time that governments pass laws and policies and when they actually implement them. Relatively few countries are on track to meet their human rights commitments.

Stigma and discrimination

AIDS-related stigma remains one of the greatest obstacles to people living with HIV being able to fulfil their human rights. Stigma is also a major barrier to creating and implementing HIV programming. Stigma is a multi-layered process of devaluation that tends to reinforce negative connotations by associating HIV and AIDS with already-marginalized groups. Stigma lies at the root of discriminatory actions that exclude people who need AIDS-related services.

Discrimination is an infringement of human rights that often leads to people being subjected to various forms of abuse. For instance, the Asia-Pacific Network of People Living with HIV/AIDS carried out research among HIV-positive people in India, Indonesia, the Philippines and Thailand. The research found a wide and persistent range of discrimination against people living with or perceived to be living with HIV. This included discrimination by friends and employees in workplace and health-care settings, as well as exclusion from social functions and being denied benefits, privileges or services.

Similar research in four Nigerian states found discriminatory and unethical AIDS-related behaviour among doctors, nurses and midwives. Abuses included denial of care, breaches of confidentiality, and HIV testing without consent. One in ten care providers reported refusing to care for HIV-positive patients, and 10% reported refusing them admission to a hospital. Furthermore, 65% reported seeing other health-care workers refusing to care for an HIV or AIDS patient. Some 20% felt that many people living with HIV had behaved immorally and deserved to be infected.

These studies confirm that creating and enforcing anti-discrimination policies and legislation are necessary. But they need to be accompanied by other measures such as in-service training and providing adequate resources for the health sector.

Denial of women's property and inheritance rights

About half of all people living with HIV are women; they face a variety of human rights concerns in the context of the epidemic. Two issues that need urgent action by governments are property and inheritance rights. When a woman's husband or father dies, other relatives may seize all property and evict orphans and widows. Women in this situation are sometimes stripped of their possessions and forced to engage in sex work or transactional sex in exchange for survival items such as food, protection and cash.

This gender inequality puts women at a much higher risk of HIV infection than men. It continues despite the fact that States are bound by the principles of the UN Charter, the Universal Declaration of Human Rights, the Convention on the Elimination of All Forms of Discrimination against Women and the Convention on the Rights of the Child.

Sexual exploitation of children

Sexual exploitation of children is a persistent flagrant violation of human rights. In the AIDS era, young girls have proven to be especially vulnerable to violence, or to being trafficked or coerced into sex work, since their youth and perceived virginity are associated with freedom from disease. Rates of HIV infection among sexually exploited children are unknown. But in 1999, country research in Asia found that 69% of sexually exploited children in Bangladesh and 70% of those in Viet Nam were infected with a sexually transmitted infection.

Ensuring a rights-based approach

As AIDS responses are scaled up worldwide, they need to be grounded in sound public health practice and they also need to respect, protect and fulfil human rights norms and standards. This is particularly important when it comes to HIV testing as a prerequisite for expanded access to treatment (see 'Prevention' chapter).

The concept that HIV testing must remain voluntary is at the heart of all HIV policies and programmes. Voluntary testing complies with human rights principles and ensures sustained public health benefits. The following mutually reinforcing key factors need to be addressed simultaneously:

1. Ensuring an ethical process for conducting the testing: this includes defining the purpose of the test and benefits to the individuals being tested and assuring there are links between the site where the test is conducted and relevant treatment, care and other services. Furthermore, testing needs to take place in an environment that guarantees confidentiality of all medical information.
2. Addressing the implications of a positive test result: people who test HIV-positive should not face discrimination and should have access to sustainable treatment.
3. Reducing AIDS-related stigma and discrimination at all levels, notably within health-care settings.
4. Ensuring a supportive legal and policy framework for scaling up the response, including safeguarding the human rights of people seeking AIDS-related services.
5. Ensuring that health-care infrastructure is adequate to address the above issues and that there is enough trained staff to meet the increased demand for testing, treatment and related services.

Source: UNAIDS Global Reference Group on HIV/AIDS and Human Rights

Reappearance of restrictive policies and laws

In recent years, a number of policies and laws have emerged that restrict the human rights of people living with HIV or AIDS, or those assumed to be infected.

Experience has confirmed that protecting people's human rights decreases their vulnerability to HIV and reduces the negative impacts of HIV and AIDS. Much progress has been achieved, but the world now needs to be vigilant to prevent backsliding toward practices that are not rights-based.

Financing the response to AIDS

6

The care economy

AIDS has thrown a harsh spotlight on the unequal divisions of household labour, particularly on the burden of AIDS care. When the male head of a household becomes ill, wives provide care and take on additional duties to support the family. When women fall sick, older or younger women step in to care for them and take responsibility for AIDS-affected children.

For example, in South Asia, the region's highly unequal gender relations impose most of the AIDS-related care burden on women (UNDP, 2003). In Viet Nam, recent household surveys reveal women are 75% of all caregivers for persons living with HIV. Mothers account for 51% of the total, while fathers make up 10% (UNDP, 2003a).

The value of the time, energy and resources required to cook, clean, shop, wash or care for the family's young, sick and elderly is called the 'care economy'. It is vast and essential to economic life. For example, in sub-Saharan Africa, an estimated 90% of AIDS care happens at home (Ogden and Esim, 2003). However, because this work is unpaid, it is often taken for granted and undervalued.

The burden of rural women

In low- and middle-income countries, having 'AIDS in the family' poses strains on women in agricultural communities. In addition to their household work, many rural women play a significant role in the economic activities that put food on their families' tables. Caring for the sick disrupts this work. In Tanzania, women with sick husbands spend up to 45% less time doing agricultural or income-earning work than before their husbands became ill.

The burden is made even heavier when activities such as fetching water and washing clothes are done far from the home. A 2002 survey of South African HIV-affected households found less than half had running water in the dwelling and almost a quarter of rural households had no toilet (Steinberg et al., 2002). Yet, South Africa is the continent's most-developed country.

Lessening the burden on women

It is crucial to recognize and support the care economy with adequate resources and enabling policies. Ways to ease women's disproportionate care burden in AIDS-affected households are available—many are similar to those used for more generalized gender inequalities. In many places, informal women's support groups have developed. Some fulfil an important advocacy function such as providing a platform for demanding health resources for communities. Still, these support groups have serious limitations: they are voluntary; make even more work for already overworked women; and do not change gender attitudes or men's care responsibilities.

Possible options for resolving problems related to the care economy include:

- cooperative day care and nutrition centres that assist women with their workload;
- nutritional and educational assistance for orphans;
- home care for people living with or affected by HIV, including orphans;
- labour-sharing and income-generating projects;
- savings clubs and credit schemes for funeral benefits;
- improving rural households' access to labour, land, capital, management skills; and
- improved technologies to make the best use of available resources.

In low- and middle-income countries, income-generating initiatives are an integral component of the AIDS response. Access to these initiatives should be increased. Recent innovations include death insurance for terminally ill patients, flexible saving arrangements and emergency loans.

Financing the response to AIDS

Ensuring there are adequate funds to mount an effective global response to the AIDS epidemic has proven difficult. However, in recent years, there has been an unprecedented increase in global financial resources. In 1996, when UNAIDS was launched, available AIDS funding in low- and middle-income countries totalled US$ 300 million. This amount represented contributions by bilateral donors, international nongovernmental organizations (NGOs), and the UN system, notably the World Bank.

By 2002, this amount had jumped to US$ 1.7 billion. By 2003, an estimated US$ 4.7 billion was available for the AIDS response that year. The latter figure also includes the steadily increasing funding that comes from country governments, and from the 'out-of-pocket' spending by directly affected individuals and families. Yet, this amount is less than half of what is required by 2005, and only a quarter of what will be required by 2007 to mount a comprehensive response to AIDS in low- and middle-income countries.

At the same time, even though more and more money has become available to respond to AIDS, in many heavily affected countries it is clear there are serious bottlenecks to spending it effectively. These blockages include lack of human and institutional capacity, the persistent negative effects of stigma and discrimination, shortfalls in political commitment, slow transfer of funds from national to local and community levels, inadequate accounting and auditing mechanisms, and inconsistent bureaucratic funding processes of the global donor community.

The ongoing funding shortage, and structural and policy deficiencies, are primarily responsible for the still inadequate AIDS response. Less than 20% of people in low- and middle-income countries who need prevention programmes have access to them; funds are not channelled to those who can use them most effectively in the AIDS response; and only 7% of people in these countries who need antiretroviral treatment receive it. For instance, only 3% of those who need treatment in sub-Saharan Africa can obtain it.

These experiences carry one crucial message for the world: increase resources to match the need and remove the bottlenecks, or the AIDS epidemic will not be reversed and stopped.

AIDS spending disparities

AIDS spending in the Latin America and Caribbean region looks large compared to that of sub-Saharan Africa, but it is small compared to spending in the United States of America. In 2000, the United States Government spent US$ 10.8 billion domestically on AIDS, which represents over US$ 13 000 per person living with HIV; per person spending rises to over US$ 30 000 when private expenditure is added (WHO, 2000; WHO, 2001). A check on the credibility of this seemingly high spending level is provided by an analysis of spending on AIDS patients in the United States, which projected that expenditure would average

Progress update on the global response to the AIDS epidemic, 2004

Finances for the AIDS response still fall far short of the amount needed

- Important progress has been made in raising additional funds to respond to the AIDS epidemic. But current annual global spending is less than half of the US$ 12 billion needed by 2005, and less than one-quarter of the amount needed in 2007.
- National governments of low- and middle-income countries spent an estimated US$ 1 billion on AIDS programmes in 2002, an amount that continues to rise. In Africa, it accounts for 6–10% of total AIDS expenditure. Bilateral/multilateral assistance contributed 50% and the remainder came from development banks such as the World Bank, and substantial out-of-pocket spending by individuals and families.
- In 2003, the Global Fund to Fight AIDS, Tuberculosis and Malaria committed US$ 2.1 billion through 227 grants in 124 countries. Pledges to the Global Fund through 2008 more than doubled in 2003 and the number of countries giving financial support continues to grow. However, this will meet only a small percentage of global resource needs for the response to HIV and AIDS.
- Vaccines and microbicides are global public goods requiring both private and public sector investment. Expenditure in 2002 on AIDS vaccine research was US$ 570 million while US$ 79 million was spent on microbicide research in 2003.

Source: *Progress report on the global response to the HIV/AIDS epidemic,* UNAIDS 2003; *Coverage of selected services for HIV/AIDS prevention and care in low- and middle-income countries in 2003,* UNAIDS/USAID/WHO/CDC and the Policy Project,2004; IAVI and the Alliance for Microbicide Development at the UNAIDS Consortium on Resource Tracking Meeting, 2004.

almost US$ 36 000 per patient (Graydon, 2000).

In fact, all evidence points to enormous global disparities in AIDS spending:

- Spending in sub-Saharan Africa, while increasing, is so minuscule as to leave millions without care and support;
- People living with HIV in middle-income Latin American and Caribbean countries do far better than their sub-Saharan African counterparts, but poor targeting of funds results in a less-efficient service mix than might be possible;
- Spending per person living with HIV in the United States exceeds that in the Latin America and Caribbean region by a factor of 35, and it is 1000 times higher than in Africa.

UNAIDS estimates that US$ 12 billion will need to be spent annually on AIDS in low- and middle-income countries by 2005—a figure that is expected to rise to US$ 20 billion annually by 2007 (see Figure 35) (Hankins et al., 2004). The good news is that global AIDS spending in these countries increased more than ninefold between 1996 and 2002. The challenge now is to more than double current spending within just two years, and to maintain high levels of commitment over the long term (UNAIDS, 2003a).

Total resources needed

The global resources needed by 2005 and 2007 for a comprehensive response have been estimated for each of 135 low- and middle-income countries. Such a response would include 19 prevention activities, six treatment and care services, and three types of orphan support. HIV prevalence and other epidemiological data determine the size and characteristics of the target population for each service, and help set realistic goals for coverage.

HIV prevention activities

- Mass media campaigns
- Voluntary counselling and testing
- Condom social marketing
- School-based AIDS education
- Peer education for out-of-school youth
- Outreach programmes for sex workers and their clients
- Outreach programmes for men who have sex with men
- Harm-reduction programmes for injecting drug users
- Prevention programmes for special populations (prisoners, migrants, truck drivers, etc.)
- Public sector condom promotion and distribution
- Treatment of sexually transmitted infections
- Prevention programmes for people living with HIV
- Workplace prevention programmes
- Prevention of mother-to-child transmission
- Post-exposure prophylaxis
- Safe medical injections
- Universal precautions
- Blood safety
- Other prevention programmes

AIDS treatment and care activities

- Palliative care
- Diagnosis of HIV infection
- Treatment of opportunistic infections
- Prophylaxis for opportunistic infections
- Antiretroviral therapy
- Laboratory services for monitoring treatment

Orphan support

- Community support for orphan care
- Orphanage support
- School fee support for orphans

Estimating global resources

UNAIDS, in partnership with the Futures Group and with support from the Inter-American Development Bank, the World Bank and the Asian Development Bank, organized nine regional and subregional workshops between January 2002 and April 2004 to train country teams in the methodology and models used to estimate required resources. Seventy-eight country teams at these workshops, which included over 155 specialists, provided country-specific estimates of unit costs and population sizes for key populations at higher risk of HIV exposure. Together, country specialists and UNAIDS experts estimated resource needs, revealing spending gaps and helping set new priorities.

Except for in-service training of teachers and health personnel, along with some laboratory strengthening, these estimated figures do include resources for further building human resource capacity or strengthening infrastructure required to deliver the services. Thus the country estimates, when combined, give a global figure that represents the minimum required to achieve the goals agreed at the 2001 UN General Assembly Special Session on HIV/AIDS (UNAIDS, 2003a).

Figure 35

Projected annual HIV and AIDS financing needs by region, 2004–2007 (in US$ million)

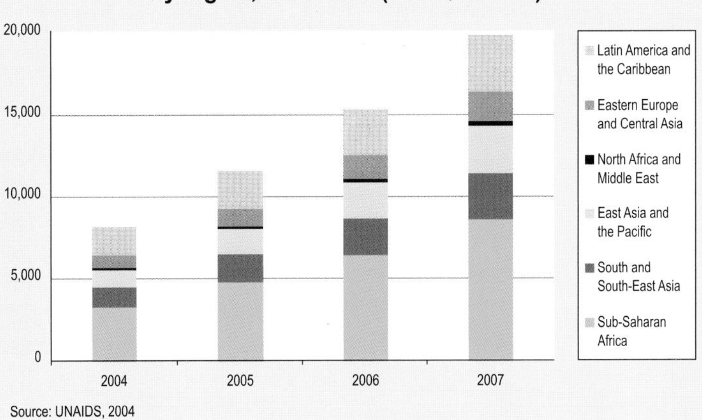

Source: UNAIDS, 2004

6

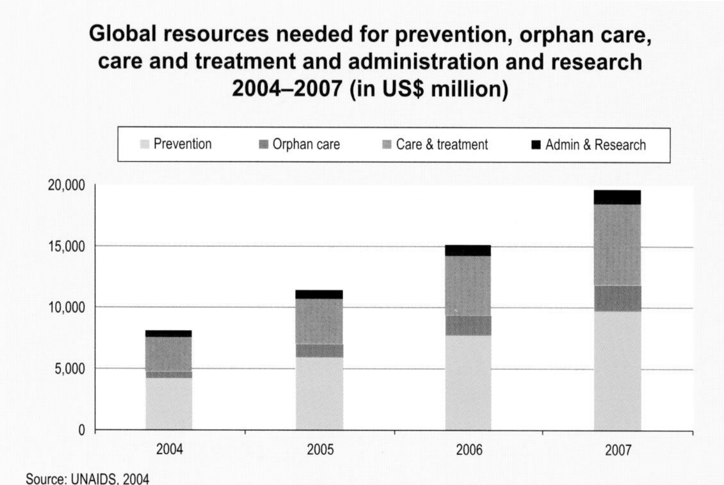

Figure 36

WHO and UNAIDS set a target for treatment

At the UN General Assembly in September 2003, the Director-General of the World Health Organization (WHO) and the Executive Director of UNAIDS called the lack of access to HIV treatment a 'global health emergency'. At that time, only 400 000 of the five to six million HIV-positive people in low- and middle-income countries who needed antiretroviral therapy were receiving it. Moreover, the slow delivery rate meant no more than one million were likely to be on treatment by 2005.

To triple this number to three million on antiretroviral therapy by the end of 2005, WHO and UNAIDS called for an international effort to build on the vision and solid foundations laid by pioneering low- and middle-income country programmes. To achieve the '3 by 5' target, US$ 5.5 billion is needed in 2004–2005—about 80% of the funds required globally for treatment and care in 2004–2005 (see 'Treatment' chapter) (Gutiérrez et al., 2004).

This amount covers direct support to the treatment programme, including:

- Patient cost—counselling and diagnostic testing, condom distribution to patients, antiretroviral drugs, treatment and prophylaxis of opportunistic infections, palliative care, and laboratory tests for patients showing signs of toxicity;
- Programme cost—strengthening in-service training and recruitment of doctors, nurses, community health workers and volunteers; supervision and monitoring; drug distribution systems; universal precautions; post-exposure prophylaxis; and, in some countries, purchase of diagnostics technology.

As of early 2004, national governments; the Global Fund to Fight AIDS, Tuberculosis and Malaria; the World Bank; the United States President's Emergency Plan for AIDS Relief, and other bilateral donors and foundations had pledged just over US$ 2 billion to scale up antiretroviral treatment access in 34 of the hardest-hit countries by the end of 2005, leaving a shortfall of US$ 3.5 billion.

However, there are huge country-level variations: some countries already have the funds to cover their proposed treatment targets, while others have large funding gaps. Further work is required to estimate the long-term costs of antiretroviral therapy, as well as the direct and indirect benefits of investing in treatment scale up, and to determine mechanisms for ensuring sustainability.

In comparison, for all low- and middle-income countries, based on 2002 spending, the annual prevention funding gap is an estimated US$ 3.8 billion for 2005 alone (Global HIV Prevention Working Group, 2003).

Paying for antiretrovirals: lack of equity

"I can take these tablets, because on the salary I earn as a judge, I am able to afford their cost ... In this I exist as a living embodiment of the inequity of drug availability and access in Africa ... My presence here embodies the injustices of AIDS in Africa because, on a continent in which 290 million Africans survive on less than one US dollar a day, I can afford monthly medication costs of about US$ 400 per month. Amidst the poverty of Africa, I stand before you because I am able to purchase health and vigour. I am here because I can afford to pay for life itself." - Mr Justice Edwin Cameron, High Court of Johannesburg, South Africa

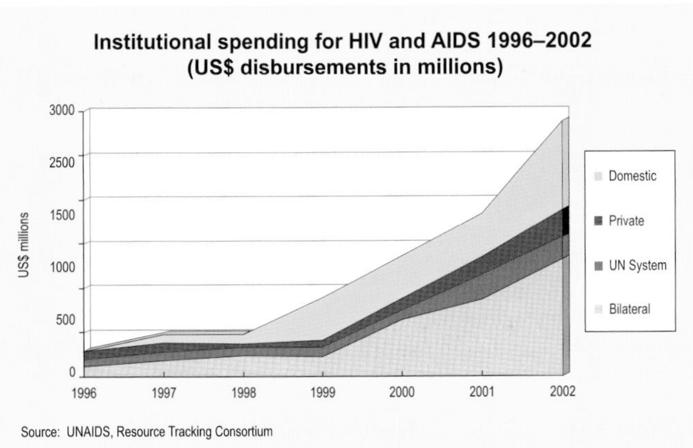

Figure 37

How to meet global resource needs

Five funding streams constitute the flow of resources needed to mount a comprehensive response to the epidemic in low- and middle-income countries: domestic spending, bilateral funding, UN-system support (including the World Bank), the Global Fund, and the private sector, including foundations. Two-thirds of global funding for 2005 and subsequent years is expected to come from the international community. Most of this money will be spent to meet the needs of the poorest and worst-affected countries of Asia and sub-Saharan Africa. Those countries will rely on external donors to meet up to 80% of their needs. Elsewhere, the major share of AIDS resources is expected to come from domestic sources, including national governments, civil society, the business sector, and out-of-pocket expenditures by affected individuals and families.

Domestic spending—both public sector and 'out-of-pocket'

Public sector

UNAIDS estimates that total domestic government spending on AIDS programmes in 2002 by 58 low- and middle-income countries reporting data for three years was about US$ 995 million—twice the amount documented in 1999 (UNAIDS, 2003c). A number of countries have increased their AIDS spending, sometimes dramatically.

For example, South Africa has the largest number of HIV-positive people in the world, and has raised AIDS spending in the national budget for 2003–2004 by 86% in nominal terms over the previous financial year (Hickey, 2004). Its provinces have also increased the proportion of discretionary health funds they spend on AIDS from 0.74% in the 2002–2003 budget to 1.22% in 2003–2004 (Hickey, 2003). China, too, has significantly increased AIDS spending. In 2001, China committed approximately US$ 300 million to dealing with the epidemic. In 2003, this rose to US$ 1.2 billion (UN/MOH China, 2003).

In Eastern Europe and Central Asia, it would take only 2–3% of total projected 2007 regional health expenditures to meet the coverage targets set for HIV prevention and treatment and care activities for that year. Although countries have embarked on radically reforming their health

Figure 38

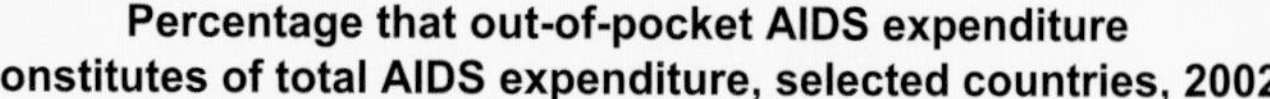

Percentage that out-of-pocket AIDS expenditure constitutes of total AIDS expenditure, selected countries, 2002

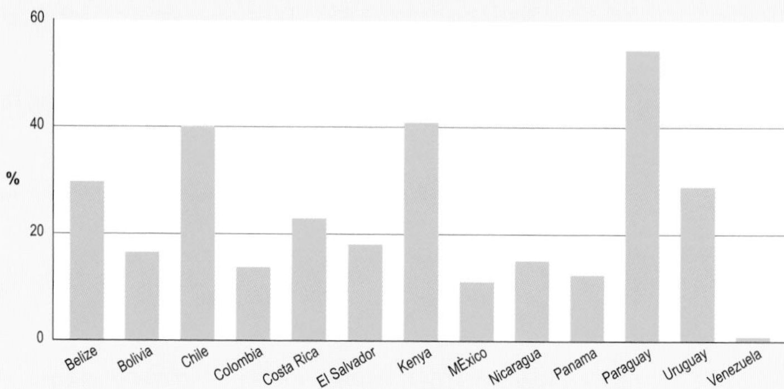

Sources: (1) For Latin America and Caribbean countries: SIDALAC, and (2) Abt Associates

systems, roughly eight out of every ten dollars spent on health is currently absorbed by a legacy of the past—an expensive and crumbling hospital-based system. This leaves few resources for prevention activities to address any disease. As things stand now, to reach the 2007 AIDS spending targets, these countries would have to increase their currently allocated funds by around 30% each year (The Futures Group, 2003).

The Global HIV Prevention Working Group estimates countries in North Africa and the Middle East need to spend about 10 times their 2002 spending to tackle the epidemic (Global HIV Prevention Working Group, 2003).

By 2000, the Latin America and Caribbean region raised 98% of its AIDS funds from domestic sources, and prospects look good for the region to pay its own way through to 2007. It would take just 1% of total health spending to meet 2007 coverage targets for HIV prevention and care. However, the region's poorest countries are likely to need substantial external donor support (Inter-American Development Bank, 2003).

6

In Africa, at the 2001 Abuja summit meeting of the Organization of African Unity, countries pledged to gradually increase their health spending to 15% of their national budgets. If this target were to be met by 2007, it would take about 3% of 2007 health spending to tackle AIDS in the region. However, in Africa, as everywhere, AIDS is just one of many competing priorities, and health spending fluctuates yearly. So far, only a few countries (Chad, the Central African Republic, Mozambique, Uganda and the United Republic of Tanzania) have met the 15% target at any point.

In many African countries, foreign aid supports the national budget, so health allocations do not necessarily represent funds raised exclusively from domestic sources. For example, a Human Sciences Research Council report states more than half of government AIDS spending in Mozambique comes from external sources (Martin, 2003).

In the final analysis, relying on external financial support for AIDS activities raises the issue of long-term sustainability—an especially important consideration for antiretroviral treatment programmes.

How much are people paying out of their own pockets?

Only a handful of countries, mostly in Latin America, have systematically collected information on out-of-pocket AIDS spending. But this information offers only a glimpse of the whole picture, and suggests massive amounts of money are spent by individual households on their own HIV-related health care. In 2002, in 14 Latin American countries, out-of-pocket spending accounted for between 17% and 24% of total AIDS spending (see Figure 38). In parts of Africa, this figure is estimated to be much higher, even though total expenditure falls far short of countries' estimated needs.

In every resource-poor country that has a generalized epidemic, out-of-pocket expenses represent a substantial share of total health

The personal cost of treatment: Rebecca's story

Rebecca lives in Kampala, Uganda, with 12 members of her extended family. In 1992, after many months of illness, her husband died of AIDS. She nursed him throughout and did not realize that he had AIDS because he denied it. But when her young son Julius got sick with tuberculosis, she and he were tested for HIV and discovered they were both infected. In 2001, Rebecca became very sick, and her family persuaded the doctors to put her on antiretrovirals; they had already lost four family members to AIDS.

Paying for the drugs is a struggle. A British woman heard of Rebecca through an NGO, and helps by sending donations whenever she can. But Rebecca still lives with chronic uncertainty as the bills keep coming. One of her recent pharmaceutical receipts is for 376 950 Ugandan shillings (US$ 190). In addition to the drugs, she has to pay 10 000 shillings (US$ 5) for each consultation, and 50 000 shillings (US$ 25) for a CD4 count test. Travel to and from the clinic costs her 3000 shillings (US$ 1.50). Julius is not yet on antiretrovirals, but requires opportunistic infection treatment from time to time, and this, too, costs money. The large family currently survives on the wages of Rebecca's brother, who is a driver, and her sister, who is a teacher. Two other married sisters living elsewhere also contribute (UNAIDS, 2003b).

expenditures on AIDS, ranging from 41% in Kenya (2002), to 93% in Rwanda (1998). These figures provide alarming evidence of the financial burden of AIDS on households. In Kenya, households with at least one HIV-positive person spend four times more on health care than unaffected households. In Rwanda, 66% of households received assistance from their church or family, 18% borrowed from family or friends, and 5% sold assets to cope with HIV-related expenditures.

Average figures mask inequities in expenditure patterns among population groups. In Rwanda, estimates of out-of-pocket expenditures on HIV and AIDS show that the wealthiest 20% of the population spend 13 times more than the poorest 20%, and men spend 2.6 times more than women. In Kenya, the wealthiest 20% of the population spend 10 times more than the poorest. These differences are reflected in wide disparities in treatment and care access.

In 2003, AIDS out-of-pocket spending is likely to have exceeded US$ 1 billion worldwide (UNAIDS, 2003a). Regional differences in the proportion of health-care resource needs met through out-of-pocket spending appear inversely related to government health-care expenditure. This means individual households are likely to pay out of their own pockets when public-health-sector infrastructure is weak.

Bilateral funding for AIDS

In 2003, high-income countries were projected to spend about US$ 3.6 billion to help low- and middle income countries tackle AIDS—20% more than 2002. In early 2003, President George W. Bush proposed that the United States commit US$ 15 billion to respond to AIDS in low- and middle-income countries over a five-year period to 2008. About US$ 9 billion of this is new money and is earmarked for 12 African countries, plus Guyana and Haiti. The rest will support ongoing AIDS activities in other low- and middle-income countries. One billion US dollars of the new money has been pledged to the Global Fund. The US President's Emergency Plan began spending the money in 2004, and allocated US$ 2.4 billion for the first year.

The benefit of investing early to avoid higher costs later is particularly obvious in the case of AIDS. Most industrialized countries will need to propose bold increases in their direct assistance to poorer countries for HIV and AIDS

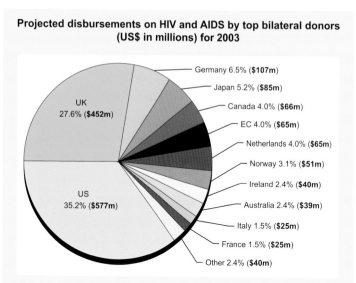

Projected disbursements on HIV and AIDS by top bilateral donors (US$ in millions) for 2003

UK 27.6% (**$452m**)
US 35.2% (**$577m**)
Germany 6.5% (**$107m**)
Japan 5.2% (**$85m**)
Canada 4.0% (**$66m**)
EC 4.0% (**$65m**)
Netherlands 4.0% (**$65m**)
Norway 3.1% (**$51m**)
Ireland 2.4% (**$40m**)
Australia 2.4% (**$39m**)
Italy 1.5% (**$25m**)
France 1.5% (**$25m**)
Other 2.4% (**$40m**)

Source: *Progress report on the global response to the HIV/AIDS epidemic, 2003. Follow-up to the 2001 United Nations General Assembly Special Session on HIV/AIDS*

Figure 39

programmes. For maximum impact, these must be additional resources, and not funds diverted from other priority development programmes aimed at reaching the Millennium Development Goals.

Forty years ago, the Organisation for Economic Co-operation and Development (OECD) called for high-income countries to contribute at least 0.7% of their gross national product to official development assistance. This move was subsequently adopted by UN Member States. However, only five countries have met this target: Denmark, Luxembourg, the Netherlands, Norway and Sweden. There has been renewed global commitment to work in partnership to achieve the Millennium Development Goals, and to overcome conditions fuelling the AIDS epidemic, such as poverty, hunger and inequality. However, the shortfall in resources remains significant.

The 2002 Monterrey Conference on Financing for Development marked a new step towards international burden-sharing to meet key global development challenges. Participating countries made pledges that would translate into an increased official development assistance resource flow from US$ 58 billion in 2002, to US$ 75 billion in 2006 (or from 0.23% to 0.29% of gross national income, which is the total domestic and foreign income claimed by the residents of the economy). This would provide significant additional funds, but it still falls abysmally short of the 0.7% commitment.

All stakeholders need to continue exploring innovative ways of raising domestic and international resources to deal with shared concerns about the developmental, economic, social and political impact of AIDS. In the most-affected countries, AIDS has taken its toll on essential development resources and capacities. However, investing in HIV prevention, AIDS treatment, and impact mitigation has proven to be good development practice and, in some countries, an imperative of national survival.

Effectively using increased official development assistance resources calls for all involved to fully recognize the developmental dimensions

Figure 40

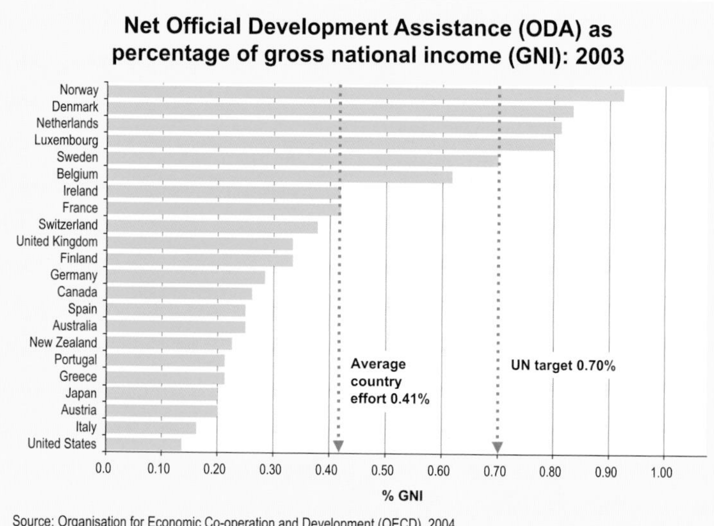

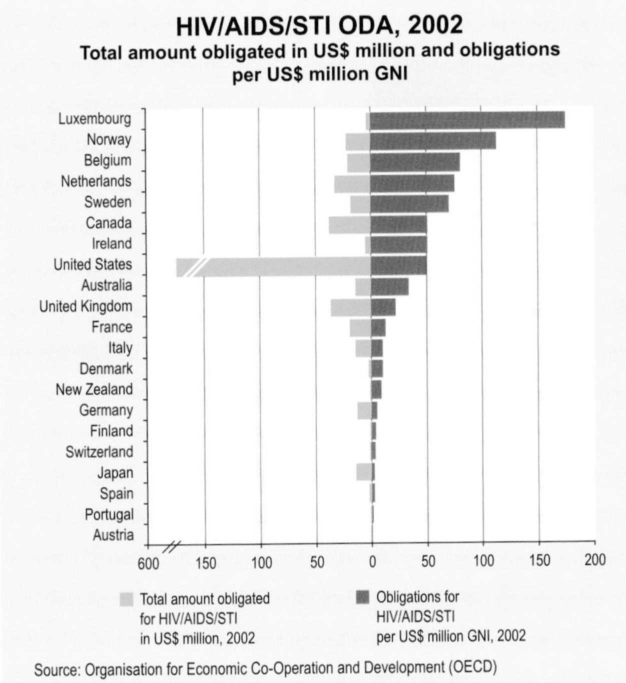

Figure 41

of AIDS, as well as the AIDS dimension of development. UNAIDS supports the need to strengthen national capacity to move towards AIDS-sensitive budgeting and to use funds efficiently and effectively. It also supports donor efforts to harmonize practices to reduce transaction costs. Regular development work forms the basis for virtually all HIV interventions: addressing poverty and inequity; strengthening physical infrastructure; and building capacity.

UN-system sources, including World Bank grants

Twenty-nine UN agencies are engaged in the AIDS response, nine of which are UNAIDS Cosponsors (see 'Overcoming AIDS' chapter). Cosponsors devote funding to AIDS and participate in the Unified Budget and Workplan of UNAIDS.

Among UN-system funding sources, the World Bank is the biggest source of AIDS funding for low-income countries. World Bank loans for HIV can be considerable, as in the cases of Brazil and India. They are considered to be domestic resources, since countries must pay them back.

World Bank grants are direct multilateral contributions to meet resource needs for a comprehensive AIDS approach. Since September 2002, International Development Association countries have received these grants. These are relatively poor countries (with less than US$ 86 in gross national income per capita per year) that need concessional resources, and have implemented social polices that promote growth and reduce poverty.

Through its Multi-Country AIDS Programme, the World Bank has approved US$ 1 billion in grants or interest-free loans to support AIDS programmes in sub-Saharan Africa. The Programme began in 2000 as the first phase of a long-term commitment to directly finance AIDS initiatives. It finds new and imaginative ways to get funds to front-line implementers. It especially emphasizes community projects and a minimum of bureaucratic hurdles. By January 2004, US$ 822.3 million had been committed to 24 countries in the region; US$ 170.6 million had been disbursed. The Programme has committed a further US$ 16.6 million to subregional and cross-border projects.

In the Caribbean, the Bank has started a similar initiative in which US$ 155 million will be disbursed in the form of five-year loans. By January 2004, more than US$ 85 million had been committed to five countries, of which nearly US$ 10.5 million had been disbursed (World Bank, 2003). In 2003, the World Bank

6

approved a US $100 million loan to Brazil for responding to AIDS and sexually transmitted infections, bringing the Bank's commitment to Brazil's epidemic to US$ 430 million. The Government of Brazil is also contributing US$ 100 million.

In addition to its Multi-Country AIDS Programme, the Bank helps finance a wide variety of AIDS programmes in 25 countries; commitments for 2003 alone amounted to just over US$ 213 million. Most of this money is given as a loan rather than a grant.

The Global Fund to Fight AIDS, Tuberculosis and Malaria
Pledges and contributions received, as of December 31, 2003

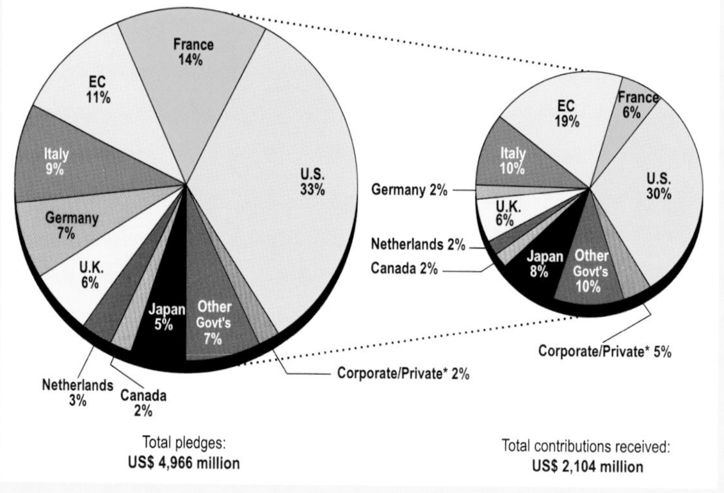

*Foundations and not-for-profit organizations, corporations, and individuals, groups and events
Source: *The Global Fund annual report, 2003.*

Figure 42

The Global Fund to Fight AIDS, Tuberculosis and Malaria

In January 2002, the Global Fund to Fight AIDS, Tuberculosis and Malaria was set up as a partnership between governments, civil society and the private sector. Its mandate is to provide new money and create new ways to disburse funds to fight the three diseases that, between them, kill more than six million people every year.

By the end of 2003, the Global Fund had approved 227 grants totalling US$ 2.1 billion in 124 countries and had already disbursed US$ 232 million (Global Fund, 2004). About 60% of these funds are earmarked for AIDS programmes, 23% go to malaria, and 17% to tuberculosis. All low- and middle-income countries have benefited, but, to date, sub-Saharan Africa has received 60% of the grant money. This region has the greatest disease burden and the scarcest resources.

By January 2004, almost US$ 5 billion had been pledged up to 2008 and beyond; US$ 2.1 billion had been actually paid into the Global Fund's bank account. In 2004, the Global Fund was due to receive another US$ 1.2 billion of the money pledged—around US$ 400 million less than it predicted would be needed to cover its commitments for the year (Global Fund, 2004a). The immediate shortfall will have to be resolved by high-income countries.

In the long run, the Global Fund is also looking to increase donations from private sector foundations and individuals to help meet its needs (Cashel and Rivers, 2003). Currently, only 2% of its funds come from the private sector; the remaining 98% are pledged by governments (Global Fund, 2003).

However, money from all sources is coming in very slowly. To help ease the uncertainty under which the Fund operates, 100 NGOs around the world started the 'Fund the Fund' coalition, a campaign for regular and committed Global Fund supporters. From 2004, the Global Fund will conduct one round of grant proposals annually, subject to funding availability.

The concept of 'additionality' is the Fund's key principle. This means its resources complement, but never replace, budgeted funding. It implies that donations are expected to be new money, not funds diverted from existing aid budgets. At the country level, donations should add to whatever has been budgeted from other sources, not used to release earmarked AIDS funds for spending on other priorities. However, this principle has not always been honoured. Sometimes, Global Fund contributions have been taken out of development assistance budgets, or have been considered by a number of African countries to be within expenditure allocations.

The private sector, including foundations and NGOs

Foundations

A 2002 survey of top United States grant-providers by Funders Concerned about AIDS affords a snapshot of foundation contributions (see Figure 43). The figures include donations to domestic and international programmes, but roughly 63% of the money from the top 10 foundations is spent abroad. Available data suggest the 2002 commitment is significantly less than in 2001—the year that saw the highest-ever commitment from international foundations. But donations are frequently intended to cover several years, so it is difficult to identify exactly what is spent in any one period.

International nongovernmental organizations

In 2002, selected international NGOs contributed an estimated US$ 95.5 million to the AIDS response. These funds come from charity donations, private households, foundations (other than the top United States grant-providers) and governments.

Figure 43

Funds committed by top 15 US grantmakers in 2002 (US$ millions)	
Gates Foundations	89.0
Bristol-Myers Squibb Foundations	16.9
The Henry J. Kaiser Family Foundation	16.2
Ford Foundation	14.0
Rockfeller Foundation	12.9
United Nations Foundation	12.3
Elizabeth Glaser Pediatric AIDS Foundations	11.8
Merck Company Foundations	11.4
Open Society Institute/Soros Foundations	7.8
Robert Wood Johnson Foundation	7.8
Abbott Laboratories Fund	6.9
M.A.C AIDS Fund	5.6
Starr Foundation	5.5
W.K. Kellogg Foundation	5.4
Broadway Cares/Equity Fight AIDS	5.4
TOTAL	**228.9**

Source: Funders concerned about AIDS, *Report on HIV/AIDS grantmaking by US philathropy, 2003.*

The business community

In countries where HIV prevalence is high, some industries are experiencing a haemorrhaging of labour and skills, as workers succumb to AIDS and drop out of employment or die. Many businesses, too, find themselves burdened with rising costs for health care, pensions and training new staff.

About 4% of global AIDS resource needs are for workplace activities. Here, too, it is difficult to assess the level of commitment because information on social spending by companies is not systematically reported. However, a recent UNAIDS-supported survey by the United Nations Research Institute for Social Development suggested 21% of the top transnational corporations have workplace AIDS programmes of some kind. Both the Global Business Coalition on HIV/AIDS and the Global Health Initiative of the World Economic Forum encourage greater private sector involvement in responding to the epidemic (see 'National Responses' and 'Treatment' chapters). Between them, they have more than 150 members (UNAIDS, 2003c; Global Business Coalition on HIV/AIDS, 2001).

Resources for vaccine and microbicide research and development

Private funding alone cannot advance research to develop prevention technologies, such as vaccines and microbicides. Such products will need to be priced so that people around the world with little disposable income can afford them. Up-front public investment is required to develop these products and ensure there are markets for the developed goods.

Products such as vaccines and microbicides are excellent examples of 'global public goods'—i.e., goods that benefit others beyond those who use them directly. Therefore, global public goods can be judged to be highly eligible for public support to complement private investment. In the case of HIV-prevention technologies, each prevented infection cuts off a potential chain of infections resulting from the primary infection.

The major public partners currently funding clinical trials research in low- and middle-income countries include the National Institutes for Health (United States of America), the Medical Research Council (the United Kingdom), the Agence nationale de recherches sur le sida (France), and the European and Developing Countries Clinical Trials Partnership.

Despite many challenges in gathering the data, the International AIDS Vaccine Initiative has established roughly how much is spent globally on researching and developing AIDS vaccines. For 2002, the latest year of its analysis, the preliminary estimate is US$ 540–570 million—an increase of around US$ 100 million on its 2001 estimate. Of this, the private sector's share is less than one-quarter; the pharmaceutical industry contributes 14%, and the biotechnology industry 7%.

According to the International AIDS Vaccine Initiative, public sector investment in vaccine research looks set to expand. However, overall funding is not keeping up with the challenges. The Initiative forecasts that investment by innovator drug companies and the biotechnology industry will decline as costs of research and development rise, the US economy struggles, and biotechnology companies have difficulty raising new venture capital (International AIDS Vaccine Initiative, 2003).

Research funding for developing microbicides is tracked by the Alliance for Microbicide Development. The microbicide field differs from others addressing neglected public-health technologies. This is because virtually all the product developers are small biotechnology companies, non-profit organizations, and academic institutions with limited funding and capacity.

Of the 40 potential microbicides being developed in 2004, only one had a major pharmaceutical company sponsor (Tibotec, a Johnson and Johnson company) which is working with the International Partnership for Microbicides. In 2003, almost US$ 79 million was committed to microbicide research, with over half coming from the United States, and the remainder from philanthropic organizations and other bilateral donors and multilateral agencies.

Figure 44

Funding for microbicide research, in US$				
SOURCE	2000	2001	2002	2003
Funding by philanthropic organizations	$26 938 920	$24 036 874	$2 993 180	$63 000 000
Funding by selected countries and agencies*	$350 000	$0	$67 435 262	$4 822 117
Funding by the United States	$34 635 492	$61 266 031	$75 280 722	$78 771 000

* Canada, Denmark, France, Ireland, Netherlands, Norway, United Kingdom, UNFPA, World Bank

Source: Lamphear TL. Funding for microbicides: An overview chart. Alliance for Microbicide Development, March 2004.

Translating funding into action–confronting programming capacity problems and funding bottlenecks

To get ahead of the epidemic, resources need to be delivered to where they are most needed and used in a 'smarter' way—more efficiently and effectively. But getting a clear picture of where AIDS funds are going, and how they are being spent, is tantamount to a forensic exercise—a matter of digging around in the financial records of government departments, institutes and organizations searching for information that is specific to AIDS. Keeping systematic records of financial in- and out-flows is vitally important for planning purposes. But tracking AIDS resources is currently a low priority in most-affected areas, and is poorly developed, or not done at all.

Tracking resource flows and linking these with monitoring and evaluation efforts

Since 1998, UNAIDS has been collecting critical data on the sources of funding and how funds are applied in responding to AIDS. The key to encouraging a regular and assured flow of funds from all sources is information which demonstrates that resources are being used efficiently, and are achieving results. In 2002, as part of this effort, UNAIDS established a Global Resource Tracking Consortium for AIDS, composed of international experts in this field. The Consortium:

- develops strategies to improve the process of collecting data on global resource flows to meet targets in the 2001 UN Declaration of Commitment on AIDS, and the Millennium Development Goals;
- identifies gaps, duplication of efforts, and comparative advantages between organizations collecting data;
- identifies key strategic priorities for tracking resource flows in the future;
- reaches consensus on methodologies and definitions used in collecting AIDS resource flow data;
- streamlines the interpretation and communication of data;
- ensures that methods and data sources used for estimating global resource flows are consistent and complementary with those used for economic and epidemiological modelling.

At the same time, UNAIDS has called for increased country and global focus and investment to monitor the implementation and impact of prevention, treatment and mitigation programmes. Within this advocacy role, UNAIDS works closely with international partners to identify, harmonize and consistently measure the most useful information. It also works with countries to develop Country Response Information Systems to monitor progress. The 2001 UN Declaration of Commitment on HIV/AIDS stimulated the global community to monitor and compare progress across regions and in individual countries. Linking impact with cost will become an ever more important tool as we learn how financial resources can best be spent.

SIDALAC, the regional AIDS initiative for Latin America and the Caribbean, and Abt Associates—Partners for Health Reform, facilitate decision-making by tracking resources spent in countries to prevent HIV spread and to treat HIV-related disease. In South Africa, the Institute for Democracy is working to encourage similar processes in the African region, and has undertaken a comparative analysis of budgets and tracking of AIDS funds in five African and five Latin American countries. The project trains local NGOs to independently monitor public expenditure on AIDS.

The limitations of programming capacity

Countries encounter significant problems when trying to scale up the response to HIV. There are many factors that limit programming capacity in low- and middle-income countries. These can be grouped into three broad categories of problems: overwhelming and competing demands for scarce resources; the struggle to overcome stigma and discrimination; and poor coordination among both domestic and external partners.

Clearly, the scale of the new financing needed for a comprehensive response to the HIV epidemic will require a very significant increase in current levels of domestic spending in affected countries. In many of these countries, it is very likely that scaling up AIDS expenditure will encounter capacity problems.

As Dr Ndwapi Ndwapi, head of the antiretroviral programme at Botswana's Princess Marina Hospital has said, "Many think that accessing the funds to put the plan into action is the biggest challenge. But once you have the money, you suddenly find there are seemingly insurmountable challenges. The gross inefficiencies in the system, that have been a problem for some time, become so apparent when you try to ask the system to do something this big ... like putting 100 000 people on treatment" (IRIN, 2004).

Human capacity in Africa

Many African countries have seen improvements in economic growth and health provision, but many face a growing human and institutional capacity crisis that hinders their ability to implement their development strategies and programmes to make progress on important development goals.

The health and education sectors face shortages in personnel, a weak institutional environment, and problems with recruiting and deploying staff to rural areas. Wealthier countries are attracting qualified and experienced workers from poorer nations, which makes their capacity problems worse (see 'National Responses' chapter). In addition to this, a decade of cutbacks in social spending under structural-adjustment programmes has reduced the number of social sector staff, leaving these sectors unable to respond rapidly to the demands of AIDS. The resulting high workload for existing personnel has meant poor working conditions leading to low staff morale.

Most African countries need more human capacity in every sector—public, private, and in civil society. Building this capacity in Africa is now almost universally seen as a prerequisite for meeting the Millennium Development Goals in general, and for overcoming AIDS in particular.

The extent of human capacity problems critically depends on the way in which funds are allocated, both between countries and within countries. An equitable strategy would direct expenditure towards identified funding gaps – i.e., it would be needs-based. Currently, there is a temptation to direct funding primarily to countries perceived as having greater capacity to spend the money in the short term. But this would leave out some countries that are most needy precisely because of the greater impact of AIDS. A more equitable strategy is to address capacity problems in the countries with greatest need through targeted investments in both human capital and physical infrastructure.

If funding is targeted towards overcoming capacity constraints in the most needy countries, it will yield long-term tangible and sustainable benefits for the well-being of partner countries.

The problem of displacement of funding and expenditure ceilings

It is an unfortunate reality that budgeting procedures too often may mean that new funds for HIV and AIDS can draw resources away from other activities, either at country level, or at donor level. Therefore, all parties need to commit themselves to the principle that *additional* funding for HIV and AIDS is to be used for *additional* spending, otherwise displacement is inevitable to the detriment of overall development.

Public expenditure ceilings are limits to expenditure within different sectors of an economy. In the 1970s and 1980s, caps on social spending, in particular, were a principal feature of structural adjustment programmes called for by the International Monetary Fund and the World Bank as a condition for concessional borrowing of money by low- and middle-income countries. Caps were considered a necessary discipline to mend ailing economies, promote growth and ease poverty in the long run by curbing inflation. But when they were seen to intensify the hardship of the poor, they came under intense criticism and were dropped as a specific condition for financial assistance.

Nevertheless they exist de facto in many countries as a by-product of Medium Term Expenditure Frameworks. These frameworks are countries' detailed financial plans, required to show the Fund and World Bank that they can balance their books and keep the macro-economy on track. They are often included in, or referred to, by Poverty Reduction Strategy Papers, which are the basis on which public debt relief is granted and much foreign aid is given. Low- and middle-income country governments are caught in conflicting pressures. They are exhorted to limit social spending in order to avoid damaging inflationary consequences, and yet are expected to ignore such pressures in the case of Global Fund or other earmarked money.

It is time to radically rethink how best to fund comprehensive country HIV programming. International financial institutions need to create mechanisms that alleviate countries' debt-service payments so they can devote additional resources to their AIDS response. The short-term inflationary effects of increased and additional resources applied in tackling the HIV epidemic pale in comparison with what will be the long-term effects of half-hearted responses on the economies of hard-hit countries. AIDS is an exceptional disease; it requires an exceptional response.

The issue of stigma and discrimination—a demand constraint

The problem of stigma and discrimination has long been recognized as a constraint to identifying who needs prevention, care or treatment services. Most people infected with HIV are not aware of their HIV status. Social stigma inhibits people from wanting to know their status and it prevents them from acting on prevention messages for fear of being identified as HIV positive. Countries such as Botswana, which introduced a programme of free treatment, found initially that fewer people than expected came forward for treatment services.

Further, stigma acts as a constraint on funds getting to where they are needed. Data from Latin America, the Caribbean, and Eastern Europe suggest that public attitudes and legal constraints may hinder activity-funding from being channelled to people working with stigmatized groups. This compounds the major hurdle of proposal writing experienced by community groups that have little knowledge or experience of how the system works. This hurdle is made worse when donors keep changing their rules and demands.

Such groups often have difficulty, too, in meeting requirements for accounting and record keeping, and many lack the capacity to efficiently use the money that comes their way. It is also true that major donors are rarely geared up to disburse the kind of tiny sums that are all that are required, or can be managed, by very many people on the front line of the epidemic—the woman running a home for a few of her neighbours' orphaned children; the man offering apprenticeships to youngsters who have had to drop out of school; or the hairdresser wanting to print leaflets on HIV to hand out in her salon.

The problems of stigma and social attitudes can be overcome. Concerted efforts in Brazil have clearly shown that a sustained campaign of access to treatment can reduce stigma by providing people with hope. The experience of Uganda further shows that stigma can be reduced by committed leadership. These are vital components of a strategy to increase programming capacity.

The issue of coordination: the 'Three Ones'

Tracking resource flows is critical to understanding how resources are being used, and for identifying key blockages. Blockages can occur when the responsibility for disbursing AIDS funds rests with a department that lacks financial and programme management skills, or which is understaffed and overworked and where AIDS comes up against competing priorities. Substantial delays can result if there are no clear plans for AIDS activities or financing mechanisms in place, or no one detailed or trained to take special responsibility for AIDS (Hickey et al., 2003).

Problems with administrative capacity can also be donor-created or exacerbated, particularly

The problem of donor-driven agendas

"In AIDS as elsewhere, program managers are often little more than data processors for donors, spending obscene amounts of time trying to satisfy dozens of duplicative reporting requirements, and hosting repetitive review missions month after month. Donor-driven agendas are raising transaction costs and reducing programme effectiveness. It is a bit rich for donors to complain of absorptive capacity when they are the ones absorbing much of it." -*Dr Peter Piot, Executive Director, UNAIDS*

when governments and donors do not work effectively to harmonize their support to the greatest extent possible. Minimizing duplication in fiduciary arrangements, monitoring procedures and reporting mechanisms, as well as conducting joint country missions can streamline funding and reporting flows, and enhance country capacity to use funds in the most effective and timely way possible.

Lack of harmonization among donors at country levels means that resources are wasted and people who need help do not receive it. In effect, lack of harmonization kills people.

Applying the 'Three Ones' principles (see 'National Responses' chapter) will result in adaptations that are appropriate to each country, situation and institution. These principles are fully compatible with the Rome Declaration on Harmonization of 25 February, 2003 and the work on aid effectiveness and donor practices of the Development Assistance Committee of the Organisation for Economic Co-operation and Development. Inherent to these principles is a shared vision of the urgent need to respond to AIDS in an exceptional way, which supports inclusive national ownership and clearly defined accountability.

Mechanisms to overcome constraints and to channel funding to the programming level

Streamlining procedures

All domestic or international funding entities have a common goal. It is to ensure their funds are used effectively—to make the greatest possible difference in the everyday lives of people who need HIV prevention, treatment and care services, and of people who also need measures to reduce the impact of AIDS on their lives. However, in reality, most funding efforts confront bottlenecks at different levels.

But there are many examples of efforts to streamline procedures, remove barriers and facilitate funding flows to the programming level. Both the World Bank's Multi-Country AIDS Programme and the more recent Global Fund to Fight AIDS, Tuberculosis and Malaria have given a good deal of thought to how they fund activities, and to easing or bypassing common blockages in the pipelines. The World Bank has pioneered new ways of channelling money swiftly to the front line, with 40% to 60% of grants currently going directly to the community (Cashel, 2003).

The Bank emphasizes giving support to a wide range of participants at all levels in order to implement national action plans, and to create 'financial plumbing systems' to deliver funding quickly and efficiently. Countries applying to the Global Fund have set up Country Coordinating Mechanisms composed of representatives of interest groups from all levels of society under government leadership. The Mechanisms shape grant applications, make an initial selection of projects and programmes, and put forward proposals to the Fund. Monies are sent directly to a 'Principal Recipient' responsible for accounting and reporting to the Fund, and for disbursing money to organizations doing the work on the front line. The Principal Recipient is key to facilitating the efficient flow of funds.

The challenge for governments is to streamline official channels by identifying the bottlenecks, and investing in the administrative and programming capacity needed to use resources more effectively. Important steps in this regard include the fact that key stakeholders now recognize the importance of the 'Three Ones', and also that countries are moving towards better national programme coordination.

Reallocating resources: the potential of debt relief

More than one-third of the world's HIV infected people—or 14 million—live in countries classified by the World Bank as heavily burdened by debt. In 2002, the 42 poorest and most indebted countries—34 in sub-Saharan Africa—together owed US$ 213 billion (Hardstaff, 2003). Many of these countries regularly pay out more to rich world creditors to service their debts than they receive in foreign aid. In fact, debt repayments take a larger slice of their budgets than public health (Boyce, 2002; Oxfam, 2002).

Countries with AIDS components in their Poverty Reduction Strategy Papers include Burkina Faso, Cameroon, Guinea, Malawi,

A question of priorities: the cost of servicing debt

- Zambia has almost one million HIV-positive people, and spends 30% more on servicing its debt than on health. In 2000, the proportion of government revenue absorbed by debt was 20%; this was expected to rise to 32% in 2004 (Oxfam, 2002; World Bank/IMF/IDA, 2003).
- Cameroon spends 3.5 times as much on debt repayment as on health, and Mali spends 1.6 times as much (Oxfam, 2002).
- Kenya spends US$ 0.76 per capita on AIDS, and US$ 12.92 per capita on debt repayments (Kimalu, 2002).
- The cost of implementing Malawi's national strategic plan for AIDS is around US$ 2.40 per capita per year. In 2002 the country transferred US$ 5 per capita to foreign creditors (Oxfam, 2002).
- The first 14 countries identified as key recipients of the United States President's Emergency Plan for AIDS Relief together spent US$ 9.1 billion in servicing their debt in 2001 (Ogden and Esim, 2003).

Mozambique, Uganda and Zambia. Debt relief may be a useful mechanism for programming funds within existing expenditure frameworks. However, it is usually counted as part of official development assistance at its full nominal value, and therefore is often not additional. Debt relief cannot play a meaningful role in reducing the funding gap for AIDS unless it is *genuinely additional* to existing levels of foreign aid.

Challenges of the 'Next Agenda'

Turning the tide of the epidemic in low- and middle-income countries means mobilizing adequate funds to mount a comprehensive response to HIV. It means enhancing country capacity to determine resource needs in prevention, treatment and care, and impact alleviation. It means close and accurate resource tracking at country level and globally to monitor the gap between funds and resource needs. Civil society organizations, especially at the grassroots level where needs are the greatest, require support to access and effectively use funds. In addition, the global community needs to invest in the global public goods that new prevention technologies represent.

Turning the tide also demands more concerted and more effective action on a much larger scale than is currently the case. Donors need to assess carefully their fair share of contributions to the global HIV response. The international community needs to determine the relative importance and complementarity of the major funding streams available for channelling resources. There should also be agreement on respective national and international responsibilities for financing various aspects of the response. International financial institutions should think broadly and creatively about mechanisms to place more funds in the hands of countries now facing large debt-service payments. At the same time, action on AIDS should not further increase debt burdens.

The need to act quickly against an epidemic that is still outstripping the global response means that everyone must 'learn by doing'. Certain critical elements must not get lost in the shuffle of urgent action, including the need to document learning so that others can take advantage of it, and ensuring that procedures are in place to facilitate fine-tuning of working methods.

Advocacy is crucial to ensure that adequate and sustainable financial resources are mobilized to scale up the AIDS response. But success depends on demonstrating that programming capacity issues can be creatively overcome, monies can be effectively used, the epidemic can be slowed, the quality of life of millions of people currently living with HIV substantially improved, and the impact on households, communities and countries alleviated. Future challenges include:

- Increasing the resources committed to the AIDS pandemic from all sources to the required US$ 12 billion annually by 2005, agreeing on 'fair share' and creating mechanisms that allow funds to be spent effectively.
- Prompting the international community and countries in need to demonstrate the increased political commitment required to turn the epidemic around by:

—mobilizing public opinion in donor countries through the World AIDS Campaign and other advocacy;

—working out ways and means for countries to invest more domestic funds in AIDS and to support secure future development through using mechanisms such as debt relief;

—mobilizing increased commitment of funds and efforts to combat poverty, discrimination, powerlessness and other socioeconomic determinants of vulnerability to HIV, and the effects of the AIDS epidemic.

- Identifying and removing potential bottlenecks in funding flows, radically improving mechanisms for delivering funds through all levels—international, national, regional, community and local—and harmonizing processes through the 'Three Ones'.
- Building programme capacity to demonstrate results by using funds efficiently and effectively, and monitoring performance and impact (spending smarter).
- Incorporating the concept of AIDS 'exceptionality' into financing the AIDS response in countries in desperate need. It is time to rewrite the rules to create a careful programme of exceptions to the normal modes of financing that protect countries' long-term economic prospects while facilitating urgent, effective country responses to AIDS.

National responses to AIDS: more action needed

7

The gender factor within national AIDS responses

UN Member States pledged in the 2001 UN Declaration of Commitment on HIV/AIDS that by 2005 they would implement national strategies that empower women to make decisions relating to their sexuality, and ensure women's access to HIV prevention, AIDS care and related services, including sexual and reproductive health. The 2003 UNAIDS *Progress report on the global response to the HIV/AIDS epidemic* reported 69% of countries have policies ensuring women's equal access to HIV prevention, AIDS care and related services. On a more practical level, the Progress Report asked countries for gender breakdowns for a number of key indicators. These included: accurate diagnosis of sexually transmitted infections; antiretroviral coverage; young people's prevention knowledge; condom use; and the percentage of HIV-infected young people. Less than one in five countries provided these gender-related data—an indication that gender concerns are a minimal pre-occupation in many countries' AIDS responses.

Leadership and legislation needed

National progress on gender depends on courageous leadership, carefully drafted legislation, spirited advocacy, and serious investment of resources. One positive leadership example is Ethiopia's recent launch of the Women's Coalition Against HIV/AIDS. At a ceremony attended by some of Ethiopia's leading female figures, Prime Minister Meles Zenawi spoke out about the need to change Ethiopians' gender attitudes and practices to stop the epidemic (IRIN, 2003).

Worldwide, there are many examples of legislative reform that reduce women's vulnerability to HIV and AIDS. Benin's 2003 comprehensive Law on Reproductive and Sexual Health guarantees several basic reproductive rights, including: equality of men and women in reproductive health matters; free choice in matters of marriage; access to reproductive and sexual health-care services, information and education; non-discrimination in health-care access and personal security. Care and non-discrimination are guaranteed to people with sexually transmitted infections, particularly HIV. Finally, the law criminalizes all forms of sexual violence targeting women and children, including female genital mutilation and forced marriage (NWMI, 2003).

Other countries have concentrated on policy development. For example, Cambodia's Ministry of Women's and Veteran's Affairs promotes the rights of women and girls at risk of HIV. The Ministry also spearheads gender mainstreaming within national development management. Its policies are closely related to initiatives such as the Partnership for Gender Equity Programme that brings the country more firmly in line with the Convention of the Elimination of All Forms of Discrimination against Women (UNDP, 2003).

National leadership on gender is not confined to the state. Since 1988, the Society for Women and AIDS in Africa has advocated on behalf of women, children and families in the AIDS response. Through its semi-autonomous country offices, the Society strengthens the capacities of women's groups, local nongovernmental organizations (NGOs) and communities to prevent, control and mitigate the epidemic's impact.

AIDS and education for girls: a convergence of national priorities

Young people's reproductive and sexual health education is a key strategy of the 2001 UN Declaration of Commitment on HIV/AIDS. Some 88% of countries say they have a policy to promote such efforts. However, these policies will miss large numbers of children—particularly girls—if they do not actually have access to schools. Female enrolment is rising, but girls still comprise 57% of children not in school (UNESCO, 2003).

Universal access to education is essential for national development, and has been entrenched in the goals of the 1990 Education for All Declaration and the 2000 Millennium Declaration. Both include a call for universal primary education by 2015 (United Nations, 2001). However, attaining this goal is under threat. The United Nations Educational, Scientific and Cultural Organization (UNESCO) estimates 55 of the world's poorest nations are unlikely to reach universal primary enrolment by 2015 (UNESCO, 2002).

Twenty-eight of these are countries experiencing severe AIDS epidemics that further constrain education efforts. A recent World Bank study estimated about US$ 2.5 billion is needed annually from the international community to meet the 2015 Education for All universal primary education goal. In 33 African countries, the AIDS burden means an estimated additional US$ 450–560 million will be needed annually if the goal is to be met (Mingat and Bruns, 2002). This figure does not include care for orphans and vulnerable children or HIV-prevention efforts.

National responses to AIDS: more action needed

Low- and middle-income countries face four fundamental issues as they build their AIDS responses. These include the need for:

- strong leadership and concrete commitment from all sectors of government and society;
- coherence and efficiency as national and external resources are committed, used and accounted for;
- a strengthening of national capacity to absorb resources and mount effective AIDS responses; and
- the production and use of strategic information to guide policy and programming decisions.

Since the turn of the millennium, AIDS leadership and resources have markedly increased. But the challenge is great; for two decades the epidemic has been tightening its grip on development. Lack of resources in low- and middle-income countries has hindered their ability to develop effective national responses to the AIDS epidemic. To this day, the epidemic is growing at a faster rate than funds can be raised to respond to it. In many countries with generalized epidemics, the challenge has shifted from finding additional resources to ensuring that new resources are efficiently absorbed into a growing and sustainable national AIDS response. A major roadblock is the lack of national capacity to scale up AIDS initiatives to critical coverage levels. In the hardest-hit countries, AIDS-related migration, illness and death are draining precious governmental capacities. This, in turn, contributes to the epidemic's spread, causes other development efforts to fail, and creates a vicious circle.

In every country, HIV prevention and AIDS treatment and care are complex problems that exceed the capability of any one sector. An effective response requires combining strong national leadership and ownership, ensuring good governance, resource mobilization, multisectoral planning and coordination, reinforcing capacity to absorb resources and implement programmes, closely monitoring and evaluating the AIDS response, and significantly involving communities, civil society and the private sector.

Bilateral and multilateral donors face their own challenges. An effective sustainable AIDS response cannot be achieved merely by giving countries multimillion-dollar grants, or by providing foreign specialists. National AIDS commissions frequently complain of 'donor-driven' agendas that favour narrow, short-term results, and ignore broader, long-term national planning and needs. They also say human resources are further stretched by individual donor-reporting requirements that create burdensome paperwork. As more external stakeholders offer assistance, it is increasingly important to create donor harmonization and coherence around national structures, strategic plans, and monitoring and evaluation systems.

Globalizing leadership on AIDS

Over the years, one of the greatest obstacles to developing effective national AIDS responses is a lack of political will to tackle, or even talk

Progress update on the global response to the AIDS epidemic, 2004

National responses: improving, but still short of what is needed

- Nearly one-third of countries lack policies that ensure women's equal access to critical prevention and care services.
- Most countries have ratified international conventions on human rights, but effective implementation of these agreements is weak. Only 40% of countries have legal measures in place to prohibit discrimination against populations vulnerable to HIV. Only 50% of countries in sub-Saharan Africa have adopted legislation to prevent discrimination against people living with HIV.
- Three-quarters of countries report that national activity and progress monitoring and evaluation remain major challenges. Only 43% of countries have a national monitoring and evaluation plan and only 24% report having a national monitoring and evaluation budget.
- Only 20% of transnational companies have adopted comprehensive workplace policies addressing HIV and AIDS. At the country level, implementation of workplace policies is generally inadequate.
- Many senior political leaders, from countries where HIV prevalence is low and the epidemic is concentrated in key populations at higher risk, remain detached from the response to HIV and AIDS.

Source: *Progress report on the global response to the HIV/AIDS epidemic,* UNAIDS, 2003; *Coverage of selected services for HIV/AIDS prevention and care in low- and middle-income countries in 2003,* Policy Project, 2004; *The level of effort in the national response to HIV/AIDS: The AIDS program effort index (API),* 2003, Round, UNAIDS/USAID/WHO and the Policy Project.

about, the AIDS epidemic. Political commitment has recently increased in the hardest-hit countries. Still, in many countries where HIV is quickly spreading, such as those in Asia and Eastern Europe, a lack of leadership raises fears these countries will not adequately address the epidemic until it is too late.

In sub-Saharan Africa, the epidemic's scale is convincing more leaders to take personal responsibility for implementing the national AIDS response. For example, Kenya's President Mwai Kibaki is chairing a new Cabinet Action Committee on AIDS and enlisting leaders from Kenya's major religions to deal with stigma and discrimination. The government has also abolished school fees, which immediately helped tens of thousands of Kenyan children orphaned by AIDS.

Botswana's President Festus Mogae was instrumental in the decision to provide free antiretroviral medicines and develop a national prevention of mother-to-child-transmission programme. Malawi's president, Bakili Muluzi, appointed a Minister for AIDS Health to improve coordination of the national response. In Lesotho, in March 2004, Prime Minister Pakalitha Mosisili and more than 80 senior civil servants were publicly tested for HIV to help break the stigma that discourages voluntary counselling and testing.

Elsewhere, in 2003, the world's two most populous countries made leadership breakthroughs. On World AIDS Day, Chinese Premier Wen Jiabao made an unprecedented hospital visit during which he met AIDS patients and promised the government would protect their rights, provide free schooling for their children, and offer free treatment for poor patients. In July, India's first National Convention of the Parliamentary Forum on AIDS stressed the need to overcome stigma. Prime Minister Atal Bihari Vajpayee said it was more urgent than ever to deal with India's epidemic, and he called for 'openness and a complete absence of prejudice towards affected persons' (Kaiser Daily AIDS Report, 2003).

The Association of South-East Asian Nations devised a Work Programme on HIV/AIDS for 2003–2005. Governments and donors are supporting and implementing the Programme's key initiatives, including intercountry activities on mobile populations and stigma and discrimination. In September 2003, ministers and senior officials from 62 countries and territories of the United Nations Economic and Social Commission for Asia and the Pacific adopted a resolution to tackle AIDS as a development challenge.

In the Caribbean, one example of activism is Denzil Douglas, Prime Minister of Saint Kitts and Nevis and leader of the Pan Caribbean Partnership against HIV/AIDS. He is particularly active in international negotiations, promoting reductions in the cost of health-care services, and increased access to antiretroviral therapy.

In the Commonwealth of Independent States (CIS), two Heads of Government summits (in Moscow and Moldova in 2002) endorsed a Programme of Urgent Response of the CIS Member States to the AIDS Epidemic, which created national coordinators for multisectoral responses. In February 2004, high-level government representatives from 53 countries attended the European Union's 'Breaking the Barriers' Conference in Dublin, and pledged to achieve concrete targets to reduce HIV and AIDS within Europe and Central Asia.

Traditional leaders can also make an impact. In Fiji, the Great Council of Chiefs (a constitutional body of 50 hereditary leaders) co-hosted the 'Accelerating Action against AIDS in the Pacific' Conference. The President of Fiji and the Chiefs committed themselves to the country's AIDS response and called on community, business and religious leaders to follow suit.

Strategies, policies, legislation and action

Ultimately, leadership must translate into concrete action. UNAIDS monitors the progress of the global AIDS response in various ways, and its AIDS Programme Effort Index is one tool for measuring country-level commitment. The Index was developed by the United States Agency for International Development, the UNAIDS Secretariat, the World Health Organization (WHO), and the United States-based Policy Project. It tracks a country's effort in 10 different programme categories but does not measure actual output, such as coverage of a specific service.

Figure 45

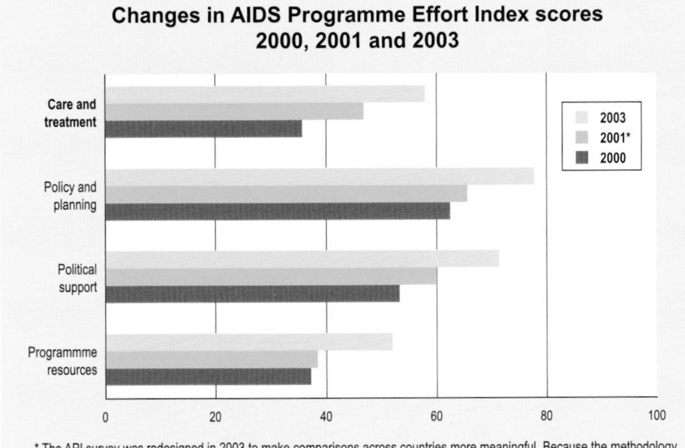

* The API survey was redesigned in 2003 to make comparisons across countries more meaningful. Because the methodology had changed, respondents in 2003 were asked to score each item twice, once for 2003 and once for 2001. The inclusion of the 2001 data facilitated efforts to gauge progress since 2000.

Source: UNAIDS, USAID, Policy Project – API surveys

The results between 2000 (40 countries) and 2003 (54 countries) show there is a general pattern of improvement (USAID et al., 2003). Significant gains in national commitment were recorded in the categories of treatment and care, political support, policy and planning, and programme resources. Improvements in providing resources, and treatment and care, were particularly notable since these were the lowest-rated components in 2000 (see Figure 45). The creation of the Global Fund to Fight AIDS, Tuberculosis and Malaria and rising bilateral donor funding levels explain much of the resource component's increase. The increase in care-related efforts probably reflects international donors' new emphasis on treatment access.

Commitment and action

In 2003, additional data were collected from 103 countries to track *national commitment and action*, and policy development and implementation (UNAIDS, 2003b). The data show an increase in the number of countries with comprehensive, multisectoral national AIDS strategies, and government-led national AIDS coordinating bodies. However, the existence of national AIDS bodies and plans does not necessarily translate into efficient and concerted action. One striking finding was that resources were often not invested in programme areas with the greatest impact. For example, in several Latin American countries, programmes for injecting drug users and men who have sex with men were scarce even though these populations suffered from high HIV infection rates (see 'Finance' chapter).

In some countries, policy and strategic planning moved ahead, but legislation did not keep up because regressive or contradictory laws remained on the books. In the context of injecting drug use, some countries with restrictive laws have nonetheless carried out pilot projects involving needle and syringe exchanges, methadone maintenance therapy, and condom promotion at entertainment establishments. In the Russian Federation, a recent criminal-code amendment allowed for harm-reduction projects to operate legally. Unfortunately, some legal barriers remain—most notably, the ban

Better governance for more effective responses

Democratic and efficient development activities depend on good governance, full constituent participation, the rule of law, transparency, community responsiveness, consensus-building, equity, effectiveness and accountability. These are complex and interrelated issues, but they have concrete applications. For example, countries with high levels of constituent participation generally have more dynamic national AIDS responses. South Africa's recent treatment and care policy changes were spurred on by steady pressure from the country's HIV-positive community, prominent legal and health professionals, and many national and international NGOs. An open, participatory governance system allowed for civil society to provoke positive change.

Similarly, the rule of law is based on legislation and regulations, and on citizens being fully aware of their rights and how to protect them within existing legal frameworks and policies (UNDP, 2002). Applying rule of law and good governance concepts to AIDS activities inspires democratic planning and implementation. In 2002, the UN Secretary-General established a Commission on HIV/AIDS and Governance in Africa to combine applied research, policy dialogue and advocacy. The Commission is based at the Economic Commission for Africa in Addis Ababa, Ethiopia. It matches current knowledge gained from AIDS responses with knowledge gaps, and works to make good governance relevant to Africa's policy-makers and implementers.

In a similar vein, UNDP's South-East Asia HIV and Development Programme has strongly promoted good governance in AIDS responses in countries such as China, the Lao People's Democratic Republic and Viet Nam (UNDP, 2002). In Eastern Europe, UNDP promotes creating open and inclusive environments. This includes comprehensive, multisectoral policies, and innovative partnerships that build trust and reduce stigma to turn back the epidemic.

on substitution therapy (UNAIDS/Ministry of Health, 2003).

Legal obstacles exist in other areas. The 2004 report of the United Nations Development Programme (UNDP), *Reversing the epidemic: Facts and policy options—HIV/AIDS in Eastern Europe and the Commonwealth of Independent States*, notes many government agencies in the region cannot transfer funds to the accounts of nongovernmental organizations (NGOs), or subcontract programme activities to them. Furthermore, many NGOs have their own problems, including inadequate skills and capacity, high staff turnover, and a mistrust of authorities that is not always justified. To resolve these issues, the Report calls for improved staff training, dialogue between state and non-state participants, and legal frameworks for NGO activities.

Faith-based leadership comes to the fore

Political leadership on AIDS comes from all sectors of society. For example, in various parts of the world, several religious communities have made important contributions. In West Africa, Muslim authorities enlisted the moral weight of local imams. In Mali, backed by Population Service International and USAID, the Malian League of Imams and Islamic Scholars created four lessons for the imams' Friday prayers, including prevention guidance and messages of compassion for people living with HIV (Development Gateway, 2003).

Meanwhile, an Argentinian Lutheran pastor, Lisandro Orlov, is urging Latin American churches to adopt more inclusive approaches to sexuality and HIV. In Nepal, at the 2003 South Asia Inter-Faith Consultation on Children, Young People and AIDS, various faith-based communities made a commitment to join the front-line AIDS response, and pledged to provide care, protection and support to those infected with and affected by HIV.

The South African Anglican Church has been a consistent advocate on AIDS issues. At major events, Anglican Archbishop Njongonkulu Ndungane has challenged the South African Government's policies on antiretroviral drugs and AIDS in prisons. Meanwhile, the NGO Positive Muslims responds to stigma and discrimination within the larger South African community.

Religious groups have also emerged as leaders in care. In Durban, South Africa, Swami Saradananda, of the Ramakrishna Centre, has counselled and cared for people living with HIV or AIDS for many years, regardless of their religious background. These activities have spread to other Hindu clinics, and the Hindu Council of Africa now works on AIDS-related issues. Another example is the Samaritan Ministry home-care programme in Nassau, Bahamas. The programme is an interfaith activity that trains community volunteers to reach out to people living with HIV, along with their families and loved ones. It is now in its 14th year, and has trained more than 300 volunteers.

Civil society and community mobilization

Community groups and civil society organizations that emerge in the AIDS response reflect the diversity of those affected by the epidemic. All have a key role to play. Civil society organizations often have innovative approaches to the epidemic, and can channel funds to communities, augment state service delivery, and monitor national government policies. People living with HIV particularly need to be involved in all aspects of the response, from planning and decision-making, to implementation and review (see 'People living with AIDS' focus).

For instance, the International Federation of Red Cross and Red Crescent Societies has formed a partnership with the Global Network of People Living with HIV/AIDS. Their joint activities focus on eradicating stigma through forming links between national and local Red Cross and Red Crescent Societies and HIV-positive organizations. The arrangement also ensures that people living with HIV play a major role in antiretroviral treatment programmes, particularly in helping people gain access to care and in assisting patients with treatment adherence.

Civil society organizations are most valuable and effective if they work with, rather than in parallel to, governments. Both sides need to be open to partnerships, and it is up to governments to provide a positive environment. Factors that enable these groups to contribute include legal recognition, tax incentives, streamlined contracting regulations, and agreed ground rules to involve them in decision-making and information sharing. In addition, both sides need to adopt measures to ensure accountability and transparency.

At the community level, governments' administrative procedures must be flexible enough to include local NGOs. In India, an evaluation of targeted interventions showed some state agencies found it almost impossible to work with community-based organizations because of rigid agency costing and accountability guidelines. For example, grant applications must include copies of the organization's official registration certificates, annual reports, and audited financial reports for the previous three years. Few community groups can provide this information (Lenton et al., 2003).

Some governments have successfully enhanced communities' capacity to use their own resources and talents in AIDS activities. For example, Malawi's national strategy on children orphaned by AIDS encouraged community-based groups to care for orphaned children. The country now has 97 community-based orphan-care groups, and some offer educational support to enrolled children (UNAIDS, 2003b).

Working in partnerships to respond to AIDS

National AIDS authorities are increasingly turning to formal partnership forums to stimulate nongovernmental participation, broaden national ownership of the response and increase transparency. This approach was first developed in Africa, under the International Partnership against AIDS in Africa. The concept is now more widespread, but its best examples are still in sub-Saharan Africa. For example, the Uganda AIDS Partnership is a national coordinating mechanism of nine 'constituencies' working on AIDS that represent all stakeholders at all levels. They share information and jointly plan and coordinate activities.

In neighbouring Kenya, an annual Joint AIDS Programme Review by all stakeholders supports the country's multisectoral response. The review was first conducted in May 2002 by the National AIDS Control Council, civil society groups, donors and other stakeholders. Among other advantages, the review provides the government with a way of linking its strategic plan and other important policy-making processes.

Both the World Bank Multi-Country HIV/AIDS Programme and the Global Fund to Fight AIDS, Tuberculosis and Malaria aim to involve civil society in direct ways. The Programme works through its financing channels to NGOs, while the Global Fund explicitly requires NGOs to participate in its Country Coordinating Mechanisms that prepare proposals for AIDS-related projects. For instance, in Morocco national NGOs have direct responsibility for managing 30% of the monies provided by the Fund. They participate in many Ministry of Health activities, and work with civil society organizations in providing local services.

Working with civil society is a constant process of learning and adapting for everyone involved. A recent International AIDS Alliance paper assessed NGO participation in the Global Fund's first round of granting funds. The paper revealed that government commitment to working with NGOs appeared to be somewhat hollow. Many appeared to cooperate with NGOs only to secure funding, and afterwards lost interest in collaborating. The study also found most NGOs invited to participate in Country Coordinating Mechanisms were based in capital cities. Rurally based organizations and those working with marginalized populations were under-represented. Furthermore, several countries said their national AIDS committees lacked the capacity to handle Global Fund disbursement to NGOs.

At the same time, many NGOs did not have enough resources or technical and managerial skills. Some NGOs were more focused on competing with each other rather than forging a cohesive voice within the NGO community. All of these factors had a negative impact on NGOs' abilities to participate in the Global Fund process. The Alliance paper recommended that NGOs receive technical and financial support to improve their networking and participating capacity. It also called on governmental partners to adopt more positive attitudes about working with NGOs (International AIDS Alliance, 2002).

Private sector engagement

Businesses can contribute to the AIDS response at different levels, depending on their size, industry and location. Their three main contributions are in the form of workplace programmes, leadership and advocacy for AIDS work, and partnerships with the community and government for a strengthened response to the epidemic. To engage the private sector at different levels, UNAIDS provides technical guidance, brokers partnerships, and develops mechanisms and tools. Its strategy is to build on what works.

The Global Business Coalition on HIV/AIDS: a corporate leader in responding to AIDS

The AIDS epidemic is profoundly affecting global businesses through its impact on workers, customers and markets. A key player in this domain is the Global Business Coalition on HIV/AIDS, which works to increase business involvement in the global AIDS response. The Coalition works with the Global Fund, UNAIDS and other partners. Its more than 130 corporate members come from varied sectors, including mining, consumer products, electronics, energy, finance, steel production, and media and communications.

The Coalition helps companies to: implement workplace, employee and community prevention, care and support programmes; use business innovation and flexibility to make AIDS programmes more effective; and carry out business advocacy and leadership to promote greater AIDS action and partnerships with governments and communities. In 2003, the Coalition and nine of its members announced a new initiative to expand AIDS-related workplace programmes into communities where companies operate, and to transfer corporate know-how to the public sector to expand access to services and reduce start-up and running costs.

Involving membership associations is a key focus. These include business organizations, such as the Global Business Coalition on HIV/AIDS and the World Economic Forum; civic organizations and such as the Rotary Club; business associations and coalitions; chambers of commerce; and trade unions.

In countries hard-hit by HIV, workplace AIDS programmes are increasing; however, employers and trade unions could still play a much larger role in the global AIDS response. To date, most workplace projects focus on prevention, and have yielded valuable experience. For example, in Indonesia, the International Labour Organization (ILO) and Aksi Stop AIDS (a Family Health International project) have set up an AIDS-in-the-world-of-work campaign targeting workers, employers and government. By the end of 2004, the campaign aims to bring HIV-prevention activities to more than 900 000 workers.

Some multinational corporations are implementing workplace programmes with a global reach. One is Standard Chartered Bank, which has some 30 000 employees in more than 50 countries. It is the largest international bank in China and India, and employs over 5000 people in 13 African countries. Its current peer-education programme, 'Living with HIV', is delivered by volunteer 'champions', and focuses on HIV-positive employees. It helps them discuss what they can do to live positively, and how they can gain access to practical and emotional support.

In high-prevalence countries, workplace efforts are integrating prevention and treatment strategies. In South Africa, mining and other companies have been leaders in providing medicines to workers. Initiatives are springing up in other parts of Africa, as well. In Cameroon, the National AIDS Commission and the country's employers' association help companies obtain essential medicines, condoms, low-cost antiretrovirals and other supplies for their employees. This partnership received a four-year credit from the World Bank Multi-Country HIV/AIDS Programme, and companies also committed their own funds to it (UNAIDS, 2003).

Business leadership, advocacy and partnerships

Some businesses go further than their own workplace and become wider AIDS advocates. A business can influence its sourcing partners and distributors, companies in other sectors, consumer groups, communities and governments. The Thailand Business Coalition on HIV/AIDS, American International Assurance (Thailand), and the Population Council have directly encouraged 125 Thai businesses to implement HIV-prevention programmes by providing life insurance premium bonuses of 5–10% to companies with workplace prevention activities.

The Global Reporting Initiative is linking the world of work to wider questions of governance. It has chosen South Africa for the first phase of its efforts to develop international standards for AIDS reporting by businesses and other organizations. Project partners include the Johannesburg Securities Exchange, the South African Institute of Chartered Accountants, the Actuarial Society of South Africa, some of the country's major companies, and representatives from other interested parties such as labour, government and the Treatment Action Campaign (Cape Argus, 2003; GRI, 2003).

In recent years, public-private partnerships have emerged as a way of redressing the AIDS-related resource imbalance between low- and middle-income and industrialized countries. The Accelerating Access Initiative, the Global Alliance for Vaccines and Immunization, the International AIDS Vaccine Initiative, the

Survey on the business impact of AIDS

In 2004, the World Economic Forum released results of a global survey on business leaders' perceptions and responses on the impact of AIDS on their businesses. The Forum/UNAIDS/Harvard University survey was called '*Business and AIDS: Who, me?*' Key findings revealed that:

- fewer than 6% of firms have formally approved, written HIV policies;
- 47% of firms felt AIDS is having, or will have, some impact on their business;
- 20% of firms believe AIDS is affecting, or will seriously affect, their communities;
- 16% of all firms provide information about the risks of HIV infection; and
- 5% say they provide antiretrovirals for all HIV-positive staff.

Only 28% of executives believe their response to the epidemic is lacking in any way. However, 56% of those who expect the epidemic to have a serious impact on their business are dissatisfied with their companies' responses. The report concluded that:

- companies are not particularly active in tackling AIDS, even when they expect the epidemic to cause serious problems for their business;
- businesses appear to be making decisions based on an incomplete assessment of the risks they face;
- companies seem to favour a broad social response to the epidemic, but only a small number of businesses currently see themselves as an integral part of that response.

Full report: www.weforum.org/site/homepublic.nsf/Content/Global+Health+Initiative%5CGHI+Global+Business+Survey

International HIV Treatment Access Coalition, and the Stop TB Partnership are examples of such international partnerships.

At national and regional levels, the most visible public-private AIDS partnerships involved major pharmaceutical companies. In Botswana, the Ministry of Health, the Bill and Melinda Gates Foundation, and the Merck Company Foundation formed an antiretroviral treatment programme known as *Masa*, a Setswana word meaning 'new dawn'. By early 2004, more than 14 000 patients were receiving antiretrovirals through the programme (see 'Treatment' chapter).

In Romania, a public-private partnership involving the government and six major pharmaceutical companies (Abbott Laboratories, Boehringer Ingelheim, Bristol-Myers Squibb, GlaxoSmithKline, Hoffman-La Roche, and Merck and Co.) has worked on the country's national plan for access to AIDS treatment and care. Under the plan, the Romanian Government supports AIDS-patient treatment and care costs from national budgets. The companies have agreed to reduce certain drug prices by between 25% and 87%, or to donate drugs and equipment to measure viral load and CD4 counts.

Businesses are also forming AIDS response partnerships with civil society organizations. For instance, in Namibia, Namdeb Diamond Corporation provides support to the *Lironga Eparu* ('learn to survive') organization of people living with HIV.

Making multisectorality work

Adhering to the principle of multisectorality through involving public, private and civil society sectors maximizes resources—financial and otherwise—for the response to AIDS in countries. It allows countries to move away from depending on external support for AIDS activities, and towards national autonomy. The 2001 UN Declaration of Commitment on HIV/AIDS urges diverse stakeholders to be actively involved in national responses. By

2003, countries were expected to establish and strengthen national-response mechanisms by involving the private sector, civil society partners, people living with HIV, and key vulnerable populations.

UNAIDS monitoring shows more than 90% of reporting countries have created national multisectoral bodies to facilitate AIDS coordination between the government, the private sector and civil society. The growth of national AIDS commissions, government-led partnership forums and working groups, expanded UN Theme Groups on HIV/AIDS and the Global Fund's Country Coordinating Mechanisms attests to the unprecedented efforts to involve diverse participants in the national response.

Nonetheless, in many countries, poorly defined roles between ministries of health and national AIDS councils have caused confusion and conflict, which has slowed national strategy implementation. Government ministries often have little incentive to follow the guidance of national coordinating mechanisms. Many perceive cooperation as a threat because they may lose influence and budgetary control. This has sometimes led to outright jurisdictional battles between national AIDS councils and health ministries. Furthermore, in far too many countries, civil society representatives still do not participate in high-level decision-making.

For instance, the Bangladesh National AIDS Committee was set up as a multisectoral body. But it is led by the Ministry of Health and Family Welfare, and has no clear policy or management framework. Other ministries saw the Committee as an extension of the Health Ministry, and did not agree to be part of the coordination process. Without any real influence, the Committee did not function effectively; it last met in 2002.

In Sri Lanka, a similar situation is unfolding. The National AIDS Commission is run by the Ministry of Health and focuses on health-related implementation issues. Participation by other ministries is low and sporadic. The Bangladesh and Sri Lanka experiences show that national leaders at the highest level need to support AIDS councils politically and legally. Equally, when bilateral and multilateral donors support and communicate with AIDS coordinating bodies, they reinforce the bodies' position as leaders of multisectoral responses.

Firm donor support also increases AIDS authorities' capacities to create a national monitoring and evaluation system, and to produce strategic information. The Global Fund and the World Bank have promoted this concept in their AIDS work, but bilateral support is more uneven. A 2004 UNAIDS Secretariat survey found 71% of African national AIDS authorities had formal relationships with bilateral initiatives. But in Asia, these links were established in only 56% of surveyed countries; in Eastern Europe, in only 43% (see Figure 46).

Figure 46

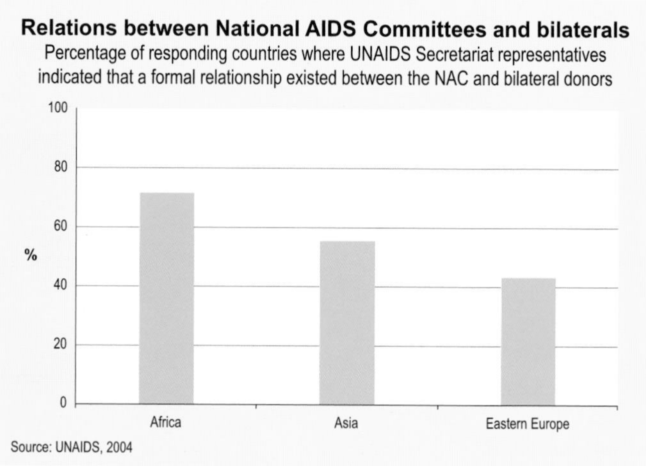

The support of bilateral donors is critical to the functioning of true national coordinating bodies. This is a particularly important principle since ministries of health will play a central role in the global scale up of antiretroviral treatment. Health ministries cannot handle this massive task alone. To rapidly expand antiretroviral access, national AIDS councils need to play a strong coordinating role, and to involve local governments and civil society.

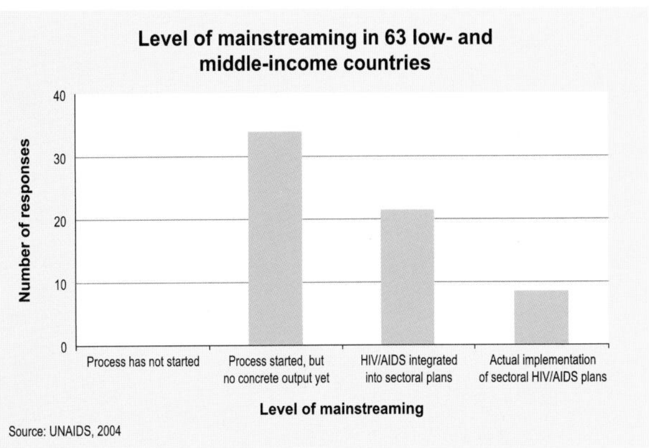

Figure 47

Mainstreaming AIDS into all institutional activities

Institutions ideally address AIDS-related issues through 'mainstreaming', ensuring that every relevant activity they carry out has an AIDS component. Mainstreaming addresses sectoral links to the AIDS response, as well as the root causes of the epidemic's spread. For example, education ministries need to provide AIDS education in schools. They also need to ensure young girls have equal access to a broader education to empower them in society, and thus decrease their vulnerability to HIV infection.

Mainstreaming is a key strategy in converting global commitments into national development agendas. The Millennium Development Goals and the 2001 UN Declaration of Commitment on HIV/AIDS have set the global agenda. To boost mainstreaming implementation, in 2001, the International Monetary Fund and the World Bank declared it was a priority to mainstream AIDS into major development frameworks. However, in early 2004, in 44% of the African countries surveyed by the UNAIDS Secretariat, there was no involvement of national AIDS commissions in the preparation of the Poverty Reduction Strategy Papers, which are prerequisites for World Bank and International Monetary Fund debt relief.

Even in countries that reported a link, it is often tenuous at best. Additional analysis carried out by UNAIDS clearly indicates a need to ensure AIDS is factored into Poverty Reduction Strategy Papers. In late 2003, a UNAIDS survey in 63 countries found all respondents reported key sectors had started mainstreaming, but only 13% had actually made progress in implementing sectoral plans (see Figure 47).

Another chronic problem is inadequate funding for multisectoral work. The highest levels of government need to protect AIDS budgets, and ministries of finance need to ensure monies are budgeted and allocated to priority ministries. Burkina Faso, Cameroon, Guinea, Malawi, Mozambique, Uganda and Zambia have AIDS components in their Poverty Reduction Strategy Papers. But AIDS initiatives are often addressed in a cursory manner. In the UNAIDS survey, only 15 countries had Poverty Reduction Strategy Papers that included HIV and AIDS indicators.

In Zambia, mainstreaming AIDS into all government sectors is a priority. For example, the government recently began training Ministry of Agriculture and Cooperatives staff to encourage them to incorporate AIDS concerns into their work. The UN's Food and

Agriculture Organization is also involved, helping to change the perception that AIDS is entirely the Ministry of Health's responsibility. The training emphasizes the epidemic's role in eroding food security, and focuses on how agricultural officials can mitigate that impact with labour-saving technologies and practices. In addition, the training shows staff members how to preserve knowledge, enhance gender equality, improve nutrition for agricultural workers living with HIV, and promote economic and food safety nets (FAO and Government of Zambia, 2003).

In Ghana, an innovative mainstreaming arrangement places different sectoral AIDS funds in the hands of the Ghana AIDS Commission. Each ministry is required to devote 5% of its AIDS budget to mainstreaming. The Ghana AIDS Commission releases the remaining 95% of the budget only after sector managers have agreed to this. This arrangement ensures there is 'buy-in' from the ministries to the mainstreaming process (Elsey and Kutengule, 2003).

But multisectorality is not a one-size-fits-all formula. The epidemic's highly varied nature rules out resolving it through detailed global guidelines. In high-prevalence countries, the epidemic touches all of society. National AIDS commissions and other coordinating bodies need to act like 'councils of war', and directly involve the head of state. Countries with lower prevalence also require strong multisectoral prevention and care responses, and they need to use the comparative advantages of individual ministries in addressing the epidemic.

In several low-prevalence countries of Asia and Eastern Europe, health ministers still consider AIDS their 'turf'. But they do not have the will or strength to catalyse, leverage or lead the necessary comprehensive response. In these regions, there are many examples of interministerial AIDS commissions, but they usually only have an advisory role.

Decentralization—empowering regions, communities and districts

Decentralization is one of the chief strategies used to improve good governance and development programme implementation. In this process, central governments devolve powers and responsibilities to lower administrative institutions. Decentralization aims to make decision-making more democratic, equitable and locally responsive. As a result, the process inspires 'national ownership', along with civil society and private sector involvement in policy-planning.

However, AIDS-response decentralization has often faltered (Lubben et al., 2002). Governments are used to working within strict hierarchical structures, and the benefits of involving communities are not always clear. At the same time, communities often do not have the necessary representative structures or administrative capacity to participate effectively. A great deal of training and facilitation may be necessary on both sides if they are to work effectively with each other (Mpanju-Shumbusho, 2003).

Despite the problems, AIDS-related decentralization is a reality in several countries. Papua New Guinea, Uganda and the United Republic of Tanzania have successfully decentralized their national responses to community and household levels. Similarly, in Morocco, multisectoral regional and provincial AIDS committees were established to develop local strategic plans, coordinate activities and monitor implementation. In Burkina Faso, Ethiopia, Kenya and Uganda, the World Bank Multi-Country

HIV/AIDS Programme has helped prevention and care programmes to reach communities and households. In Ghana, the Programme is funding the country's District Response Initiative, which is decentralizing the AIDS response in 27 districts.

The UNDP also emphasizes decentralizing AIDS efforts. In Cambodia, its Community Enhancement Programme works with the Ministry of Rural Affairs to encourage communes (local districts) to prepare development plans rather than have the government allocate a set amount of funding to each commune for uniform activities. This Programme includes building local capacity to collect and analyse AIDS data used to support planning and monitoring. In a recent planning cycle, most Commune Councillors identified AIDS as a local priority, and said they were willing to create detailed care and prevention plans.

Various country experiences show that strong financial and political investment is needed to create effective district and local coordination bodies. At the local level, capacity gaps pose challenges, much as they do at the national level. There is now an urgent need to develop innovative ways of addressing capacity issues at all levels of health systems, particularly at lower staff levels. This situation is becoming even more urgent as access to antiretroviral therapy expands.

Harmonization and coherence

The relationships between donors and recipient countries, and between the donors themselves, can have a powerful impact on how the national response is implemented. Some donors pursue their own agendas without reference to national priorities, or to other donors' actions. However, this is changing, particularly when countries and donors engage in constructive dialogue. In February 2003, a watershed understanding was reached when senior officials of about 50 countries and more than 20 multilateral and bilateral development institutions issued the Rome Declaration on Harmonization, which recognized that donor aid imposes high transaction costs on recipients.

Donors can alleviate this problem by coordinating their strategies and reporting requirements, and helping partner countries to lead their own development processes. Harmonization is facilitated by creating national AIDS action frameworks that align all partners. Sector-wide approaches often have shown promise in developing the health, education and agriculture sectors. These approaches coordinate investments around a jointly developed national strategic plan with an agreed financial administrative framework and reporting system.

In Malawi, AIDS-funding mechanisms have recently improved a great deal—most notably, in June 2003, when the government and four international donors (Canada, Norway, the United Kingdom and the World Bank) created a 'pooled' funding arrangement of US$ 72 million for 2003–2008. It operates alongside the traditional 'earmarked' donor-funding system. Within it, the National AIDS Commission can allocate funds to its national priority areas.

If there is a need to reallocate funds to accommodate unforeseen changes in plans, donor transactional costs are reduced because all participants are working from a common workplan, financing mechanism and technical-reporting format. For the first time, Malawi's arrangement has allowed the World Bank to pool AIDS funds. It is hoped the National AIDS Commission's dual system of pooled and earmarked funding will provide sufficient checks and balances, which will help create a more effective national AIDS-funding mechanism.

In Myanmar, the Joint Programme for HIV/AIDS proves that funding from multiple donors can be secured, harmonized and disbursed even under difficult political circumstances. The country's ruling party and political opposition consider AIDS a social emergency and have called for donor funding. Because of its unique position, the UN system led the way in creating the 2003–2005 Joint Programme, and the related Fund for HIV/AIDS in Myanmar. Together, the programmes are channelling US$ 24 million (mostly from Norway, Sweden and the United Kingdom) into AIDS projects that are part of an integrated workplan designed and implemented by government bodies, civil society and UN agencies.

Managing the flow of funds

More funds are flowing into the global AIDS response, and using them effectively is increasingly important (see 'Finance' chapter). This is an integral part of improving governance—particularly transparency (seeing how and why decisions are made) and accountability (making decision-makers answerable for their decisions and their consequences).

In many countries, multisectoral AIDS-funding arrangements have met with serious problems. They have been plagued by poor planning and a lack of clearly defined roles and working arrangements between national AIDS coordinating bodies, the ministries responsible for implementing most HIV programming (typically Health and Education), and the Ministry of Finance, which holds the purse strings. The result is that many action plans are not fully funded and, thus, never fully implemented.

Another problem is rigid or outmoded allocation practices, which contribute to the 'money-shaping programmes' phenomenon. For example, in some former Soviet countries, government accounting practices have not fully evolved since the Soviet era. In several Central Asian countries, only government health resources can be spent in government hospitals and clinics. Therefore, NGO outreach programmes cannot procure or distribute individual HIV-prevention tools such as clean syringes, needles, condoms, disinfectants and test kits.

For instance, in Kazakhstan, much of the central and local governments' AIDS funds are still swallowed by mass testing programmes. This is despite the fact that the 2001–2005 National AIDS Response Programme calls for balancing HIV prevention, testing and treatment activities. This discrepancy occurs because there is no budgetary classification for prevention; changing this requires a specific government decree. Therefore, government-funded prevention activities cannot be implemented. A related issue is the tendency of many AIDS service organizations to focus on testing—the only activity that receives government funding. Recent additional extrabudgetary funds, including a two-year, US$ 6.5 million Global Fund grant that includes prevention activities, have helped, but the overall imbalance persists.

If financing is to be effective, it needs to be continuous. In Paraguay, the National AIDS Programme currently provides antiretroviral therapy to 300 people. However, for several months each year, funding shortfalls stop treatment (UNAIDS, 2003b). In the Indian state of Andhra Pradesh, a recent evaluation showed that NGOs there face serious funding delays (Lenton et al., 2003).

The 'Three Ones'

In April 2004, at a meeting in Washington DC, co-chaired by UNAIDS, the United Kingdom and the United States, a historic agreement was reached by donors and low- and middle-income countries to work more effectively together in scaling up national AIDS responses. They adopted three core principles for concerted country-level action—the 'Three Ones'.

- one agreed AIDS Action Framework that provides the basis for coordinating the work of all partners;
- one National AIDS Coordinating Authority with a broad-based multisectoral mandate;
- one agreed country-level Monitoring and Evaluation system.

The concepts of national ownership, multisectorality, mainstreaming, harmonization and coherence have been combined into these principles, which aim to increase the pace of the AIDS response and promote using resources more effectively by clarifying relevant roles and relationships. The blueprint begins with one agreed AIDS action framework, which is a nationally devised strategic plan for coordination across partnerships and funding mechanisms.

The national AIDS coordinating body needs to have legal status, a strong, broad-based multisectoral mandate, and a democratic oversight mechanism to function effectively. It is responsible for managing partners' actions within the framework. The coordination body also requires overarching national policy leadership in order to facilitate the partnership arrangements that allow for implementing and reviewing the action framework. Many countries state that national AIDS councils and national strategic plans exist, but only a few meet the specific criteria described above.

Even rarer is the existence of one agreed monitoring and evaluation system that provides a single mechanism to account for various funding arrangements, monitors AIDS programme effectiveness, and provides the strategic information needed to adjust the action framework (UNAIDS, 2003).

Strengthening capacity

The AIDS epidemic works in a vicious circle, striking hardest in those countries with the weakest capacity to respond to it. In many countries, AIDS is currently depleting technical and administrative capacity faster than it can be replenished. This is creating an unparalleled crisis in human resources, and is reversing many of the development gains made in previous decades. In parts of Uganda and Malawi, the World Bank reports that nearly one-third of all teachers are HIV-positive. In the Central African Republic, AIDS was responsible for 85% of the 340 deaths among teachers between 1996 and 1998.

Even before HIV emerged, public service systems in low- and middle-income countries were struggling to meet their citizens' needs. In the health-care sector, problems included poor delivery infrastructure; inadequate human resources; poorly defined services, functions, skills and protocols; and inadequate management and administration. In much of sub-Saharan Africa, AIDS has turned these weaknesses into crises. In Malawi, a recent impact study found a total of 1462 health-sector employees died between 1990 and 2000. In a 2004 review of 50 low- and middle-income countries, 95% of UNAIDS Secretariat offices in African countries said a lack of health personnel was severely hindering the AIDS response (see Figure 48).

In Asia, 67% of representatives reported health resource difficulties, versus 47% in Latin

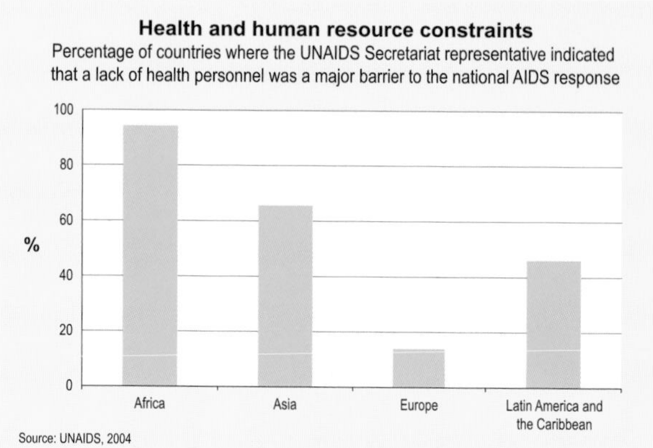

Figure 48

American and the Caribbean (see Figure 48). These countries face a significant increase in demand for health services. They also face a greater disease burden with the resurgence of other related health issues such as tuberculosis, malnutrition, diarrhoea and pneumonia. Indeed, some countries in sub-Saharan Africa report HIV patients occupy 60–70% of hospital beds. This makes it very difficult for patients with other conditions to receive the treatment and care they need.

Maintaining existing capacity and stopping the brain drain

Capacity-building requires funding and political commitment, but it also calls for a broader vision that combines short-term emergency measures with long-term, sustained strengthening of the fundamental institutions of modern statehood. The most immediate requirement is to preserve existing capacity by keeping people alive and healthy. In the worst-affected African countries, no other measure will so quickly and directly arrest the decline in national capacity as providing treatment and care (Piot, 2003). At the same time, efforts will need to focus on using existing capacity to its fullest as HIV-treatment initiatives get up to speed. A wide range of untapped community resources (particularly people living with HIV) will need to compensate for formal skills gaps.

Furthermore, additional efforts are required to minimize the 'brain drain'—the migration of trained civil servants to higher-income countries. This phenomenon is most obvious in the health sectors of Southern Africa, where doctors and nurses are emigrating to Australia, Europe, the Gulf countries, Japan and the United States. These countries offer these workers an attractive alternative to the poor conditions and low pay that characterize their own health-care systems.

South Africa is particularly hard-hit by an exodus of doctors and nurses leaving for higher-paid jobs overseas (Thomson, 2003; IOM, 2003). The South African Medical Association estimates as many as 5000 doctors have left the country in recent years. The Democratic Nursing Organization of South Africa says 300 trained nurses leave each month. Zambia is another hard-hit country; it has only 400 practising doctors. Once, it had 1600 (Lauring, 2002).

Some countries, such as the United Kingdom, have established codes of conduct to prevent 'poaching'. Improving working conditions and wages in affected countries can also keep health professionals from moving abroad. An International Organization for Migration programme, called 'Migration for Development in Africa', helps African countries to encourage their qualified expatriates to return, and to retain professionals who might otherwise be tempted to leave. The programme operates in Benin, Cape Verde, Ghana, Kenya, Rwanda and Uganda (IOM, 2003).

Rebuilding and increasing capacity

Inadequate training of new health professionals is another major issue. In some cases, the pre-service training system in hard-hit countries has completely broken down. For example, in Malawi, the state-run nursing school closed in 2003 due to a lack of funds, and the medical school faced a similar budget crisis. UNDP's Southern Africa Capacity Initiative is exploring ways to build sustainable capacity across sectors. The Initiative has a training component that supports local institutions in training professionals in key sectors. Information technology is also helping health systems to do more with fewer trained staff. UNDP also advocates non-traditional approaches to stemming the loss of workers in all sectors. Examples include franchising out public-service delivery to civil society organizations or international NGOs to achieve greater quality and higher motivation. Similarly, the private sector can be contracted to provide public services.

In Botswana, a variety of strategies underpin the *Masa* antiretroviral treatment programme. The country does not have enough qualified professionals to cope with expanding services. Foreign professionals are hired to provide much-needed treatment and care, and to build local capacity through a training programme carried out in partnership with the Botswana-Harvard AIDS Institute Partnership. Botswana's Ministry of Health also has a training programme called *Kitso* ('knowledge' in Setswana). By mid-2003, over 700 people at all levels (approximately 10% of the public health-sector workforce) had received AIDS-specific training. Private practitioners and health personnel at hospitals run by large mining companies have also been trained. In addition, a 'preceptorship' programme brings HIV experts from top international institutions to mentor national staff (UNAIDS, 2003).

South-South cooperation: Brazil leads the way

Cooperation between low- and middle-income countries ('South-South' cooperation) can provide key support to national responses, particularly in capacity-building. Brazil excels at this type of cooperation, particularly among the Portuguese-speaking countries of Africa and among Central and South American nations. In 2001, the Brazilian Cooperation Agency established a partnership with the United Nations to transfer Brazilian experience in reproductive health and in preventing and treating HIV and sexually transmitted infections to other low- and middle-income countries (SELA, 2003).

One example is a three-year project with Mozambique to improve the quality of AIDS and reproductive health information for young people, particularly through youth associations and institutions that work with them. The project is supported by the United Nations Educational Scientific and Cultural Organization (UNESCO), the United Nations Population Fund (UNFPA), the United Nations Children's Fund (UNICEF), and the United States Agency for International Development (USAID), and has a number of NGO and bilateral partners.

Brazil is also working with Bolivia, Colombia, the Dominican Republic, El Salvador and Paraguay, and has helped them receive antiretroviral drugs worth about US$ 1 million to support pilot projects to treat people living with HIV. In June 2003, Russian officials and experts visited Brazil to learn about its experience in providing treatment and about government and civil society cooperation for school-based youth HIV-prevention programmes.

Strategic information

Investment by countries and the global community in creating and using strategic information is critical to turning the epidemic around. Policy-makers and programme planners, communities and countries need the evidence base to make informed decisions about the best courses of action.

- Strengthened surveillance systems support efforts to place AIDS clearly on countries' development agendas, and can point to where programming must be enhanced and focused to do the most good.
- Explicit operations research work detects strengths and weaknesses to improve programme delivery for the greatest impact.
- Monitoring and evaluation help countries and the global community to assess progress on goals and targets of the 2001 UN Declaration of Commitment on HIV/AIDS. They also help countries to move towards attaining the Millennium Development Goal of halting and reversing the HIV epidemic by 2015.
- Focus groups, key informant interviews, mapping of potential intervention sites, surveys, scientific literature reviews, case studies and collection of empirical evidence from programmes can be rich sources of information for decision-making.

WHO works with the German Agency for Technical Cooperation to help African and European institutions become 'knowledge hubs' in AIDS treatment and HIV prevention for regional skills transfer and training. In Uganda, a knowledge hub has been established with the Joint Clinical Research Centre and other leading training providers. So far, it has provided hands-on training to hundreds of Ugandan health workers, and has recently started providing capacity-building opportunities for other countries in the region. Similar knowledge hubs have been established in Eastern Europe and West Africa.

Strategic information for evidence-informed policy and programming

Strategic information is any information that can usefully guide policy and programming decisions. All decision-makers facing the tough choices and dilemmas presented by AIDS need evidence-informed policy guidance. For example, decisions about introducing appropriate harm-reduction strategies or mixes of combination prevention for sexual transmission need to be informed by clear evidence about what works.

For example, while needle exchange has been shown to reduce HIV transmission and bring injecting drug users into contact with health and social services, it is too soon to gauge the effectiveness of supervised injection centres, which hold the promise of reducing HIV transmission among the injecting drug users most at risk of exposure to HIV. In other cases, decisions about how to balance promoting abstinence, delaying sexual debut, reducing the number of sexual partners and encouraging condom use need to be informed by scientific evidence about the effectiveness of each strategy in different contexts, and young people's and adults' perspectives on what might work best.

If policies and programmes are to reflect the epidemic's realities, countries need the capacity to track the epidemic and analyse trends, understand behavioural patterns, measure social and economic impact, monitor programme indicators, evaluate progress and conduct operations research to refine programmes. Both the short-term and long-term effectiveness of national responses depend on knowing which data are needed, and how to collect, compile, analyse and translate them into strategic information to move policy agendas forward and ensure the most effective programming. In many parts of the world, this 'data-informing-decisions' capacity needs strengthening.

During 2003, UNAIDS worked with partners such as WHO, the US Centers for Disease Control and Prevention, Family Health International, the East-West Center and the Futures Group International to build and enhance capacity at country level for modelling and estimation of the epidemic. Over 300 representatives from national AIDS programmes and the research institutions of 130 countries have been trained in skills for capturing, validating and interpreting HIV-related data and in use of updated modelling methodologies to improve HIV and AIDS estimates.

Improving surveillance

Classic surveillance collects information such as HIV prevalence, AIDS cases and mortality. Second-generation surveillance adds risk behaviour information. Both help countries to assess the course of their epidemics and decide on strategic responses. Examples of behavioural data collection activities include India's massive 2001–2002 national behavioural survey and the UNAIDS Second-Generation Surveillance Project, funded by the European Community and carried out in partnership with WHO and eight countries in Africa, Asia, the Caribbean and Latin America.

Including NGOs in surveillance activities helps provide access to hard-to-reach populations. In Vietnam and Mexico, NGOs facilitated access to injecting drug users for behavioural research. In the Dominican Republic, the sex workers' association MODEMU, and the gay men's organization *Amigos Siempre Amigos* ('friends always') provided peer interviewers (WHO/UNAIDS, 2003).

Recently, Indonesia conducted behavioural surveillance covering nearly half its provinces and all key populations at higher risk—men who buy sex, sex workers (women, men and transgender), injecting drug users, men who have sex with men and youth at higher risk. Robust provincial estimates were developed on the number of people at risk of infection and already infected with HIV. This permitted policy-makers, community groups, NGOs and local AIDS Control Commissions to adapt existing programming to actual conditions. For example, harm reduction programmes now focus on sexual and injecting risk, since it was found that many male injectors—up to 70% in one major city—have unprotected sex with sex workers. Furthermore, condom promotion programmes have a renewed emphasis on reaching potential clients of sex workers.

Operations research

Operations research collects and analyses information as programmes are implemented and scaled up. This research uses a systematic approach to 'learning by doing' and captures information in a way that helps programme managers and designers to make the best use of it.

Key questions for treatment scale up include: how best to avoid drug stock-outs; the most useful components of community treatment literacy programmes; how to maintain adherence; the tasks care providers can undertake and the training needed; how best to keep costs down; which laboratory monitoring is essential; and how to measure the clinical effects of treatment and return to normal function. For instance, Senegal monitored antiretroviral adherence in relation to the costs born directly by patients. The more patients paid on a sliding scale by income, the less adherent they were. These findings influenced Senegal's decision to introduce a universal access, free-of-charge antiretroviral programme.

Operations research in prevention can focus on many different aspects of programming, such as comparing results of various methods of offering HIV testing and assessing the effects on stigma of prevention programming. Prevention-treatment integration can influence the effectiveness of prevention and treatment. For example, antiretroviral treatment programmes in Khayelitsha, South Africa; Masaka, Uganda; and Cange, Haiti have helped support prevention activities by documenting increased interest and willingness of community members to come forward for HIV testing (see 'Prevention' chapter).

Monitoring and evaluating national and local responses

UNAIDS' major priorities include reporting on the impact of the global response and building country capacity to carry out credible monitoring and evaluation. To drive this agenda forward, UNAIDS provides innovative links between monitoring, evaluation research and financial tracking.

Monitoring and evaluation are essential to determining whether programmes are reaching target populations and accomplishing their objectives. This information is needed to garner additional resources by showing proof of money well spent. It also helps with refining interventions for maximum impact, tracking increasing access to services and supporting the information needs of new partners, such as the Global Fund to Fight AIDS, Tuberculosis and Malaria. Yet, lack of technical capacity and resources is hindering action in this crucial area.

In September 2003, UNAIDS published its first *Progress report on the global response to the HIV/AIDS epidemic*. It reported that 75% of 103 reporting countries feel inadequate capacity is a serious obstacle to their ability to report reliably on national indicators such as HIV workplace policies, coverage of antiretroviral treatment and access to services for preventing mother-to-child transmission. Only 43% of reporting countries had a national monitoring and evaluation plan, and only 24% had a national budget dedicated to these activities (UNAIDS, 2003b).

Global initiatives

When the 2001 UN Declaration of Commitment on HIV/AIDS was drafted, UNAIDS was charged with assessing progress on achieving its defined goals and targets. In close collaboration with its partners in the UNAIDS Monitoring and Evaluation Reference Group, a set of core indicators was finalized for countries to use in measuring progress. For the first time, standardized data could be compared across countries in many critical areas: AIDS awareness levels, availability of prevention and treatment services, reduction of risk behaviour, levels of financial investments and impact on new infections.

Progress has been made in political commitment and improved policy environments, but has been lacking in human rights and human capacity. Prevention and treatment service coverage also remains extremely low. The second progress report will be released in 2005 and will measure progress made on an expanded list of service delivery targets, including the WHO and UNAIDS '3 by 5' Initiative.

Spurred on by UNAIDS, over the past three years various stakeholders have come to a consensus on global indicators for various comprehensive response interventions. But this is just a beginning. It is now time to focus on country capacity to measure these indicators, and to

The Country Response Information System (CRIS)—supporting management of national AIDS information

UNAIDS has spearheaded efforts to supply countries with a user-friendly database management tool designed to strengthen the management of strategic information and its analysis at the country level. This database tool houses indicators, project and resource tracking, and country-level research. It is housed in National AIDS Commissions (or their equivalents). From October 2002 to April 2004, an ambitious training programme, involving 18 workshops and over 100 countries, introduced CRIS as a tool within country monitoring and evaluation frameworks.

Its modular approach permits national and subnational indicators and programme information to be stored. The first indicator module is in English, French, Spanish, Russian and Chinese, and was released in June 2003. In late 2003 and early 2004, the resource tracking module was tested in Indonesia, Kenya and Uganda. The research inventory module, financially supported by the US National Institutes of Health, was tested in Bangladesh and Uganda. These modules are slated for release in mid-2004 to complete the integrated database tool.

By the end of 2003, 25 countries were already using CRIS to store and analyse data. Information from country reports will be reflected in the 2005 UN Declaration of Commitment progress report.

In partnership with other UN agencies and strategic partners, UNAIDS has led efforts to facilitate data transfer between existing and new tools. A common transmission format for indicators—an XML transfer tool—will ensure easy data transfer between CRIS, UNICEF's DevInfo and WHO's HealthMapper.

use this information to improve programmes so they work effectively.

Building country capacity

To build capacity, a comprehensive approach is needed, which includes training, technical assistance, access to improved guidelines and tools, and helping countries to recruit national expert staff for monitoring and evaluation activities. UNAIDS, and other partners such as the United States government, have conducted regional training sessions. These sessions use a standardized curriculum to teach monitoring expertise, computer database use and ways to present complex data to different audiences.

The Global AIDS Monitoring and Evaluation Team, housed at the World Bank, concentrates on helping countries to find and hire local monitoring and evaluation staff and to develop functioning monitoring and evaluation offices. To mentor and assist these efforts, UNAIDS and the US Centers for Disease Control are sending a group of experts to key countries. They will build on existing efforts and address key monitoring and evaluation information gaps.

A good example of expanding country capacity is Zimbabwe's District Response Information System, which is based at District AIDS Action Committee Offices, and is being piloted in 10 districts. It is linked to community subdistrict offices and implementing agencies (NGOs, mission hospitals and other sector ministries), as well as to the National AIDS Commission headquarters and provincial offices. At the field level, front-line workers and Village AIDS Action Committees collect village-level data which are validated at monthly meetings of all village front-line workers. The National AIDS Commission worked with UNAIDS, the US Centers for Disease Control and the

University of Zimbabwe to define a set of standardized national indicators. The System will feed indicator data into the national Country Response Information System (see box on page 173).

Challenges of the 'Next Agenda'

An effective global response will only be achieved if countries own and drive their national responses within their own borders. International financial and technical assistance from UN agencies, donors, bilateral funders, foundations and others is important. But it only works effectively if it is embedded within national responses. The cornerstones of nationally led responses to AIDS are best summed up by the concept of the 'Three Ones'.

The key to success is national leadership that involves and empowers all levels of civil society, particularly women. Time after time, national success stories are clear examples of such inclusiveness. In addition, responses only become truly effective if *all* activities are harmonized among *all* key participants. Too often, the opposite occurs, and responses at international and domestic levels are fragmented, ad hoc, or even haphazard.

Finally, bottlenecks exist within both international and domestic systems, causing delays in the transfer of funding and other resources to the key stakeholders who can best use them. Often, bureaucratic factors keep funding blocked at the national level. In other cases, attempts to involve community-level participants are mere window-dressing, because these participants may not readily have the opportunities or skills to participate in the response. Often, they are not empowered to be effectively involved in decision-making that affects them.

Ultimately, this means that the energy and commitment of people on the front lines of the response are not harnessed.

Future challenges include:

- strengthening and sustaining national leadership in the fight against AIDS;
- harmonizing multisectoral responses, donor activities, and monitoring and evaluation so that countries can succeed in their national responses;
- producing scientific data and strategic information to guide the response;
- improving countries' capacity to use the AIDS funds—national and international—at their disposal;
- establishing accountability mechanisms to track resources and demonstrate that they are being used to their fullest potential;
- creating mechanisms for civil society and business to contribute coherently to the AIDS response, through public-private partnerships;
- reviewing, and, where necessary, revising development instruments and policies (a number of internationally agreed instruments have been applied imperfectly and inconsistently—debt relief, tariff removal, Poverty Reduction Strategy Papers, etc.—and have the potential to improve health policies, governance and institutions in relation to AIDS); and
- ensuring that decentralization is a cornerstone of national AIDS responses (empowerment and capacity need to be devolved from national to regional, district and community levels).

Focus

AIDS and conflict: a growing problem worldwide

Serious armed conflicts occur regularly in many regions of the world. In 2003, more than 72 countries were identified as unstable, and various conflicts have resulted in over 42 million refugees and internally displaced people worldwide (IASC, 2003).

Populations fleeing complex emergencies such as armed conflicts generally face destitution and food shortages. Their situation is made worse because they often have no access to health care, either because systems have collapsed or simply do not exist in refugee hosting areas. For example, in the 1998–2001 war in the Democratic Republic of Congo, 80% of the estimated 2.5 million 'excess deaths' resulted from malnutrition, communicable diseases and other factors aggravated by the violent conflict (IRC, 2001).

These conflicts can also create conditions that increase the risk of contracting infections such as HIV, and may also lead to their spread. This can happen either during the conflict itself, or after it is over. In some cases, armed conflict increases HIV levels or changes HIV distribution patterns.

In other cases, conflict has appeared to serve as a brake on the epidemic. This has led to the view that greatest vulnerability may well occur during the often fragile post-conflict period. Differing scenarios show the relationship between HIV and conflict is much more complex and varied than previously thought, and is clearly context specific.

Whatever the case, countries recovering from armed conflict need to integrate an AIDS response into their recovery programmes—particularly HIV-prevention activities. Without this, and without significantly scaled-up international support, HIV infection may rapidly escalate and threaten national efforts to recover from the fighting and the displacement it causes. Likewise, HIV-related activities should be integrated into refugee assistance and other humanitarian programmes.

Factors in conflicts that may lead to the spread of HIV

Evidence shows HIV levels among certain populations and regions within a country can sometimes increase during complex emergencies such as armed conflict. In Rwanda, the 1994 genocide is believed to have contributed to the epidemic expanding to rural areas, which had previously been less affected. This came about because urban and rural populations were mixed together in refugee camps in neighbouring countries.

Armed conflict can increase the likelihood of exposure to HIV infection in several of the following ways:

- Population displacement: conflict often prompts large numbers of people to flee the fighting, which uproots them from their usual areas of residence. When people move from low-prevalence to high-prevalence HIV settings, they inevitably face increased risk of HIV exposure. In addition, rapid population movements disrupt social networks and institutions that normally protect and support people. Furthermore, displacement frequently places people in chaotic circumstances in which access to condoms and other prevention tools may be scarce.

- Breakdown of traditional sexual norms: the chaotic conditions associated with conflict often lead to the disintegration of traditional values and norms regarding sexual behaviour, which contributes to an overall increase in risk of HIV exposure (Hankins et al., 2002).
- Women and girls: armed conflict can create conditions of such severe deprivation that women and girls, in particular, are coerced into exchanging sex for money, food or protection. The presence of large numbers of armed men in uniforms often means a sex industry springs up, increasing HIV risk for sex workers and uniformed services personnel (see 'Prevention' chapter).
- Rape as a 'weapon of war': in a variety of recent conflicts—including Bosnia-Herzegovina, Democratic Republic of Congo, Liberia and Rwanda—combatants have used rape as a weapon of war. A study in Rwanda revealed 17% of women who had been raped tested HIV-positive, compared with 11% of women who had not been raped (UNAIDS/UNHCR, 2003). In some conflicts, young men and boys have also been targets of rape.
- Collapse of health systems: when armed conflict triggers health system malfunction and collapse, national blood supply safety is threatened, and HIV prevention and care programmes can disintegrate.
- Increased substance use: to cope with chaos caused by conflicts, some individuals—including children—may seek comfort in increased alcohol consumption, or turn to other psychoactive substances, including glue and illicit drugs. Drug injecting is especially likely when conflicts disrupt supply routes of drugs that are usually ingested, sniffed or smoked. This can lead to drugs being introduced that are more likely to be injected (Smith, 2002; Strathdee et al., 2002; Hankins et al., 2002).

Conflict situations: prevention among uniformed services and peacekeepers

Over 25 million people serve in armed forces around the world, although this number could be closer to 50 million if members of civil defence and paramilitary forces are taken into account. Most armed forces personnel are young men and women in their 20s and 30s and, as such, they represent one of the professional groups most affected by AIDS.

Uniformed services personnel generally have an ethos of risk-taking that can place them at higher risk of HIV infection. Often soldiers and peacekeepers are posted away from their families and communities for long periods of time, removing them from the social discipline that would normally prevail in their home communities. During conflict both consensual and non-consensual sexual encounters tend to increase, and adherence to prevention measures declines.

Data on AIDS among uniformed forces are scant. However, in general, estimates suggest that sexually transmitted infections among uniformed services personnel could be at least twice as high as in the general population. In some countries where HIV has been present for more than 10 years, armed forces report infection rates of 50–60%. Even in peaceful Botswana, one in three members of the military has tested HIV-positive. HIV prevalence in the Cambodian military was 5.9% in 1995; this figure had increased to 7% by 1997. High HIV-prevalence levels are creating substantial losses in command-level continuity, reducing military preparedness, causing high recruitment and training costs and ultimately debilitating some national uniformed services.

Countries respond

Fortunately, soldiers are also a 'captive audience'—used to learning new skills, following orders and taking initiative. This makes them potentially excellent agents for change and role models for other young people. Globally, the military and other uniformed services have begun to respond to AIDS within their ranks. An increasing number of countries, including Botswana, Chile, the Philippines, South Africa, Thailand, Ukraine and Zambia, have implemented prevention measures within their armed forces, ranging from prevention education to condom distribution. Brazil, the Dominican Republic, Mozambique, Peru and Uruguay pledged to carry out similar activities when their Ministries of Defence, Interior, and Health signed partnership declarations with UNAIDS.

A variety of approaches have been used successfully. The Ugandan Peoples' Defence Force has used 'Post Test Clubs' to increase HIV awareness and reduce stigma. These test clubs are open to everyone who has had an HIV test, regardless of the results. They aim to instill hope through providing support for people living with HIV and their families. HIV prevalence in Uganda's military fell from over 10% in 1990 to less than 7% in 2003. In Cambodia, since 1997, a brand of condoms marketed specifically to the military has helped reduce unprotected sexual contacts between Cambodian soldiers and sex workers, from 70% to 54%.

Similar projects have also been initiated among non-military staff. In Myanmar, UNAIDS, the United Nations Office on Drugs and Crime (UNODC), Care International and the Ministry of Home Affairs are working on a prevention programme targeting police personnel and their families. Lithuania is implementing similar activities among its border guards and police force.

During 2002–2003, UNAIDS actively promoted and supported similar new initiatives in over 40 countries. Meanwhile, the UNAIDS Office on AIDS, Security and Humanitarian Response has developed a comprehensive programming, training and awareness-raising package. The training focuses on increasing HIV awareness, encouraging prevention, eliminating sexual violence, and promoting gender equality, human rights, condom distribution and care and support services for HIV-positive personnel.

Prevention among peacekeepers

As of 2004, the UN Department of Peacekeeping Operations was involved in 15 missions worldwide, with some 89 countries contributing over 45 000 personnel. UNAIDS and the Department are mounting an AIDS response in all major peacekeeping operations. It is aimed at preventing HIV among personnel and helping peacekeepers to become advocates for HIV awareness wherever they are mobilized. The HIV/AIDS Awareness Card for Peacekeeping Operations is integral to the strategy developed by UNAIDS and the Department, and has been translated into 11 languages. It contains basic messages on HIV, as well as relevant codes of conduct for civil and military peacekeepers.

However, there are still several challenges to implementing AIDS strategies in peacekeeping settings. First, HIV training needs to be tailored to the wide range of cultures represented by peacekeepers. Second, training is provided for officers, but there is no mechanism to ensure that this information reaches the lower ranks.

Five new peacekeeping missions were established in 2004, and UNAIDS and the Department are working together to ensure that AIDS is addressed at mission level, and in each of the troop-contributing countries prior to deployment.

HIV and conflict: a complex relationship

Increased vulnerability during conflicts

Experts studying HIV spread within conflict situations have often believed there is a direct correlation between conflict and HIV vulnerability. However, this does not necessarily translate into increased HIV transmission. During Sierra Leone's 10-year civil war, indirect indicators suggested the increased vulnerability was indeed translating into increased HIV infections.

- Indications of high HIV levels: Sierra Leone's government estimated HIV prevalence among sex workers at 27% in 1995, and 71% in 1997 (Kaiser et al., 2002). Meanwhile, in the same period, surveillance in the country's antenatal clinics showed HIV prevalence rose from 4% to 7%. These findings echoed other studies that stated 11% of peacekeepers returning to Nigeria from Sierra Leone were HIV-positive—more than double Nigeria's then-current HIV prevalence (Smith, 2002).
- Low HIV awareness: among surveyed peacekeepers and soldiers from the national army, only 23% could cite at least three HIV-transmission routes; 38% reported not being worried about AIDS; and only 39% had used a condom during their last sexual encounter (McGinn et al., 2001).
- High levels of sexual violence: a 2001 study found 9% of women displaced by armed conflict had been sexually assaulted (UNAIDS/UNHCR, 2003). Other reports documented that rebel militia members systematically raped young girls and women (Salama et al., 1999).

Can conflict sometimes act as a brake on the epidemic?

Recently, more rigorous research has been carried out on the relationship between conflict and HIV vulnerability and risk. In a few cases, it suggests that under some conditions of conflict, HIV transmission may actually be slowed. In Sierra Leone, once hostilities ceased, the government formed a partnership with the World Bank and the US Centers for Disease Control and Prevention to carry out a national HIV prevalence and behavioural risk survey. The 2002 study confirmed low levels of HIV-related knowledge and high levels of sexual violence.

But contrary to the indirect indicators suggesting increased HIV infection, the study also found much lower HIV-infection levels (1–4%) than previously documented during the conflict. A partial explanation for this is that during the war, movement within the country, cross-border migration and trade became extremely difficult. This helped to 'insulate' Sierra Leone from the growing HIV epidemic in West Africa. In the 2002 survey, some 90% of people remained in the country as internally displaced persons; only 10% fled to neighbouring countries. Therefore, in this instance, the increased risk of HIV infection that had translated into high HIV prevalence among sex workers did not actually translate into sustained increased infection among the general population.

Experience in other countries has revealed similar findings. For example, Bosnia and Herzegovina was a war zone from 1992 to 1995, yet it continued to have a very low HIV prevalence (0.0003% of the population in 2001). This is despite the fact that the war displaced large numbers of people, and there were very high levels of sexual violence (Cavaljuga, 2002).

If HIV is not already prevalent in a country in conflict, the virus cannot take advantage of conditions conducive to its spread. In addition, conflict can make a population less mobile, and therefore possibly less likely to encounter HIV than in peacetime.

Refugees and HIV

Millions of people fleeing armed conflict find shelter in large refugee camps. Unfortunately, many of these refugees, especially women and girls, experience poverty, powerlessness, social instability and sexual abuse (Lubbers, 2003). Because refugees are vulnerable from a socio-economic and cultural standpoint, it has long been assumed they face a greater risk of HIV exposure. However, as in some prolonged conflict situations, recent evidence suggests they may not develop higher HIV-infection levels.

Between 2001 and 2003, the UN High Commissioner for Refugees (UNHCR) and its partners measured HIV prevalence among pregnant women in more than 20 camps housing some 800 000 refugees in Kenya, Rwanda, Sudan and Tanzania. The results: refugee populations in three of the four countries had significantly lower HIV prevalence than the surrounding host communities. For example, in northwestern Kenya, 5% of refugees were HIV-positive, compared with an 18% HIV prevalence in the surrounding host country population. In the fourth country, Sudan, the refugee camps and host community had comparable infection rates (Lubbers, 2003).

HIV prevalence by country of asylum and country of origin, by region, 2003

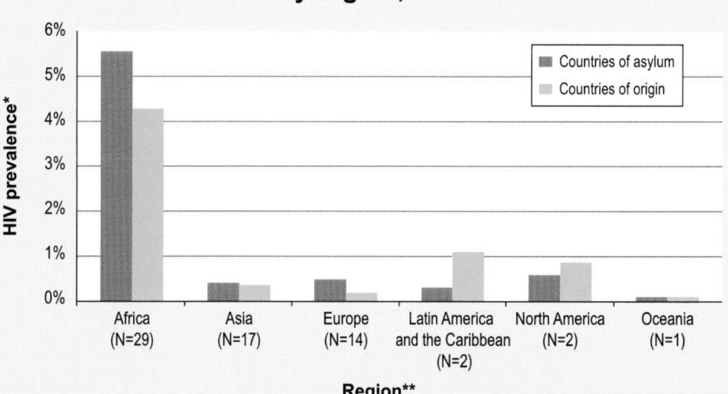

* Weighted means: country of asylum by population size, country of origin by refugee population size
** N refers to countries of asylum with ≥10,000 refugees
Source: UNHCR, 2004

Figure 49

Several explanations may underlie discrepancies in HIV prevalence between refugee and host-country populations. Historically, the home countries of most refugees in Africa and Asia have typically had lower HIV prevalence than countries hosting the refugees (see Figure 49). Refugees often live in camps in remote rural areas with limited freedom of movement, which may limit their exposure to the host country's population, especially in high-prevalence rural areas. In addition, international agencies and nongovernmental organizations (NGOs) have mounted HIV-prevention programmes targeting refugee populations. This potentially reduces risk of HIV exposure through sexual

Arriving at estimates of HIV prevalence in conflict situations

In countries with generalized epidemics, most national HIV-prevalence estimates are based on surveillance data that assess prevalence over time among pregnant women who attend selected sentinel antenatal clinics. If these are disrupted during conflict and post-conflict situations, population-based surveys may be used. These surveys may underestimate infection levels if participation is too low. However, they may better reach rural populations that generally have lower HIV levels than urban populations. These surveys also include men as well as non-pregnant women. The Sierra Leone survey (discussed on page 178) was population-based, which may partly explain why HIV prevalence appeared lower after the conflict than in previous sentinel surveillance surveys (Spiegel, 2003).

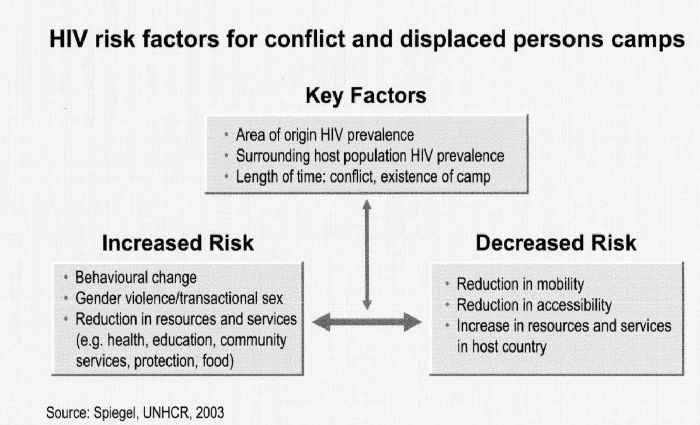

HIV risk factors for conflict and displaced persons camps
Key Factors
• Area of origin HIV prevalence
• Surrounding host population HIV prevalence
• Length of time: conflict, existence of camp
Increased Risk
• Behavioural change
• Gender violence/transactional sex
• Reduction in resources and services (e.g. health, education, community services, protection, food)
Decreased Risk
• Reduction in mobility
• Reduction in accessibility
• Increase in resources and services in host country
Source: Spiegel, UNHCR, 2003

Figure 50

activity, contaminated injection equipment and unscreened blood supplies.

Angola provides a case in point. When the Angolan conflict ended in April 2002, the country had substantially lower HIV prevalence (5–10% in Luanda and 1–3% in rural areas) than other countries in Southern Africa. Again, compared with surrounding countries, prolonged conflict may have acted as a brake on HIV spread in Angola. As refugees began repatriating from Namibia and Zambia, false rumours surfaced among the Angolan population that as many as 70% of them were HIV-positive. These rumours created great public anxiety that returning refugees would spread HIV and imperil the country's recovery.

In fact, UNHCR used indirect HIV-prevalence indicators to show that HIV prevalence among returning refugees was much lower than the surrounding host populations' prevalence in Namibia and Zambia. Strong HIV-prevention programmes in refugee camps meant that returning refugees actually had better HIV knowledge than the average Angolan. Indeed, prevention training in refugee camps may actually help the returning refugees to become an important HIV-prevention resource for Angola (Spiegel and de Jong, 2003).

HIV surveillance and emergencies

Experience in Angola and Sierra Leone shows that more and better research, surveillance and behavioural monitoring are needed in emergency situations. The growing understanding of the complex relationship between HIV and conflict means some factors that reduce HIV-related risk (e.g., reduced mobility, improved prevention targeting) may compete with factors that increase risk. Key factors in the balance between these competing forces include the degree of interaction between refugee and host country populations; the type of interaction, including the extent of sexual violence; and the respective HIV prevalence of these groups (see Figure 50). Therefore, careful monitoring is required to provide guidance on appropriate policy and programme responses in different contexts.

Improving HIV surveillance in emergency situations is a daunting task, but agencies working in such situations need to make it a priority. Effective surveillance requires knowledge of HIV prevalence in the areas where affected populations lived prior to displacement. It also needs post-displacement behavioural and biological information on HIV infections among displaced persons and surrounding host communities. Finally, there needs to be a sub-regional approach with improved coordination and information sharing; it should take into account the entire displacement cycle, including repatriation and reintegration.

Biological and behavioural surveillance help agencies better understand factors that accelerate and slow HIV transmission, and facilitate more effective programme responses. HIV surveillance is not easy to undertake during an emergency's acute phase. But it is still possible to obtain indirect estimates of HIV prevalence as blood donations are screened, and results documented by age and sex. In post-conflict situations, sentinel surveillance provides information that better reflects the general population as a whole (Spiegel, 2003).

Taking effective action

Until recently, agencies involved in conflict situations paid little attention to HIV prevention, care and surveillance in emergencies. However, the 1994 Rwandan crisis helped them realize that both non-displaced and displaced persons affected by conflict need HIV-related interventions. To underscore this point, in 2002, UNHCR began to implement its 2002–2004 HIV and Refugees Strategic Plan. In particular, it stressed the importance of initiating essential reproductive and sexual health services, including HIV and sexually transmitted infection prevention and care at the very earliest stage of a refugee crisis.

In 2003, UN agencies and NGOs reconstituted an Interagency Standing Committee Reference Group on HIV in Emergency Settings to coordinate action in emergency situations. Guidelines were produced that stressed the importance of multisectoral action. UN agencies have also supported comprehensive HIV-prevention activities in peacekeeping missions in countries such as the Democratic Republic of Congo, Eritrea, Ethiopia and Sierra Leone.

In Liberia, the Liberian Red Cross and the United Nations Population Fund (UNFPA) worked with many local NGOs to establish HIV-prevention and education programmes within camps for internally displaced persons. These included 'adolescent-friendly' corners that provided safe places for frank discussion of youth concerns about HIV. Youth teams were established to mobilize and sensitize internally displaced persons and their host communities about HIV. In addition, concerted efforts were made to maintain condom distribution for the displaced.

NGOs working in refugee camps have also recently begun to implement more comprehensive HIV programmes, such as voluntary counselling and testing, and prevention of mother-to-child transmission. For example, in Tanzania, Norwegian People's Aid started a pilot programme for refugees in Lukole and Kitali camps, and for the surrounding population. During its first three months, the programme counselled nearly 3000 pregnant women, with more than 80% of them accepting HIV testing (Norwegian People's Aid, 2002).

In Angola, now that peace has returned, UN agencies are working with the government and other partners to keep HIV prevalence low. The UN anticipated that 240 000 refugees would be repatriated from camps in the Democratic Republic of Congo, Namibia and Zambia, and developed an action plan—since endorsed by the Government of Angola. While still in refugee camps, individuals will receive HIV-prevention training and access to condoms. On arrival in Angola, reception centres will provide them with education, condoms and peer-based interventions. The action plan also calls for comprehensive HIV programmes for all Angolans who live in the areas of return. These emerging plans reflect a growing recognition of the need for subregional and integrated approaches to implementing HIV-related interventions in post-conflict repatriation and reintegration situations.

Focus

The essential role of people living with AIDS

Around the world, wherever HIV spreads, people living with HIV often quickly establish networks of self-help, support, and empowerment.

In June 1983 in Denver, United States of America, a movement of people living with HIV emerged at the Second National Forum on AIDS. The 'Denver Principles' adopted at the forum called for those living with HIV to be supported when they opposed AIDS-related stigma and discrimination. The Principles also stated that people living with HIV should "be involved at every level of decision-making [...], serve on the boards of directors of provider organizations, and participate in all AIDS meetings with as much credibility as other participants, to share their own experiences and knowledge" (Senterfitt, 1998). By 1988, the publication *AIDS Treatment News* listed more than 20 coalitions of people living with HIV across the Canada, United States, and the United Kingdom.

National and global groups emerge

In Uganda, The AIDS Support Organisation was the pioneer. It was formed in 1987 in Kampala by a group of 16 volunteers, 12 of whom were living with HIV. Such groups often form around clusters of people caring for a loved one. For example, Jamaica AIDS Support started up unofficially in 1991 as a result of a group of men helping a friend dying from AIDS. In other cases, a courageous individual has been prepared to be open about living with HIV, and has inspired others to take positive action. In 1990, Joe Muriithi in Kenya was one of the first Africans to publicly disclose his HIV-positive status, and he and his wife, Jane Muriithi, started the Know AIDS Society. In 1992, Auxillia Chimusoro—one of the founders of the International Community of Women with HIV/AIDS—was one of the first people in Zimbabwe to publicly disclose her seropositive status, and she went on to form the Batanayi support group.

In Brazil, the Grupo Pela Vidda of Rio de Janeiro was founded in 1989 by writer and civil rights activist Herbert Daniel. The group's Declaration of the Rights of People Living with HIV/AIDS was adopted unanimously by more than 50 organizations at the second National Meeting of HIV/AIDS NGOs in Porto Alegre, Brazil in 1989. In India, at a 1997 national workshop, some 35 HIV-positive individuals formed the Indian Network of Positive People. Ashok Pillai was elected General Secretary, and he assumed a public and prominent role on behalf of those living with HIV. Today, the Network has more than 1000 members from 14 states, and includes a positive women's network. Sadly, like so many other pioneers of the AIDS movement, Ashok Pillai has passed away.

Globally, an international network of people living with HIV was initially formed in 1986, and later became the Global Network of People Living with HIV/AIDS. In July 1992, the International Community of Women Living with HIV/AIDS was formed by a group of HIV-positive women from 30 different countries who were attending the 8th International

Conference on AIDS in Amsterdam. The Community drew on the growing movement of HIV-positive women in Africa, which led to a new kind of activism extending beyond the immediate concerns of creating self-help and support groups.

The GIPA principle

The principle of the Greater Involvement of People Living with HIV/AIDS (GIPA) was formally recognized at the 1994 Paris AIDS Summit, when 42 countries agreed to support an initiative to "strengthen the capacity and coordination of networks of people living with HIV/AIDS and community-based organizations". They added that, "by ensuring their full involvement in our common response to the pandemic at all—national, regional and global—levels, this initiative will, in particular, stimulate the creation of supportive political, legal and social environments".

The Paris Declaration also expressed "determination to mobilize all of society—the public and private sectors, community-based organizations and people living with HIV/AIDS—in a spirit of true partnership", as well as to fully involve "people living with HIV/AIDS in the formulation and implementation of public policies [and] ensure equal protection under the law for persons living with HIV/AIDS".

In 2001, the United Nations Declaration of Commitment on HIV/AIDS endorsed the GIPA principle, which was further upheld in the Guiding Principles of the '3 by 5' Treatment Initiative. These guiding principles state that, "The Initiative clearly places the needs and involvement of people living with HIV/AIDS in the centre of all of its programming" (WHO, 2003). UNAIDS has promoted GIPA since its beginning by involving people living with HIV at all levels, including on its Programme Coordinating Board.

Roles of people living with HIV: national leadership

Despite these endorsements, the active involvement of people living with HIV in decision-making is still far from universal. Furthermore, the involvement of HIV-positive women, youth and children has lagged far behind that of men in most parts of the world. One constraint is that, globally, only about 10% of those living with HIV know their seropositive status. Others are unable to be open about their status because they fear they will face discrimination and stigma. Nevertheless, progress is being made.

In Eastern Europe and Central Asia, the epidemic is still relatively new, but few people know their HIV status. Even fewer are willing to be open about it, and there is little tradition of civil society involvement. But, in recent years, the movement of people living with HIV has become stronger and more influential. For example, in Ukraine, the All-Ukrainian Network of Persons Living with HIV/AIDS has helped shape the National AIDS Prevention Programme, and is increasingly involved in providing HIV-related care services (UNDP, 2003).

The Cambodian People Living with HIV/AIDS Network has been actively involved in policy development. As a member of the Country Coordinating Mechanism, it helped formulate Cambodia's successful funding proposal to the Global Fund to Fight AIDS, Tuberculosis and Malaria. Similarly, partnership forums have been established in many countries, bringing together people living with HIV and other government and nongovernmental partners in shaping AIDS responses (see Figure 51).

Elsewhere, the Asia-Pacific Network for People Living with HIV/AIDS has united people from over 20 Asian countries under the United Nations Development Programme's (UNDP) 'Leadership for Results' programme. This regional network has fostered developing national organizations of people living with HIV. One of these is Spiritia, in Indonesia, which has also received UNAIDS support. In cases of more recently emerging epidemics, UN Theme Groups on HIV/AIDS have encouraged and supported AIDS activist groups that are starting up.

Figure 51

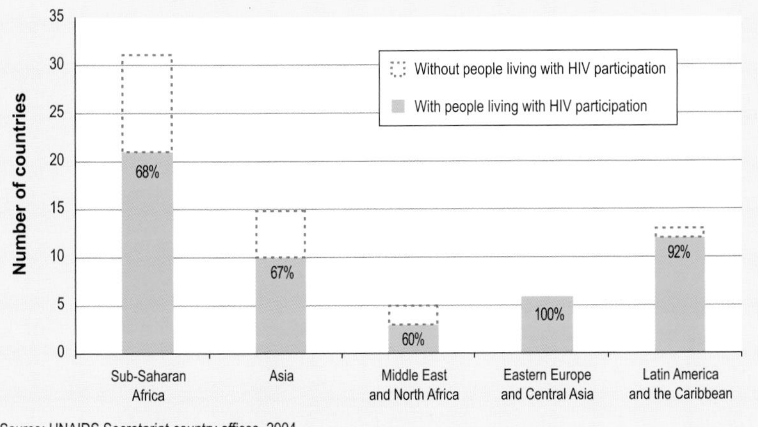

Source: UNAIDS Secretariat country offices, 2004

Providing services and encouraging local participation

In other cases, people living with HIV have long been involved in national decision-making. Increasingly, HIV-positive people are actively participating in local decision-making processes, and in providing services to others with HIV. Often, they are at the front line of care and support. For instance, in Cambodia, through the 'Friend Help Friend' units at district health centres, volunteers living with HIV provide AIDS information and support, and help people adhere to their treatment regimens.

The link between providing services and national advocacy has most prominently come into play around the issue of extending access to treatment—one of the main priorities of AIDS activism. For example, in Thailand, the Thai Network of People Living with HIV/AIDS and the Thai NGO Coalition on AIDS encouraged the government to provide antiretroviral drugs under its national health insurance scheme. In December 2001, the Thai Government announced that it would extend health care to cover these medicines, and created a panel with Network representatives to oversee implementation.

In Kazakhstan, 30% of the country's HIV-positive people live in the city of Temirtau, where, since 1998, the NGO *Shapagat* ('mercy' in Kazakh) gives them a voice. The local municipal government provides *Shapagat* with offices, an d the NGO works with its local AIDS centre, United Nations agencies, and the Open Society Foundation. *Shapagat* makes regular presentations to the local parliament and the government's executive authority. Temirtau's HIV-positive people have served on the country's National AIDS Commission, and have also participated in the Global Fund's Country Coordinating Mechanism for Kazakhstan.

Employment and workplace issues

The presence of people openly living with HIV in the workplace shows it is possible to go on living and working normally, a critical first step in successfully dealing with work-related discrimination. The United Nations Volunteers Programme has backed GIPA in Southern Africa by placing people living with HIV in mining companies, parastatal organizations, and United Nations agencies, among others. Programme participants carry out advocacy and education programmes, and actively help to develop AIDS workplace action plans. Similarly, in the Caribbean, since 2000 about 50 HIV-positive members of the United Nations Volunteers Programme have worked to counter AIDS-related discrimination in seven countries in the region.

Rarely do HIV-positive people get paid for caring for and supporting others living with the virus. One exception is Botswana, where a member of the country's Network of People Living with HIV/AIDS works as a community liaison officer with the infectious diseases clinic in the capital, Gabarone. Her personal experiences encountered in the process of living with HIV have been particularly important in helping patients (especially those who have come from distant villages) talk about the difficulties they have with adhering to their drug regimen, or the pressures that relatives exert on HIV-positive mothers to breastfeed their newborn children (UNAIDS, 2003).

Corporate, trade union and government support for AIDS workplace programmes exists in many places (see 'Impact' chapter and 'Prevention' chapter). However, the informal work sector still poses a significant challenge. India is a case in point. Some 92% of India's people work in the informal economy. The International Labour Organization (ILO), along with employers' and workers' organizations, has supported the Network of Positive People of Delhi's work in the informal sector. The Network's members provide training, job assistance, and care and support to both HIV-positive workers and the families of those who have died of AIDS.

Commitment and courage require support

Involving people living with HIV in national AIDS responses has proved extremely valuable. However, doing so effectively requires recognizing a range of needs. Many programmes depend on the commitment and courage of HIV-positive individuals. An HIV diagnosis is already a life-changing event causing shock, grief, and a sense of loss of control over one's life. Disclosing one's HIV-positive status can be traumatic, even under the best of circumstances. Doing so publicly—as many HIV-positive activists have—is never easy, even when done with the support of the organizations in which they are active. Many United Nations, governmental and NGO initiatives around the world encourage such disclosure in order to prevent further spread of the virus, but they often fail to help HIV-positive people prepare for it, and they do not provide adequate support for the ongoing work the activists do.

Financing is crucial. People living with HIV need access to antiretroviral drugs and other essential care, and they need to receive a salary or other paid compensation for their time and contributions. Otherwise, their capacity to participate in the AIDS response is seriously hindered. One example of an innovative effort to plug the gap is in Uganda. A Treatment Fund for HIV/AIDS Advocates in Uganda currently provides six advocates with antiretroviral treatment, and is funded by Rotary International, and its Belgian and Ugandan branches (Uganda AIDS Commission and UNAIDS, 2003). The Fund is co-managed by the Persons Living with HIV/AIDS Forum, which brings together all of Uganda's relevant networks and associations.

HIV-positive African women taking on activist roles have faced enormous challenges. They are frustrated over the pressures they encounter to disclose their status as part of prevention campaigns, while their own financial, medical and emotional needs are ignored. The commitment and volunteerism of people living with HIV has been exploited by NGOs and government programmes that use this cheap or free labour in place of health-care services (Manchester, 2003).

A study of 17 NGOs providing HIV and AIDS services in four countries (Burkina Faso, Ecuador, India and Zambia) revealed that failure to account for the needs of HIV-positive people reduced the effectiveness of the services provided. Involving people living with HIV in outreach education, before they receive the necessary training and ongoing support, can have a negative impact on service quality, and can also harm the individuals themselves (Horizons Program, 2002). Participation of people living with HIV at the international level can be hindered by difficulties obtaining travel insurance to cover any HIV-related illnesses or travel restrictions that many countries impose on people living with HIV.

Greater involvement comes from a supportive enabling environment

There are no simple answers to these problems. Within organizations seeking real (and not token) involvement, creating a supportive, enabling environment requires a great deal of thought and commitment. HIV-positive people need training and support so they can participate more actively, and institutions need to make their procedures more participatory and accessible to people who may not be used to the customary formality of meetings and other institutional requirements. This is especially necessary if more HIV-positive women and young people—traditionally excluded from decision-making processes—are to be empowered to contribute in a meaningful way.

All of this means it is more essential than ever to provide more funds for capacity-building, financial compensation for work performed, and treatment and psychological support for HIV-positive people involved in such work. But more formal involvement of networks and organizations of people living with HIV (as opposed to informal personal involvement) would also help in implementing the GIPA principle in a sustained manner. The transition from self-help groups to representative organizations has taken place in many countries, creating additional needs to build organizational, management, advocacy, and leadership capacities.

The theme of the September 2003 International Conference of People Living with HIV/AIDS—The Dawn of New Positive Leadership—recognized these new roles. The Conference Declaration noted that "Our communities and organizations are still starved of the resources they need to effectively fulfil their potential and perform the role that is being demanded of us". The Declaration demanded "That we are supported in our efforts to build capacity to effectively contribute as equal partners in the response".

Conclusion

Experience has shown that involving people living with HIV in a meaningful way is a core element of an effective response to the epidemic. Strengthening and sustaining this role requires:

i) **that people know their HIV status** (which, in turn, requires vastly increased access to voluntary counselling and testing facilities);

ii) **keeping people alive** with antiretroviral treatment so they can remain active in their chosen fields of work; and

iii) **creating the practical and political space for people living with HIV to expand their role and contribution** by addressing HIV-related stigma and discrimination; promoting appropriate legal and policy environments; and supporting participation with resources, including organizational development.

Already, AIDS organizations exist in many forms—from support and service-delivery bodies to advocacy and representational organizations. In the face of a long-standing but constantly changing epidemic, the range of these organizations needs to be extended even further. In particular, as more people know their HIV status, it means reaching out beyond recognized AIDS networks, to non-health-care settings—for instance, to workplaces, places of worship, schools and other institutions. Networks of people living with HIV are demonstrating their commitment to forging new partnerships; now they need help in order to enhance their organizational capacities and meet these new challenges.

Table of country-specific HIV/AIDS estimates and data, end 2003

Global surveillance of HIV/AIDS and sexually transmitted infections is a joint effort of the World Health Organization (WHO) and the Joint United Nations Programme on HIV/AIDS (UNAIDS). The UNAIDS/WHO Working Group on Global HIV/AIDS and STI Surveillance, initiated in 1996, is the main coordination and implementation mechanism through which UNAIDS and WHO compile the best information available and help improve the quality of data needed for informed decision-making and planning at national, regional and global levels. The estimates contained in this table are a product of the Working Group, and they are derived in close collaboration with national AIDS programmes and many other partners.

1. Estimated number of people living with HIV						
	Adults and children, end 2003		Adults and children, end 2001		Adults (15–49), end 2003	
Country	**Estimate**	**[low estimate - high estimate]**	**Estimate**	**[low estimate - high estimate]**	**Estimate**	**[low estimate - high estimate]**
Global Total	**37,800,000**	**[34,600,000 - 42,300,000]**	**34,900,000**	**[32,000,000 - 39,000,000]**	**35,700,000**	**[32,700,000 - 39,800,000]**
Sub-Saharan Africa	**25,000,000**	**[23,100,000 - 27,900,000]**	**23,800,000**	**[22,000,000 - 26,600,000]**	**23,100,000**	**[21,400,000 - 25,700,000]**
Angola	240,000	[97,000 - 600,000]	220,000	[86,000 - 550,000]	220,000	[88,000 - 540,000]
Benin	68,000	[38,000 - 120,000]	65,000	[36,000 - 110,000]	62,000	[35,000 - 110,000]
Botswana *	350,000	[330,000 - 380,000]	350,000	[330,000 - 380,000]	330,000	[310,000 - 340,000]
Burkina Faso *	300,000	[190,000 - 470,000]	280,000	[180,000 - 440,000]	270,000	[170,000 - 420,000]
Burundi	250,000	[170,000 - 370,000]	240,000	[160,000 - 360,000]	220,000	[150,000 - 320,000]
Cameroon *	560,000	[390,000 - 810,000]	530,000	[370,000 - 770,000]	520,000	[360,000 - 740,000]
Central African Republic	260,000	[160,000 - 410,000]	250,000	[150,000 - 400,000]	240,000	[150,000 - 380,000]
Chad	200,000	[130,000 - 300,000]	190,000	[120,000 - 290,000]	180,000	[120,000 - 270,000]
Comoros	...	...	...	...	...	...
Congo	90,000	[39,000 - 200,000]	90,000	[39,000 - 200,000]	80,000	[34,000 - 180,000]
Côte d'Ivoire	570,000	[390,000 - 820,000]	510,000	[350,000 - 740,000]	530,000	[370,000 - 750,000]
Dem. Republic of Congo **	1,100,000	[450,000 - 2,600,000]	1,100,000	[430,000 - 2,500,000]	1,000,000	[410,000 - 2,400,000]
Djibouti	9,100	[2,300 - 24,000]	8,100	[2,400 - 23,000]	8,400	[2,100 - 21,000]
Equatorial Guinea	...	...	...	...	...	...
Eritrea	60,000	[21,000 - 170,000]	61,000	[22,000 - 160,000]	55,000	[19,000 - 150,000]
Ethiopia	1,500,000	[950,000 - 2,300,000]	1,300,000	[820,000 - 2,000,000]	1,400,000	[890,000 - 2,100,000]
Gabon	48,000	[24,000 - 91,000]	39,000	[19,000 - 78,000]	45,000	[23,000 - 86,000]
Gambia	6,800	[1,800 - 24,000]	6,700	[1,800 - 24,000]	6,300	[1,700 - 23,000]
Ghana *	350,000	[210,000 - 560,000]	330,000	[200,000 - 540,000]	320,000	[200,000 - 520,000]
Guinea *	140,000	[51,000 - 360,000]	110,000	[40,000 - 310,000]	130,000	[48,000 - 330,000]
Guinea-Bissau	...	...	...	...	...	...
Kenya *	1,200,000	[820,000 - 1,700,000]	1,300,000	[890,000 - 1,800,000]	1,100,000	[760,000 - 1,600,000]
Lesotho *	320,000	[290,000 - 360,000]	320,000	[290,000 - 360,000]	300,000	[270,000 - 330,000]
Liberia	100,000	[47,000 - 220,000]	86,000	[37,000 - 190,000]	96,000	[44,000 - 200,000]
Madagascar	140,000	[68,000 - 250,000]	100,000	[50,000 - 180,000]	130,000	[66,000 - 220,000]
Malawi *	900,000	[700,000 - 1,100,000]	850,000	[660,000 - 1,100,000]	810,000	[650,000 - 1,000,000]
Mali	140,000	[44,000 - 420,000]	130,000	[40,000 - 390,000]	120,000	[40,000 - 380,000]
Mauritania	9,500	[4,500 - 17,000]	6,300	[3,000 - 11,000]	8,900	[4,400 - 15,000]
Mauritius	...	...	...	...	...	...
Mozambique	1,300,000	[980,000 - 1,700,000]	1,200,000	[930,000 - 1,600,000]	1,200,000	[910,000 - 1,500,000]
Namibia	210,000	[180,000 - 250,000]	200,000	[170,000 - 230,000]	200,000	[170,000 - 230,000]
Niger	70,000	[36,000 - 130,000]	56,000	[28,000 - 110,000]	64,000	[34,000 - 120,000]
Nigeria	3,600,000	[2,400,000 - 5,400,000]	3,400,000	[2,200,000 - 5,000,000]	3,300,000	[2,200,000 - 4,900,000]
Rwanda *	250,000	[170,000 - 380,000]	240,000	[160,000 - 360,000]	230,000	[150,000 - 350,000]
Senegal *	44,000	[22,000 - 89,000]	40,000	[20,000 - 81,000]	41,000	[21,000 - 83,000]
Sierra Leone	...	...	...	...	...	...
Somalia	...	...	...	...	...	...
South Africa *	5,300,000	[4,500,000 - 6,200,000]	5,000,000	[4,200,000 - 5,900,000]	5,100,000	[4,300,000 - 5,900,000]
Swaziland **	220,000	[210,000 - 230,000]	210,000	[190,000 - 220,000]	200,000	[190,000 - 210,000]
Togo	110,000	[67,000 - 170,000]	100,000	[65,000 - 160,000]	96,000	[61,000 - 150,000]
Uganda *	530,000	[350,000 - 880,000]	620,000	[420,000 - 980,000]	450,000	[300,000 - 730,000]
United Rep. of Tanzania *	1,600,000	[1,200,000 - 2,300,000]	1,600,000	[1,100,000 - 2,200,000]	1,500,000	[1,100,000 - 2,000,000]
Zambia	920,000	[730,000 - 1,100,000]	890,000	[710,000 - 1,100,000]	830,000	[680,000 - 1,000,000]
Zimbabwe	1,800,000	[1,500,000 - 2,000,000]	1,700,000	[1,500,000 - 2,000,000]	1,600,000	[1,400,000 - 1,900,000]
East Asia	**900,000**	**[450,000 - 1,500,000]**	**680,000**	**[340,000 - 1,100,000]**	**900,000**	**[450,000 - 1,500,000]**
China	840,000	[430,000 - 1,500,000]	660,000	[320,000 - 1,100,000]	830,000	[430,000 - 1,400,000]
Hong Kong SAR	2,600	[1,300 - 4,400]	2,700	[1,300 - 4,400]	2,600	[1,300 - 4,300]
Dem. Peo. Rep. of Korea	...	...	...	...	...	...
Japan	12,000	[5,700 - 19,000]	12,000	[5,800 - 20,000]	12,000	[5,700 - 19,000]
Mongolia	<500	[<1,000]	<200	[<400]	<500	[<1,000]
Republic of Korea	8,300	[2,700 - 16,000]	5,600	[1,800 - 11,000]	8,300	[2,700 - 16,000]
Oceania	**32,000**	**[21,000 - 46,000]**	**24,000**	**[16,000 - 35,000]**	**31,000**	**[21,000 - 45,000]**
Australia	14,000	[6,800 - 22,000]	12,000	[6,000 - 20,000]	14,000	[6,600 - 22,000]
Fiji	600	[200 - 1,300]	<500	[<1,000]	600	[200 - 1,200]
New Zealand	1,400	[480 - 2,800]	1,200	[420 - 2,400]	1,400	[500 - 2,800]
Papua New Guinea	16,000	[7,800 - 28,000]	10,000	[4,900 - 17,000]	16,000	[7,700 - 26,000]

1. Estimated number of people living with HIV (continued)								
	Adults (15–49), end 2001		Adults (15–49) rate (%) end 2003		Adults (15–49) rate (%) end 2001		Women (15–49), end 2003	
Country	Estimate	[low estimate - high estimate]	Estimate	[low estimate - high estimate]	Estimate	[low estimate - high estimate]	Estimate	[low estimate - high estimate]
Global Total	**32,900,000**	**[30,200,000 - 36,700,000]**	**1.1**	**[1.0 - 1.2]**	**1.0**	**[0.9 - 1.1]**	**17,000,000**	**[15,800,000 - 18,800,000]**
Sub-Saharan Africa	**22,000,000**	**[20,400,000 - 24,500,000]**	**7.5**	**[6.9 - 8.3]**	**7.6**	**[7.0 - 8.5]**	**13,100,000**	**[12,200,000 - 14,600,000]**
Angola	200,000	[78,000 - 490,000]	3.9	[1.6 - 9.4]	3.7	[1.5 - 9.1]	130,000	[50,000 - 300,000]
Benin	59,000	[34,000 - 100,000]	1.9	[1.1 - 3.3]	1.9	[1.1 - 3.4]	35,000	[20,000 - 62,000]
Botswana *	330,000	[320,000 - 340,000]	37.3	[35.5 - 39.1]	38.0	[36.3 - 39.7]	190,000	[180,000 - 190,000]
Burkina Faso *	250,000	[160,000 - 390,000]	4.2	[2.7 - 6.5]	4.2	[2.7 - 6.5]	150,000	[98,000 - 240,000]
Burundi	220,000	[150,000 - 310,000]	6.0	[4.1 - 8.8]	6.2	[4.3 - 9.0]	130,000	[85,000 - 180,000]
Cameroon *	500,000	[350,000 - 700,000]	6.9	[4.8 - 9.8]	7.0	[4.9 - 9.9]	290,000	[200,000 - 420,000]
Central African Republic	230,000	[140,000 - 360,000]	13.5	[8.3 - 21.2]	13.5	[8.3 - 21.2]	130,000	[83,000 - 210,000]
Chad	170,000	[110,000 - 260,000]	4.8	[3.1 - 7.2]	4.9	[3.2 - 7.4]	100,000	[66,000 - 150,000]
Comoros	...	...	...	...	...	...	...	...
Congo	80,000	[35,000 - 170,000]	4.9	[2.1 - 11.0]	5.3	[2.3 - 11.5]	45,000	[19,000 - 100,000]
Côte d'Ivoire	480,000	[330,000 - 680,000]	7.0	[4.9 - 10.0]	6.7	[4.7 - 9.6]	300,000	[210,000 - 420,000]
Dem. Republic of Congo **	950,000	[390,000 - 2,200,000]	4.2	[1.7 - 9.9]	4.2	[1.7 - 10.0]	570,000	[230,000 - 1,300,000]
Djibouti	7,500	[2,200 - 21,000]	2.9	[0.7 - 7.5]	2.8	[0.8 - 7.9]	4,700	[1,200 - 12,000]
Equatorial Guinea	...	...	...	...	...	...	...	...
Eritrea	55,000	[20,000 - 150,000]	2.7	[0.9 - 7.3]	2.8	[1.0 - 7.6]	31,000	[11,000 - 85,000]
Ethiopia	1,200,000	[760,000 - 1,900,000]	4.4	[2.8 - 6.7]	4.1	[2.6 - 6.3]	770,000	[500,000 - 1,200,000]
Gabon	37,000	[18,000 - 73,000]	8.1	[4.1 - 15.3]	6.9	[3.3 - 13.7]	26,000	[13,000 - 48,000]
Gambia	6,300	[1,700 - 22,000]	1.2	[0.3 - 4.2]	1.2	[0.3 - 4.3]	3,600	[970 - 13,000]
Ghana *	310,000	[190,000 - 500,000]	3.1	[1.9 - 5.0]	3.1	[1.9 - 5.1]	180,000	[110,000 - 300,000]
Guinea *	100,000	[37,000 - 280,000]	3.2	[1.2 - 8.2]	2.8	[1.0 - 7.5]	72,000	[27,000 - 190,000]
Guinea-Bissau	...	...	...	...	...	...	...	...
Kenya	1,200,000	[830,000 - 1,600,000]	6.7	[4.7 - 9.6]	8.0	[5.8 - 11.1]	720,000	[500,000 - 1,000,000]
Lesotho *	300,000	[270,000 - 330,000]	28.9	[26.3 - 31.7]	29.6	[27.0 - 32.3]	170,000	[150,000 - 190,000]
Liberia	80,000	[35,000 - 180,000]	5.9	[2.7 - 12.4]	5.1	[2.2 - 11.3]	54,000	[25,000 - 110,000]
Madagascar	98,000	[48,000 - 160,000]	1.7	[0.8 - 2.7]	1.3	[0.6 - 2.1]	76,000	[37,000 - 120,000]
Malawi *	770,000	[610,000 - 960,000]	14.2	[11.3 - 17.7]	14.3	[11.4 - 17.9]	460,000	[370,000 - 570,000]
Mali	120,000	[37,000 - 350,000]	1.9	[0.6 - 5.9]	1.9	[0.6 - 5.8]	71,000	[23,000 - 210,000]
Mauritania	5,900	[2,900 - 9,700]	0.6	[0.3 - 1.1]	0.5	[0.2 - 0.7]	5,100	[2,500 - 8,300]
Mauritius	...	...	...	...	...	...	...	...
Mozambique	1,100,000	[870,000 - 1,500,000]	12.2	[9.4 - 15.7]	12.1	[9.4 - 15.6]	670,000	[520,000 - 860,000]
Namibia	190,000	[160,000 - 220,000]	21.3	[18.2 - 24.7]	21.3	[18.2 - 24.7]	110,000	[94,000 - 130,000]
Niger	51,000	[26,000 - 98,000]	1.2	[0.7 - 2.3]	1.1	[0.5 - 2.0]	36,000	[19,000 - 68,000]
Nigeria	3,100,000	[2,100,000 - 4,600,000]	5.4	[3.6 - 8.0]	5.5	[3.7 - 8.1]	1,900,000	[1,200,000 - 2,700,000]
Rwanda *	220,000	[140,000 - 320,000]	5.1	[3.4 - 7.6]	5.1	[3.4 - 7.6]	130,000	[86,000 - 200,000]
Senegal *	38,000	[19,000 - 76,000]	0.8	[0.4 - 1.7]	0.8	[0.4 - 1.6]	23,000	[12,000 - 47,000]
Sierra Leone	...	...	...	...	...	...	...	...
Somalia	...	...	...	...	...	...	...	...
South Africa *	4,800,000	[4,100,000 - 5,600,000]	21.5	[18.5 - 24.9]	20.9	[17.8 - 24.3]	2,900,000	[2,500,000 - 3,300,000]
Swaziland **	190,000	[180,000 - 200,000]	38.8	[37.2 - 40.4]	38.2	[36.5 - 39.8]	110,000	[110,000 - 120,000]
Togo	94,000	[61,000 - 140,000]	4.1	[2.7 - 6.4]	4.3	[2.8 - 6.6]	54,000	[35,000 - 84,000]
Uganda *	520,000	[370,000 - 810,000]	4.1	[2.8 - 6.6]	5.1	[3.5 - 7.9]	270,000	[170,000 - 410,000]
United Rep. of Tanzania *	1,400,000	[1,100,000 - 2,000,000]	8.8	[6.4 - 11.9]	9.0	[6.6 - 12.2]	840,000	[610,000 - 1,100,000]
Zambia	800,000	[660,000 - 970,000]	16.5	[13.5 - 20.0]	16.7	[13.6 - 20.2]	470,000	[380,000 - 570,000]
Zimbabwe	1,600,000	[1,400,000 - 1,800,000]	24.6	[21.7 - 27.8]	24.9	[22.0 - 28.1]	930,000	[820,000 - 1,000,000]
East Asia	**670,000**	**[340,000 - 1,100,000]**	**0.1**	**[0.1 - 0.2]**	**0.1**	**[0.1 - 0.2]**	**200,000**	**[100,000 - 320,000]**
China	650,000	[320,000 - 1,100,000]	0.1	[0.1 - 0.2]	0.1	[0.0 - 0.2]	190,000	[95,000 - 320,000]
Hong Kong SAR	2,600	[1,300 - 4,300]	0.1	[<0.2]	0.1	[<0.2]	900	[400 - 1,400]
Dem. Peo. Rep. of Korea	...	...	...	...	...	...	...	...
Japan	12,000	[5,800 - 19,000]	<0.1	[<0.2]	<0.1	[<0.2]	2,900	[1,400 - 4,800]
Mongolia	<200	[<400]	<0.1	[<0.2]	<0.1	[<0.2]	<200	[<400]
Republic of Korea	5,600	[1,800 - 11,000]	<0.1	[<0.2]	<0.1	[<0.2]	900	[300 - 1,800]
Oceania	**24,000**	**[16,000 - 34,000]**	**0.2**	**[0.1 - 0.3]**	**0.2**	**[0.1 - 0.3]**	**6,100**	**[3,600 - 9,200]**
Australia	12,000	[5,900 - 20,000]	0.1	[0.1 - 0.2]	0.1	[0.1 - 0.2]	1,000	[500 - 1,600]
Fiji	500	[200 - 900]	0.1	[0.0 - 0.2]	0.1	[0.0 - 0.2]	<200	[<400]
New Zealand	1,200	[400 - 2,400]	0.1	[<0.2]	0.1	[<0.2]	<200	[<400]
Papua New Guinea	10,000	[4,900 - 16,000]	0.6	[0.3 - 1.0]	0.4	[0.2 - 0.7]	4,800	[2,400 - 7,900]

	1. Estimated number of people living with HIV (continued)					
	Women (15–49), end 2001		Children (0–14), end 2003		Children (0–14), end 2001	
Country	Estimate	[low estimate - high estimate]	Estimate	[low estimate - high estimate]	Estimate	[low estimate - high estimate]
Global Total	**15,700,000**	**[14,600,000 - 17,400,000]**	**2,100,000**	**[1,900,000 - 2,500,000]**	**2,000,000**	**[1,800,000 - 2,300,000]**
Sub-Saharan Africa	**12,500,000**	**[11,600,000 - 13,900,000]**	**1,900,000**	**[1,700,000 - 2,200,000]**	**1,800,000**	**[1,600,000 - 2,100,000]**
Angola	110,000	[44,000 - 280,000]	23,000	[8,600 - 61,000]	20,000	[7,500 - 54,000]
Benin	34,000	[19,000 - 59,000]	5,700	[2,900 - 11,000]	5,100	[2,600 - 10,000]
Botswana *	190,000	[180,000 - 190,000]	25,000	[17,000 - 36,000]	22,000	[15,000 - 33,000]
Burkina Faso *	140,000	[91,000 - 220,000]	31,000	[18,000 - 56,000]	31,000	[18,000 - 56,000]
Burundi	120,000	[84,000 - 180,000]	27,000	[16,000 - 45,000]	26,000	[15,000 - 44,000]
Cameroon *	280,000	[200,000 - 400,000]	43,000	[26,000 - 72,000]	39,000	[23,000 - 64,000]
Central African Republic	130,000	[80,000 - 200,000]	21,000	[11,000 - 38,000]	19,000	[10,000 - 35,000]
Chad	97,000	[64,000 - 150,000]	18,000	[10,000 - 32,000]	16,000	[9,400 - 29,000]
Comoros	...	...	...	...	...	...
Congo	45,000	[20,000 - 99,000]	10,000	[4,200 - 26,000]	11,000	[4,400 - 26,000]
Côte d'Ivoire	270,000	[190,000 - 380,000]	40,000	[24,000 - 67,000]	38,000	[23,000 - 64,000]
Dem. Republic of Congo **	540,000	[220,000 - 1,300,000]	110,000	[42,000 - 280,000]	100,000	[40,000 - 270,000]
Djibouti	4,200	[1,200 - 12,000]	680	[210 - 2,400]	570	[200 - 2,300]
Equatorial Guinea	...	...	...	...	...	...
Eritrea	31,000	[11,000 - 84,000]	5,600	[1,900 - 17,000]	5,400	[1,800 - 16,000]
Ethiopia	670,000	[430,000 - 1,000,000]	120,000	[69,000 - 220,000]	110,000	[60,000 - 190,000]
Gabon	21,000	[10,000 - 41,000]	2,500	[1,200 - 5,300]	2,000	[900 - 4,400]
Gambia	3,500	[1,000 - 12,000]	500	[100 - 1,900]	<500	[<1,600]
Ghana *	170,000	[110,000 - 280,000]	24,000	[9,600 - 36,000]	22,000	[12,000 - 41,000]
Guinea *	59,000	[21,000 - 160,000]	9,200	[3,300 - 26,000]	7,300	[2,500 - 22,000]
Guinea-Bissau	...	...	...	...	...	...
Kenya	750,000	[540,000 - 1,000,000]	100,000	[61,000 - 170,000]	100,000	[63,000 - 170,000]
Lesotho *	170,000	[150,000 - 180,000]	22,000	[15,000 - 32,000]	20,000	[13,000 - 29,000]
Liberia	45,000	[20,000 - 99,000]	8,000	[3,400 - 19,000]	6,400	[2,600 - 16,000]
Madagascar	55,000	[27,000 - 91,000]	8,600	[2,500 - 30,000]	6,000	[1,600 - 22,000]
Malawi *	440,000	[350,000 - 540,000]	83,000	[54,000 - 130,000]	77,000	[50,000 - 120,000]
Mali	65,000	[21,000 - 200,000]	13,000	[3,900 - 42,000]	12,000	[3,500 - 38,000]
Mauritania	3,300	[1,600 - 5,500]	...	...	...	...
Mauritius	...	...	...	...	...	...
Mozambique	640,000	[490,000 - 820,000]	99,000	[63,000 - 160,000]	87,000	[55,000 - 140,000]
Namibia	100,000	[90,000 - 120,000]	15,000	[10,000 - 22,000]	12,000	[8,200 - 18,000]
Niger	29,000	[15,000 - 56,000]	5,900	[2,800 - 12,000]	4,500	[2,100 - 9,700]
Nigeria	1,800,000	[1,200,000 - 2,600,000]	290,000	[170,000 - 500,000]	260,000	[150,000 - 450,000]
Rwanda *	120,000	[81,000 - 180,000]	22,000	[12,000 - 37,000]	20,000	[12,000 - 35,000]
Senegal *	21,000	[10,000 - 43,000]	3,100	[1,400 - 6,800]	2,700	[1,200 - 5,900]
Sierra Leone	...	...	...	...	...	...
Somalia	...	...	...	...	...	...
South Africa *	2,700,000	[2,300,000 - 3,200,000]	230,000	[150,000 - 340,000]	190,000	[130,000 - 280,000]
Swaziland **	110,000	[100,000 - 110,000]	16,000	[11,000 - 23,000]	14,000	[9,400 - 20,000]
Togo	53,000	[34,000 - 82,000]	9,300	[5,200 - 17,000]	8,700	[4,900 - 15,000]
Uganda *	310,000	[210,000 - 460,000]	84,000	[46,000 - 150,000]	97,000	[54,000 - 160,000]
United Rep. of Tanzania *	820,000	[600,000 - 1,100,000]	140,000	[85,000 - 230,000]	130,000	[83,000 - 220,000]
Zambia	450,000	[370,000 - 550,000]	85,000	[56,000 - 130,000]	84,000	[55,000 - 130,000]
Zimbabwe	900,000	[790,000 - 1,000,000]	120,000	[84,000 - 180,000]	120,000	[83,000 - 180,000]
East Asia	**140,000**	**[69,000 - 220,000]**	**7,700**	**[2,700 - 22,000]**	**5,300**	**[1,800 - 16,000]**
China	130,000	[65,000 - 220,000]	...	...	...	...
Hong Kong SAR	800	[400 - 1,300]	...	...	...	...
Dem. Peo. Rep. of Korea	...	...	...	...	...	...
Japan	2,700	[1,300 - 4,500]	...	...	...	...
Mongolia	<200	[<400]	...	...	...	...
Republic of Korea	600	[200 - 1,100]	...	...	...	...
Oceania	**4,000**	**[2,400 - 5,900]**	**600**	**[<2,000]**	**400**	**[<1,200]**
Australia	800	[400 - 1,300]	...	...	...	...
Fiji	<200	[<400]	...	...	...	...
New Zealand	<200	[<400]	...	...	...	...
Papua New Guinea	2,900	[1,400 - 4,800]	...	...	...	...

	2. AIDS deaths				3. Orphans due to AIDS			
	Deaths in adults and children, end 2003		Deaths in adults and children, end 2001		Orphans (0–17), living 2003		Orphans (0–17), living in 2001	
Country	Estimate	[low estimate - high estimate]	Estimate	[low estimate - high estimate]	Estimate	[low estimate - high estimate]	Estimate	[low estimate - high estimate]
Global Total	**2,900,000**	**[2,600,000 - 3,300,000]**	**2,500,000**	**[2,300,000 - 2,800,000]**	**15,000,000**	**[13,000,000 - 18,000,000]**	**11,500,000**	**[10,000,000 - 14,000,000]**
Sub-Saharan Africa	**2,200,000**	**[2,000,000 - 2,500,000]**	**1,900,000**	**[1,700,000 - 2,200,000]**	**12,100,000**	**[11,000,000 - 13,400,000]**	**9,600,000**	**[8,800,000 - 10,700,000]**
Angola	21,000	[9,600 - 45,000]	18,000	[8,500 - 40,000]	110,000	[74,000 - 160,000]	87,000	[58,000 - 120,000]
Benin	5,800	[3,400 - 10,000]	4,900	[2,800 - 8,600]	34,000	[23,000 - 48,000]	25,000	[17,000 - 36,000]
Botswana *	33,000	[25,000 - 43,000]	28,000	[21,000 - 37,000]	120,000	[84,000 - 180,000]	95,000	[63,000 - 140,000]
Burkina Faso *	29,000	[18,000 - 47,000]	30,000	[19,000 - 48,000]	260,000	[180,000 - 370,000]	240,000	[160,000 - 340,000]
Burundi	25,000	[16,000 - 39,000]	25,000	[16,000 - 38,000]	200,000	[130,000 - 280,000]	170,000	[120,000 - 250,000]
Cameroon *	49,000	[32,000 - 74,000]	41,000	[26,000 - 63,000]	240,000	[160,000 - 340,000]	170,000	[110,000 - 240,000]
Central African Republic	23,000	[13,000 - 40,000]	20,000	[12,000 - 35,000]	110,000	[77,000 - 160,000]	90,000	[60,000 - 130,000]
Chad	18,000	[11,000 - 28,000]	16,000	[9,900 - 25,000]	96,000	[64,000 - 140,000]	73,000	[49,000 - 100,000]
Comoros	...	...	...	...	...	...	...	...
Congo	9,700	[4,900 - 20,000]	10,000	[5,100 - 20,000]	97,000	[65,000 - 140,000]	87,000	[59,000 - 120,000]
Côte d'Ivoire	47,000	[30,000 - 72,000]	43,000	[28,000 - 66,000]	310,000	[200,000 - 440,000]	270,000	[180,000 - 390,000]
Dem. Republic of Congo **	100,000	[50,000 - 220,000]	100,000	[48,000 - 210,000]	770,000	[520,000 - 1,100,000]	680,000	[450,000 - 970,000]
Djibouti	690	[320 - 1,900]	550	[300 - 1,800]	5,000	[3,400 - 7,200]	4,100	[2,700 - 5,800]
Equatorial Guinea	...	...	...	...	...	...	...	...
Eritrea	6,300	[2,900 - 14,000]	5,800	[2,700 - 13,000]	39,000	[26,000 - 55,000]	28,000	[19,000 - 41,000]
Ethiopia	120,000	[74,000 - 190,000]	100,000	[58,000 - 180,000]	720,000	[480,000 - 1,000,000]	560,000	[370,000 - 790,000]
Gabon	3,000	[1,500 - 5,700]	2,200	[1,100 - 4,500]	14,000	[9,300 - 20,000]	10,000	[6,900 - 15,000]
Gambia	600	[200 - 1,500]	<500	[<1,200]	2,000	[1,500 - 3,200]	1,500	[990 - 2,100]
Ghana *	30,000	[18,000 - 49,000]	26,000	[16,000 - 42,000]	170,000	[120,000 - 250,000]	140,000	[91,000 - 190,000]
Guinea *	9,000	[4,000 - 20,000]	6,900	[3,000 - 16,000]	35,000	[23,000 - 50,000]	25,000	[17,000 - 35,000]
Guinea-Bissau	...	...	...	...	...	...	...	...
Kenya	150,000	[89,000 - 200,000]	140,000	[87,000 - 190,000]	650,000	[430,000 - 930,000]	500,000	[340,000 - 720,000]
Lesotho *	29,000	[22,000 - 39,000]	24,000	[18,000 - 33,000]	100,000	[68,000 - 150,000]	68,000	[46,000 - 97,000]
Liberia	7,200	[3,500 - 15,000]	5,900	[2,800 - 12,000]	36,000	[24,000 - 52,000]	28,000	[19,000 - 40,000]
Madagascar	7,500	[3,200 - 16,000]	4,900	[2,100 - 11,000]	30,000	[20,000 - 42,000]	18,000	[12,000 - 25,000]
Malawi *	84,000	[58,000 - 120,000]	75,000	[52,000 - 110,000]	500,000	[330,000 - 710,000]	390,000	[260,000 - 560,000]
Mali	12,000	[5,100 - 29,000]	11,000	[4,500 - 26,000]	75,000	[50,000 - 110,000]	59,000	[40,000 - 85,000]
Mauritania	<500	[<1,000]	<500	[<1,000]	2,000	[1,100 - 2,300]	1,000	[700 - 1,400]
Mauritius	...	...	...	...	...	...	...	...
Mozambique	110,000	[74,000 - 160,000]	89,000	[60,000 - 130,000]	470,000	[310,000 - 670,000]	330,000	[220,000 - 470,000]
Namibia	16,000	[11,000 - 22,000]	11,000	[7,900 - 16,000]	57,000	[38,000 - 81,000]	33,000	[22,000 - 48,000]
Niger	4,800	[2,300 - 9,800]	3,600	[1,700 - 7,600]	24,000	[16,000 - 35,000]	16,000	[11,000 - 23,000]
Nigeria	310,000	[200,000 - 490,000]	260,000	[160,000 - 410,000]	1,800,000	[1,200,000 - 2,600,000]	1,300,000	[890,000 - 1,900,000]
Rwanda *	22,000	[14,000 - 36,000]	21,000	[14,000 - 34,000]	160,000	[110,000 - 240,000]	160,000	[110,000 - 230,000]
Senegal *	3,500	[1,900 - 6,500]	2,800	[1,500 - 5,300]	17,000	[12,000 - 25,000]	12,000	[8,200 - 18,000]
Sierra Leone	...	...	...	...	...	...	...	...
Somalia	...	...	...	...	...	...	...	...
South Africa *	370,000	[270,000 - 520,000]	270,000	[190,000 - 390,000]	1,100,000	[710,000 - 1,500,000]	660,000	[440,000 - 940,000]
Swaziland **	17,000	[13,000 - 23,000]	13,000	[9,900 - 18,000]	65,000	[43,000 - 93,000]	44,000	[30,000 - 63,000]
Togo	10,000	[6,400 - 16,000]	8,900	[5,600 - 14,000]	54,000	[36,000 - 77,000]	37,000	[25,000 - 53,000]
Uganda *	78,000	[54,000 - 120,000]	94,000	[66,000 - 140,000]	940,000	[630,000 - 1,400,000]	910,000	[610,000 - 1,300,000]
United Rep. of Tanzania *	160,000	[110,000 - 230,000]	150,000	[98,000 - 220,000]	980,000	[660,000 - 1,400,000]	790,000	[530,000 - 1,100,000]
Zambia	89,000	[63,000 - 130,000]	88,000	[62,000 - 120,000]	630,000	[420,000 - 910,000]	570,000	[380,000 - 810,000]
Zimbabwe	170,000	[130,000 - 230,000]	160,000	[120,000 - 220,000]	980,000	[660,000 - 1,400,000]	830,000	[560,000 - 1,200,000]
East Asia	**44,000**	**[22,000 - 75,000]**	**31,000**	**[15,000 - 52,000]**				
China	44,000	[21,000 - 75,000]	30,000	[15,000 - 51,000]	...	...	...	...
Hong Kong SAR	<200	[<400]	<200	[<400]	...	...	...	...
Dem. Peo. Rep. of Korea	...	...	...	...	...	...	...	...
Japan	<500	[<1,000]	<500	[<1,000]	...	...	...	...
Mongolia	<200	[<400]	<200	[<400]	...	...	...	...
Republic of Korea	<200	[<400]	<200	[<400]	...	...	...	...
Oceania	**700**	**[<1,300]**	**400**	**[<800]**				
Australia	<200	[<400]	<200	[<400]	...	...	...	...
Fiji	<200	[<400]	<200	[<400]	...	...	...	...
New Zealand	<200	[<400]	<200	[<400]	...	...	...	...
Papua New Guinea	600	[200 - 1,200]	<500	[<1,000]	...	...	...	...

	4. HIV prevalence (%) in young pregnant women (15–24) in capital city		5. HIV prevalence (%) in groups with high-risk behaviour in capital city						6. Knowledge and behaviour indicators	
			Injecting drug users		Sex workers		Men who have sex with men		Know a healthy-looking person can have HIV (%) (15–24)	
Country	**Year**	**Median**	**Year**	**Median**	**Year**	**Median**	**Year**	**Median**	**Female**	**Male**
Global Total										
Sub-Saharan Africa										
Angola	...	...	...	...	2002	33.3	...	...	...	...
Benin	2002	2.3	...	...	2001	60.5	...	...	56	69
Botswana *	2003	32.9	...	...	...	...	...	...	81	76
Burkina Faso *	2002	2.3	...	...	...	...	...	...	42 v	64 v
Burundi	2002	13.6	...	...	...	...	...	...	66	...
Cameroon *	2002	7.0	...	...	...	...	...	...	57	63
Central African Republic	2002	14.0	...	...	...	...	...	...	46	...
Chad	2003	4.8	...	...	...	...	...	...	28	...
Comoros	...	...	...	...	...	...	...	...	55	...
Congo	...	...	...	...	...	...	...	...	...	...
Côte d'Ivoire	2002	5.2	...	...	...	...	...	...	64	67
Dem. Republic of Congo **	...	...	...	...	...	...	...	...	...	...
Djibouti	...	...	...	...	...	...	...	...	...	...
Equatorial Guinea	...	...	...	...	...	...	...	...	46	...
Eritrea	...	...	...	...	...	...	...	...	79	...
Ethiopia	2003	11.7	...	...	...	...	...	...	39	54
Gabon	...	...	...	...	...	...	...	...	72	81
Gambia	...	...	...	...	...	...	...	...	53	...
Ghana *	2003	3.9	...	...	...	...	...	...	71	77
Guinea *	...	...	...	...	2001	39.7	...	...	60	56
Guinea-Bissau	...	...	...	...	...	...	...	...	31	...
Kenya	...	...	...	...	2000	25.5	...	...	74	80
Lesotho *	2003	27.8	...	...	...	...	...	...	46	...
Liberia	...	...	...	...	...	...	...	...	...	...
Madagascar	...	...	...	...	2001	0.2	...	...	27	...
Malawi *	2003	18.0	...	...	...	...	...	...	84	89
Mali	2003	2.2	...	...	2000	21.0	...	...	46	59
Mauritania	...	...	...	...	...	...	...	...	30	39
Mauritius	...	...	...	...	...	...	...	...	...	...
Mozambique	2002	14.7	...	...	...	...	...	...	62	71
Namibia	...	...	...	...	...	...	...	...	82	87
Niger	...	...	...	...	...	...	...	...	37	41
Nigeria	2003	4.2	...	...	...	...	...	...	45	51
Rwanda *	2002	11.6	...	...	...	...	...	...	64	69
Senegal *	2002	1.1	...	...	2002	14.2	...	...	46	...
Sierra Leone	...	...	...	...	...	...	...	...	35	...
Somalia	...	...	...	...	...	...	...	...	13	...
South Africa *	2002	24.0	...	...	...	...	...	...	54	...
Swaziland **	2002	39.0	...	...	...	...	...	...	81	...
Togo	2003	9.1	...	...	...	...	...	...	66	73
Uganda *	2001	10.0	...	...	...	...	...	...	76	83
United Rep. of Tanzania *	2002	7.0	...	...	...	...	...	...	65	68
Zambia	2002	22.1	...	...	...	...	...	...	74	73
Zimbabwe	...	...	...	...	...	...	...	...	74	83
East Asia										
China	...	...	2000	0.0	2000	0.2	...	...	...	...
Hong Kong SAR	...	...	...	...	...	...	...	...	...	...
Dem. Peo. Rep. of Korea	...	...	...	...	...	...	...	...	...	...
Japan	...	...	...	...	...	...	2000	2.9	...	...
Mongolia	...	...	...	...	...	...	...	...	57	...
Republic of Korea	...	...	...	...	...	...	...	...	...	...
Oceania										
Australia	...	...	...	...	...	...	...	...	...	...
Fiji	...	...	...	...	...	...	...	...	...	...
New Zealand	...	...	...	...	...	...	...	...	...	...
Papua New Guinea	...	...	...	...	2000	16.0	...	...	...	...

6. Knowledge and behaviour indicators

Country	Can identify two prevention methods and reject three misconceptions (%) (15–24)		Had sex before age 15 (%) (15–19)		Reported higher-risk sex in the last year (%) (15–24)		Used a condom the last time they had higher-risk sex, of those who had high-risk sex in the last year (%) (15–24)		Year
	Female	Male	Female	Male	Female	Male	Female	Male	
Global Total									
Sub-Saharan Africa									
Angola	...	...	...	...	...	...	...	...	...
Benin	8	14	16	24	36	90	19	34	2001 d
Botswana *	40	33	...	...	...	...	75 x	88 x	2001 b
Burkina Faso *	...	...	12	8	19	82	41	55	1999 d
Burundi	24	...	...	...	...	...	...	...	2000 c
Cameroon *	16 c,x	...	26	18	41	86	16	31	1998 d
Central African Republic	5	...	...	...	...	...	...	...	2000 c
Chad	5	...	...	...	...	...	...	...	2000 c
Comoros	10	...	...	...	...	...	...	...	2000 c
Congo	...	...	...	...	...	...	...	...	...
Côte d'Ivoire	16 c,x	...	22	14	51	91	25	56	1998 d
Dem. Republic of Congo **	...	...	...	...	...	...	...	...	...
Djibouti	...	...	...	...	...	...	...	...	...
Equatorial Guinea	4	...	...	...	...	...	...	...	2000 c
Eritrea	...	...	9	...	...	...	...	...	2002 d
Ethiopia	...	...	14	5	7	64	17	30	2000 d
Gabon	24	22	24	48	53	75	33	48	2000 d
Gambia	15	...	...	...	...	...	...	...	2000 c
Ghana *	...	...	7	4	...	...	...	...	1998 d
Guinea *	...	...	27	20	23	92	17	32	1999 d
Guinea-Bissau	8	...	...	...	...	...	...	...	2000 c
Kenya	26 c,x	...	15	32	39	92	14	43	1998 d
Lesotho *	18	...	...	...	...	...	...	...	2000 c
Liberia	...	...	32	12	...	...	...	...	1999 d
Madagascar	...	...	...	...	...	...	...	...	2000 c
Malawi *	34	41	17	29	17	71	32	38	2000 d
Mali	9	15	26	11	18	85	14	30	2001 d
Mauritania	...	...	13	2	...	...	...	...	2000 d
Mauritius	...	...	...	...	...	...	...	...	...
Mozambique	...	...	...	...	...	...	...	...	2001 e
Namibia	31	41	10	31	80	85	48	69	2000 d
Niger	5 c,x	...	28	10	4	56	7	30	1998 d
Nigeria	...	...	16	8	...	...	...	...	1999 d
Rwanda *	23	20	3	...	10	42	23	55	2000 d
Senegal *	...	...	...	...	...	...	...	...	2000 c
Sierra Leone	16	...	...	...	...	...	...	...	2000 c
Somalia	0	...	...	...	...	...	...	...	2000 c
South Africa *	20	...	9	...	...	...	20	...	1998 d
Swaziland **	27	...	...	...	...	...	...	...	2000 c
Togo	20 c,x	...	20	...	51	89	22	41	1998 d
Uganda *	28	40	14	16	22	59	44	62	2000 d
United Rep. of Tanzania *	26	29	15	24	40	87	21	31	1999 d
Zambia	31	33	18	27	19	50	33	42	2001 d
Zimbabwe	...	...	3	6	20	82	42	69	1999 d
East Asia									
China	...	...	...	...	...	...	...	...	...
Hong Kong SAR	...	...	...	...	...	...	...	...	...
Dem. Peo. Rep. of Korea	...	...	...	...	...	...	...	...	...
Japan	...	...	...	...	...	...	...	...	...
Mongolia	32	...	...	...	...	...	...	...	2000 c
Republic of Korea	...	...	...	...	...	...	...	...	...
Oceania									
Australia	...	...	...	...	...	...	...	...	...
Fiji	...	...	...	...	...	...	...	...	...
New Zealand	...	...	...	...	...	...	...	...	...
Papua New Guinea	...	...	...	...	...	...	...	...	...

	1. Estimated number of people living with HIV					
	Adults and children, end 2003		Adults and children, end 2001		Adults (15–49), end 2003	
Country	Estimate	[low estimate - high estimate]	Estimate	[low estimate - high estimate]	Estimate	[low estimate - high estimate]
South & South-East Asia	**6,500,000**	**[4,100,000 - 9,600,000]**	**5,900,000**	**[3,700,000 - 8,700,000]**	**6,300,000**	**[4,000,000 - 9,300,000]**
Afghanistan	...	...	...	...	...	...
Bangladesh **	...	[2,500 - 15,000]	...	[2,200 - 13,000]	...	[2,400 - 15,000]
Bhutan	...	...	...	...	...	...
Brunei Darussalam	<200	[<400]	<200	[<400]	<200	[<400]
Cambodia	170,000	[100,000 - 290,000]	170,000	[100,000 - 270,000]	170,000	[99,000 - 280,000]
India	...	[2,200,000 - 7,600,000]	...	[2,000,000 - 6,900,000]	...	[2,200,000 - 7,300,000]
Indonesia	110,000	[53,000 - 180,000]	58,000	[28,000 - 95,000]	110,000	[53,000 - 180,000]
Iran (Islamic Republic of)	31,000	[10,000 - 61,000]	18,000	[6,000 - 36,000]	31,000	[10,000 - 60,000]
Lao People's Dem. Rep.	1,700	[600 - 3,600]	800	[300 - 1,600]	1,700	[550 - 3,300]
Malaysia	52,000	[25,000 - 86,000]	42,000	[20,000 - 70,000]	51,000	[25,000 - 84,000]
Maldives	...	...	...	...	...	...
Myanmar **	330,000	[170,000 - 620,000]	280,000	[150,000 - 510,000]	320,000	[170,000 - 610,000]
Nepal	61,000	[29,000 - 110,000]	45,000	[22,000 - 78,000]	60,000	[29,000 - 98,000]
Pakistan	74,000	[24,000 - 150,000]	63,000	[21,000 - 130,000]	73,000	[24,000 - 140,000]
Philippines	9,000	[3,000 - 18,000]	4,400	[1,400 - 8,700]	8,900	[2,900 - 18,000]
Singapore	4,100	[1,300 - 8,000]	3,400	[1,100 - 6,700]	4,100	[1,300 - 8,000]
Sri Lanka	3,500	[1,200 - 6,900]	2,200	[700 - 4,300]	3,500	[1,100 - 6,800]
Thailand	570,000	[310,000 - 1,000,000]	630,000	[360,000 - 1,100,000]	560,000	[310,000 - 1,000,000]
Viet Nam	220,000	[110,000 - 360,000]	150,000	[75,000 - 250,000]	200,000	[100,000 - 350,000]
Eastern Europe & Central Asia	**1,300,000**	**[860,000 - 1,900,000]**	**890,000**	**[570,000 - 1,300,000]**	**1,300,000**	**[850,000 - 1,900,000]**
Armenia	2,600	[1,200 - 4,300]	2,000	[990 - 3,400]	2,500	[1,200 - 4,100]
Azerbaijan	1,400	[500 - 2,800]	...	...	1,400	[500 - 2,800]
Belarus	...	[12,000 - 42,000]	...	[10,000 - 39,000]	...	[12,000 - 40,000]
Bosnia and Herzegovina	900	[300 - 1,800]	...	...	900	[300 - 1,800]
Bulgaria	<500	[<1,000]	...	...	<500	[<1,000]
Croatia	<200	[<400]	...	...	<200	[<400]
Czech Republic	2,500	[800 - 4,900]	2,100	[750 - 4,700]	2,500	[820 - 4,900]
Estonia	7,800	[2,600 - 15,000]	5,100	[1,700 - 10,000]	7,700	[2,500 - 15,000]
Georgia	3,000	[2,000 - 12,000]	1,500	[660 - 4,000]	3,000	[2,000 - 12,000]
Hungary	2,800	[900 - 5,500]	...	...	2,800	[900 - 5,500]
Kazakhstan	16,500	[5,800 - 35,000]	10,400	[5,000 - 30,000]	16,400	[5,700 - 34,000]
Kyrgyzstan	3,900	[1,500 - 8,000]	1,500	[700 - 4,000]	3,900	[1,500 - 8,000]
Latvia	7,600	[3,700 - 12,000]	6,000	[2,900 - 9,800]	7,500	[3,700 - 12,000]
Lithuania	1,300	[400 - 2,600]	1,100	[400 - 2,200]	1,300	[400 - 2,600]
Poland	14,000	[6,900 - 23,000]	...	...	14,000	[6,900 - 23,000]
Republic of Moldova	5,500	[2,700 - 9,000]	...	...	5,500	[2,700 - 9,000]
Romania	6,500	[4,800 - 8,900]	4,000	[4,000 - 4,000]	2,500	[800 - 4,900]
Russian Federation	860,000	[420,000 - 1,400,000]	530,000	[260,000 - 870,000]	860,000	[420,000 - 1,400,000]
Slovakia	<200	[<400]	...	...	<200	[<400]
Tajikistan	<200	[<400]	...	...	<200	[<400]
Turkmenistan	<200	[<400]	...	...	<200	[<400]
Ukraine	360,000	[180,000 - 590,000]	300,000	[150,000 - 490,000]	360,000	[170,000 - 580,000]
Uzbekistan	11,000	[4,900 - 30,000]	3,000	[1,900 - 12,000]	11,000	[4,900 - 29,000]
Western Europe	**580,000**	**[460,000 - 730,000]**	**540,000**	**[430,000 - 690,000]**	**570,000**	**[450,000 - 720,000]**
Albania	...	...	...	...	...	...
Austria	10,000	[5,000 - 16,000]	10,000	[4,900 - 16,000]	10,000	[4,900 - 16,000]
Belgium	10,000	[5,300 - 17,000]	8,400	[4,300 - 14,000]	10,000	[4,900 - 16,000]
Denmark	5,000	[2,500 - 8,200]	4,600	[2,300 - 7,600]	5,000	[2,500 - 8,200]
Finland	1,500	[500 - 3,000]	1,200	[400 - 2,400]	1,500	[500 - 3,000]
France	120,000	[60,000 - 200,000]	110,000	[56,000 - 190,000]	120,000	[59,000 - 200,000]
Germany	43,000	[21,000 - 71,000]	41,000	[20,000 - 68,000]	43,000	[21,000 - 71,000]
Greece	9,100	[4,500 - 15,000]	8,900	[4,400 - 14,000]	9,000	[4,400 - 15,000]
Iceland	<500	[<1,000]	<500	[<1,000]	<200	[<400]
Ireland	2,800	[1,100 - 5,300]	2,400	[800 - 4,900]	2,600	[900 - 5,100]
Italy	140,000	[67,000 - 220,000]	130,000	[65,000 - 210,000]	140,000	[66,000 - 220,000]
Luxembourg	<500	[<1,000]	<500	[<1,000]	<500	[<1,000]
Malta	<500	[<1,000]	<500	[<1,000]	<500	[<1,000]
Netherlands	19,000	[9,500 - 31,000]	17,000	[8,500 - 28,000]	19,000	[9,300 - 31,000]
Norway	2,100	[700 - 4,000]	1,900	[600 - 3,600]	2,000	[700 - 3,900]
Portugal	22,000	[11,000 - 36,000]	21,000	[11,000 - 35,000]	22,000	[11,000 - 35,000]

1. Estimated number of people living with HIV (continued)								
	Adults (15–49), end 2001		Adults (15–49) rate (%) end 2003		Adults (15–49) rate (%) end 2001		Women (15–49), end 2003	
Country	Estimate	[low estimate - high estimate]	Estimate	[low estimate - high estimate]	Estimate	[low estimate - high estimate]	Estimate	[low estimate - high estimate]
South & South-East Asia	**5,800,000**	**[3,700,000 - 8,400,000]**	**0.6**	**[0.4 - 0.9]**	**0.6**	**[0.4 - 0.9]**	**1,800,000**	**[1,200,000 - 2,700,000]**
Afghanistan	...	...	...	...	...	...	...	...
Bangladesh **	...	[2,200 - 13,000]	...	[<0.2]	...	[<0.2]	...	[400 - 2,500]
Bhutan	...	...	...	...	...	...	...	...
Brunei Darussalam	<200	[<400]	<0.1	[<0.2]	<0.1	[<0.2]	<200	[<400]
Cambodia	160,000	[100,000 - 260,000]	2.6	[1.5 - 4.4]	2.7	[1.7 - 4.3]	51,000	[31,000 - 86,000]
India	...	[2,000,000 - 6,700,000]	...	[0.4 - 1.3]	...	[0.4 - 1.3]	...	[630,000 - 2,100,000]
Indonesia	57,000	[28,000 - 94,000]	0.1	[0.0 - 0.2]	0.1	[<0.2]	15,000	[7,100 - 24,000]
Iran (Islamic Republic of)	18,000	[6,000 - 36,000]	0.1	[0.0 - 0.2]	0.1	[<0.2]	3,800	[1,200 - 7,400]
Lao People's Dem. Rep.	800	[300 - 1,500]	0.1	[<0.2]	<0.1	<0.2	<500	[<1,000]
Malaysia	41,000	[20,000 - 68,000]	0.4	[0.2 - 0.7]	0.4	[0.2 - 0.6]	8,500	[4,100 - 14,000]
Maldives	...	...	...	...	...	...	...	...
Myanmar **	270,000	[140,000 - 500,000]	1.2	[0.6 - 2.2]	1.0	[0.6 - 1.9]	97,000	[51,000 - 180,000]
Nepal	44,000	[22,000 - 72,000]	0.5	[0.3 - 0.9]	0.4	[0.2 - 0.6]	16,000	[7,200 - 24,000]
Pakistan	62,000	[20,000 - 120,000]	0.1	[0.0 - 0.2]	0.1	[0.0 - 0.2]	8,900	[3,000 - 18,000]
Philippines	4,300	[1,400 - 8,500]	<0.1	[<0.2]	<0.1	[<0.2]	2,000	[700 - 4,000]
Singapore	3,400	[1,100 - 6,600]	0.2	[0.1 - 0.5]	0.2	[0.1 - 0.4]	1,000	[300 - 2,000]
Sri Lanka	2,200	[700 - 4,300]	<0.1	[<0.2]	<0.1	[<0.2]	600	[200 - 1,200]
Thailand	620,000	[360,000 - 1,100,000]	1.5	[0.8 - 2.8]	1.7	[1.0 - 2.9]	200,000	[110,000 - 370,000]
Viet Nam	150,000	[75,000 - 250,000]	0.4	[0.2 - 0.8]	0.3	[0.2 - 0.6]	65,000	[31,000 - 110,000]
Eastern Europe & Central Asia	**880,000**	**[570,000 - 1,300,000]**	**0.6**	**[0.4 - 0.9]**	**0.4**	**[0.3 - 0.6]**	**440,000**	**[280,000 - 650,000]**
Armenia	2,000	[1,000 - 3,300]	0.1	[0.1 - 0.2]	0.1	[0.0 - 0.2]	900	[400 - 1,400]
Azerbaijan	...	...	<0.1	[<0.2]	...	...	...	...
Belarus	...	[10,000 - 38,000]	...	[0.2 - 0.8]	...	[0.2 - 0.7]	...	[3,100 - 14,000]
Bosnia and Herzegovina	...	...	<0.1	[<0.2]	...	...	...	...
Bulgaria	...	...	<0.1	[<0.2]	...	...	...	...
Croatia	...	...	<0.1	[<0.2]	...	...	...	...
Czech Republic	2,100	[750 - 4,700]	0.1	[<0.2]	<0.1	[<0.2]	800	[300 - 1,700]
Estonia	5,000	[1,700 - 9,900]	1.1	[0.4 - 2.1]	0.7	[0.2 - 1.3]	2,600	[900 - 5,200]
Georgia	1,500	[700 - 3,900]	0.1	[0.1 - 0.4]	<0.1	[<0.2]	1,000	[700 - 4,000]
Hungary	...	...	0.1	[0.0 - 0.2]	...	...	...	...
Kazakhstan	10,300	[5,000 - 30,000]	0.2	[0.1 - 0.3]	0.1	[<0.2]	5,500	[2,000 - 12,000]
Kyrgyzstan	1,500	[700 - 4,000]	0.1	[<0.2]	<0.1	[<0.2]	<800	[<1,500]
Latvia	5,900	[2,900 - 9,700]	0.6	[0.3 - 1.0]	0.5	[0.2 - 0.8]	2,500	[1,200 - 4,100]
Lithuania	1,100	[400 - 2,200]	0.1	[<0.2]	0.1	[<0.2]	<500	[<1,000]
Poland	...	...	0.1	[0.1 - 0.2]	...	...	...	...
Republic of Moldova	...	...	0.2	[0.1 - 0.3]	...	...	...	...
Romania	...	...	<0.1	[<0.2]	...	...	...	...
Russian Federation	530,000	[260,000 - 870,000]	1.1	[0.6 - 1.9]	0.7	[0.3 - 1.2]	290,000	[140,000 - 480,000]
Slovakia	...	...	<0.1	[<0.2]	...	...	...	...
Tajikistan	...	...	<0.1	[<0.2]	...	...	...	...
Turkmenistan	...	...	<0.1	[<0.2]	...	...	...	...
Ukraine	300,000	[150,000 - 490,000]	1.4	[0.7 - 2.3]	1.2	[0.6 - 1.9]	120,000	[59,000 - 200,000]
Uzbekistan	3,000	[1,900 - 11,000]	0.1	[0.0 - 0.2]	<0.1	<0.2	3,700	[1,700 - 9,900]
Western Europe	**540,000**	**[420,000 - 680,000]**	**0.3**	**[0.2 - 0.4]**	**0.3**	**[0.2 - 0.4]**	**150,000**	**[110,000 - 190,000]**
Albania	...	...	...	...	...	...	...	...
Austria	9,900	[4,900 - 16,000]	0.3	[0.1 - 0.4]	0.2	[0.1 - 0.4]	2,200	[1,100 - 3,600]
Belgium	8,100	[4,000 - 13,000]	0.2	[0.1 - 0.3]	0.2	[0.1 - 0.3]	3,500	[1,700 - 5,700]
Denmark	4,600	[2,300 - 7,500]	0.2	[0.1 - 0.3]	0.2	[0.1 - 0.3]	900	[400 - 1,500]
Finland	1,200	[400 - 2,400]	0.1	[<0.2]	0.1	[<0.2]	<500	[<1,000]
France	110,000	[55,000 - 180,000]	0.4	[0.2 - 0.7]	0.4	[0.2 - 0.6]	32,000	[16,000 - 52,000]
Germany	41,000	[20,000 - 67,000]	0.1	[0.1 - 0.2]	0.1	[0.1 - 0.2]	9,500	[4,700 - 16,000]
Greece	8,800	[4,300 - 14,000]	0.2	[0.1 - 0.3]	0.2	[0.1 - 0.3]	1,800	[900 - 3,000]
Iceland	<200	[<400]	0.2	[0.1 - 0.3]	0.2	[0.1 - 0.3]	<200	[<400]
Ireland	2,200	[700 - 4,300]	0.1	[0.0 - 0.3]	0.1	[0.0 - 0.2]	800	[300 - 1,500]
Italy	130,000	[64,000 - 210,000]	0.5	[0.2 - 0.8]	0.5	[0.2 - 0.8]	45,000	[22,000 - 74,000]
Luxembourg	<500	[<1,000]	0.2	[0.1 - 0.4]	0.2	[0.1 - 0.3]	...	...
Malta	<500	[<1,000]	0.2	[0.1 - 0.3]	0.1	[0.0 - 0.2]	...	...
Netherlands	17,000	[8,300 - 28,000]	0.2	[0.1 - 0.4]	0.2	[0.1 - 0.3]	3,800	[1,900 - 6,200]
Norway	1,800	[600 - 3,500]	0.1	[0.0 - 0.2]	0.1	[0.0 - 0.2]	<500	[<1,000]
Portugal	21,000	[10,000 - 34,000]	0.4	[0.2 - 0.7]	0.4	[0.2 - 0.7]	4,300	[2,100 - 7,100]

1. Estimated number of people living with HIV (continued)						
	Women (15–49), end 2001		Children (0–14), end 2003		Children (0–14), end 2001	
Country	Estimate	[low estimate - high estimate]	Estimate	[low estimate - high estimate]	Estimate	[low estimate - high estimate]
South & South-East Asia	**1,600,000**	**[1,000,000 - 2,300,000]**	**160,000**	**[91,000 - 300,000]**	**130,000**	**[77,000 - 260,000]**
Afghanistan	...	...	...	...	...	...
Bangladesh **	...	[300 - 2,100]	...	...	...	...
Bhutan	...	...	...	...	...	...
Brunei Darussalam	<200	[<400]	...	...	...	...
Cambodia	48,000	[30,000 - 77,000]	7,300	[3,800 - 14,000]	6,400	[3,500 - 12,000]
India	...	[550,000 - 1,800,000]	...	[54,000 - 270,000]	...	[46,000 - 230,000]
Indonesia	6,900	[3,400 - 11,000]	...	...	...	...
Iran (Islamic Republic of)	1,900	[600 - 3,800]	...	...	...	...
Lao People's Dem. Rep.	<200	[<400]	...	...	...	...
Malaysia	6,300	[3,100 - 10,000]	...	...	...	...
Maldives	...	...	...	...	...	...
Myanmar **	78,000	[42,000 - 140,000]	7,600	[3,600 - 16,000]	5,700	[2,800 - 12,000]
Nepal	9,100	[4,500 - 15,000]	...	...	...	...
Pakistan	4,300	[1,400 - 8,500]	...	...	...	...
Philippines	900	[300 - 1,800]	...	...	...	...
Singapore	800	[300 - 1,500]	...	...	...	...
Sri Lanka	<500	[<1,000]	...	...	...	...
Thailand	200,000	[110,000 - 340,000]	12,000	[5,700 - 24,000]	12,000	[6,200 - 23,000]
Viet Nam	41,000	[21,000 - 69,000]	...	...	...	...
Eastern Europe & Central Asia	**280,000**	**[180,000 - 410,000]**	**8,100**	**[6,600 - 12,000]**	**7,000**	**[5,800 - 9,700]**
Armenia	700	[300 - 1,100]	...	...	...	...
Azerbaijan	...	...	...	...	...	...
Belarus	...	[2,800 - 12,000]	...	...	...	...
Bosnia and Herzegovina	...	...	...	...	...	...
Bulgaria	...	...	...	...	...	...
Croatia	...	...	...	...	...	...
Czech Republic	700	[300 - 1,600]	...	...	...	...
Estonia	1,600	[500 - 3,200]	...	...	...	...
Georgia	<600	[200 - 1,300]	...	...	...	...
Hungary	...	...	...	...	...	...
Kazakhstan	3,500	[1,000 - 7,000]	...	...	...	...
Kyrgyzstan	<500	[<1,000]	...	...	...	...
Latvia	1,900	[900 - 3,100]	...	...	...	...
Lithuania	<500	[<1,000]	...	...	...	...
Poland	...	...	...	...	...	...
Republic of Moldova	...	...	...	...	...	...
Romania	...	...	...	...	...	...
Russian Federation	170,000	[85,000 - 280,000]	...	...	...	...
Slovakia	...	...	...	...	...	...
Tajikistan	...	...	...	...	...	...
Turkmenistan	...	...	...	...	...	...
Ukraine	96,000	[47,000 - 160,000]	...	...	...	...
Uzbekistan	1,000	[600 - 3,600]	...	...	...	...
Western Europe	**130,000**	**[100,000 - 170,000]**	**6,200**	**[4,900 - 7,900]**	**5,800**	**[4,600 - 7,400]**
Albania	...	...	...	...	...	...
Austria	2,200	[1,100 - 3,600]	...	...	...	...
Belgium	2,900	[1,400 - 4,800]	...	...	...	...
Denmark	800	[400 - 1,300]	...	...	...	...
Finland	<500	[<1,000]	...	...	...	...
France	30,000	[15,000 - 49,000]	...	...	...	...
Germany	8,100	[4,000 - 13,000]	...	...	...	...
Greece	1,800	[900 - 3,000]	...	...	...	...
Iceland	<200	[<400]	...	...	...	...
Ireland	700	[200 - 1,300]	...	...	...	...
Italy	42,000	[21,000 - 69,000]	...	...	...	...
Luxembourg	...	...	...	...	...	...
Malta	...	...	...	...	...	...
Netherlands	3,300	[1,600 - 5,400]	...	...	...	...
Norway	<500	[<1,000]	...	...	...	...
Portugal	4,200	[2,100 - 6,900]	...	...	...	...

	2. AIDS deaths				3. Orphans due to AIDS			
	Deaths in adults and children, end 2003		Deaths in adults and children, end 2001		Orphans (0–17), living 2003		Orphans (0–17), living in 2001	
Country	**Estimate**	**[low estimate - high estimate]**	**Estimate**	**[low estimate - high estimate]**	**Estimate**	**[low estimate - high estimate]**	**Estimate**	**[low estimate - high estimate]**
South & South-East Asia	**460,000**	**[290,000 - 700,000]**	**390,000**	**[240,000 - 590,000]**				
Afghanistan	...	...	...	...	...	...	...	...
Bangladesh **	...	[<400]	...	[<400]	...	...	...	...
Bhutan	...	...	...	...	...	...	...	...
Brunei Darussalam	<200	[<400]	<200	[<400]	...	...	...	...
Cambodia	15,000	[9,100 - 25,000]	13,000	[7,800 - 21,000]	...	...	...	...
India	...	[160,000 - 560,000]	...	[140,000 - 480,000]	...	...	...	...
Indonesia	2,400	[1,100 - 4,100]	600	[300 - 1,000]	...	...	...	...
Iran (Islamic Republic of)	800	[300 - 1,600]	<500	[<1,000]	...	...	...	...
Lao People's Dem. Rep.	<200	[<400]	<200	[<400]	...	...	...	...
Malaysia	2,000	[1,000 - 3,600]	1,500	[700 - 2,900]	...	...	...	...
Maldives	...	...	...	...	...	...	...	...
Myanmar **	20,000	[11,000 - 35,000]	14,000	[7,800 - 26,000]	...	...	...	...
Nepal	3,100	[1,000 - 6,400]	2,000	[900 - 4,200]	...	...	...	...
Pakistan	4,900	[1,600 - 11,000]	3,900	[1,300 - 8,500]	...	...	...	...
Philippines	<500	[<1,000]	<200	[<400]	...	...	...	...
Singapore	<200	[<400]	<200	[<400]	...	...	...	...
Sri Lanka	<200	[<400]	<200	[<400]	...	...	...	...
Thailand	58,000	[34,000 - 97,000]	58,000	[34,000 - 96,000]	...	...	...	...
Viet Nam	9,000	[4,500 - 16,000]	5,000	[3,000 - 9,100]	...	...	...	...
Eastern Europe & Central Asia	**49,000**	**[32,000 - 71,000]**	**31,000**	**[21,000 - 45,000]**				
Armenia	<200	[<400]	<200	[<400]	...	...	...	...
Azerbaijan	...	...	...	...	...	...	...	...
Belarus	...	[900 - 3,300]	...	[800 - 3,000]	...	...	...	...
Bosnia and Herzegovina	...	...	...	...	...	...	...	...
Bulgaria	...	...	...	...	...	...	...	...
Croatia	...	...	...	...	...	...	...	...
Czech Republic	...	...	...	...	...	...	...	...
Estonia	<200	[<400]	<200	[<400]	...	...	...	...
Georgia	<200	[<400]	<200	[<400]	...	...	...	...
Hungary	...	...	...	...	...	...	...	...
Kazakhstan	<200	[<400]	<200	[<400]	...	...	...	...
Kyrgyzstan	<200	[<400]	<200	[<400]	...	...	...	...
Latvia	<500	[<1,000]	<200	[<400]	...	...	...	...
Lithuania	<200	[<400]	<200	[<400]	...	...	...	...
Poland	...	...	...	...	...	...	...	...
Republic of Moldova	...	...	...	...	...	...	...	...
Romania	...	...	...	...	...	...	...	...
Russian Federation	...	...	...	...	...	...	...	...
Slovakia	...	...	...	...	...	...	...	...
Tajikistan	...	...	...	...	...	...	...	...
Turkmenistan	...	...	...	...	...	...	...	...
Ukraine	20,000	[9,600 - 33,000]	14,000	[7,000 - 24,000]	...	...	...	...
Uzbekistan	<500	[<1,000]	<200	[<400]	...	...	...	...
Western Europe	**6,000**	**[<8000]**	**6,000**	**[<8000]**				
Albania	...	...	...	...	...	...	...	...
Austria	<100	[<200]	<100	[<200]	...	...	...	...
Belgium	<100	[<200]	<100	[<200]	...	...	...	...
Denmark	<100	[<200]	<100	[<200]	...	...	...	...
Finland	<100	[<200]	<100	[<200]	...	...	...	...
France	<1,000	[<2,000]	<1,000	[<2,000]	...	...	...	...
Germany	<1,000	[<2,000]	<1,000	[<2,000]	...	...	...	...
Greece	<100	[<200]	<100	[<200]	...	...	...	...
Iceland	<100	[<200]	<100	[<200]	...	...	...	...
Ireland	<100	[<200]	<100	[<200]	...	...	...	...
Italy	<1000	[<2,000]	<1000	[<2,000]	...	...	...	...
Luxembourg	<100	[<200]	<100	[<200]	...	...	...	...
Malta	<100	[<200]	<100	[<200]	...	...	...	...
Netherlands	<100	[<200]	<100	[<200]	...	...	...	...
Norway	<100	[<200]	<100	[<200]	...	...	...	...
Portugal	<1000	[<2,000]	<1000	[<2,000]	...	...	...	...

	4. HIV prevalence (%) in young pregnant women (15–24) in capital city		5. HIV prevalence (%) in groups with high-risk behaviour in capital city						6. Knowledge and behaviour indicators	
			Injecting drug users		Sex workers		Men who have sex with men		Know a healthy-looking person can have HIV (%) (15–24)	
Country	**Year**	**Median**	**Year**	**Median**	**Year**	**Median**	**Year**	**Median**	**Female**	**Male**
South & South-East Asia										
Afghanistan	...	...	...	...	...	...	...	...	...	...
Bangladesh **	...	...	1999	2.5	2000	20.0	1999	0.3	...	...
Bhutan	...	...	...	...	...	...	...	...	...	...
Brunei Darussalam	...	...	...	...	...	...	...	...	...	...
Cambodia	...	...	...	...	2002	18.5	...	...	62	...
India	...	...	2002	7.2	...	...	...	...	...	...
Indonesia	...	...	...	...	2001	0.0	...	...	32	...
Iran (Islamic Republic of)	...	...	...	...	...	...	...	...	...	...
Lao People's Dem. Rep.	...	...	...	...	2001	1.1	...	...	...	...
Malaysia	...	...	...	...	...	...	...	...	...	...
Maldives	...	...	...	...	...	...	...	...	...	...
Myanmar **	...	...	2000	37.1	2000	26.0	...	...	...	...
Nepal	...	...	2000	50.0	2002	17.0	...	...	...	...
Pakistan	...	...	...	...	...	...	...	...	...	...
Philippines	...	...	...	...	...	...	...	...	67	...
Singapore	...	...	...	...	...	...	...	...	...	...
Sri Lanka	...	...	...	...	...	...	...	...	...	...
Thailand	...	...	2002	53.7	2002	2.6	...	...	...	...
Viet Nam	...	...	2001	22.3	2001	11.5	...	...	63	...
Eastern Europe & Central Asia										
Armenia	...	...	...	...	1999	7.5	...	...	53	48
Azerbaijan	...	...	...	...	...	...	...	...	35	...
Belarus	...	...	...	...	...	...	...	...	...	...
Bosnia and Herzegovina	...	...	...	...	...	...	...	...	74	...
Bulgaria	...	...	...	...	...	...	...	...	...	...
Croatia	...	...	...	...	...	...	...	...	...	...
Czech Republic	...	...	...	...	...	...	...	...	...	...
Estonia	...	...	...	...	...	...	...	...	...	...
Georgia	...	...	...	...	...	...	...	...	...	...
Hungary	...	...	2000	2.2	...	...	...	...	...	...
Kazakhstan	...	...	2002	0.0	...	...	...	...	63 x	73 x
Kyrgyzstan	...	...	...	...	...	...	...	...	...	...
Latvia	...	...	2002	17.3	...	...	...	...	...	...
Lithuania	...	...	...	...	2001	0.5	...	...	...	...
Poland	...	...	...	...	...	...	...	...	...	...
Republic of Moldova	...	...	...	...	...	...	...	...	79	...
Romania	...	...	...	...	...	...	...	...	70	77
Russian Federation	...	...	...	...	2002	3.0	...	...	...	...
Slovakia	...	...	...	...	...	...	...	...	...	...
Tajikistan	...	...	...	...	...	...	...	...	8	...
Turkmenistan	...	...	...	...	...	...	...	...	42	...
Ukraine	...	...	...	...	...	...	...	...	78	...
Uzbekistan	...	...	...	...	...	...	...	...	41	...
Western Europe										
Albania	...	...	...	...	...	...	...	...	40	...
Austria	...	...	...	...	...	...	...	...	...	...
Belgium	...	...	...	...	...	...	...	...	...	...
Denmark	...	...	...	...	...	...	...	...	...	...
Finland	...	...	...	...	...	...	...	...	...	...
France	...	...	...	...	...	...	...	...	...	...
Germany	...	...	...	...	...	...	...	...	...	...
Greece	...	...	...	...	...	...	...	...	...	...
Iceland	...	...	...	...	...	...	...	...	...	...
Ireland	...	...	...	...	...	...	...	...	...	...
Italy	...	...	...	...	...	...	...	...	...	...
Luxembourg	...	...	...	...	...	...	...	...	...	...
Malta	...	...	...	...	...	...	...	...	...	...
Netherlands	...	...	...	...	...	...	...	...	...	...
Norway	...	...	...	...	...	...	...	...	...	...
Portugal	...	...	...	...	...	...	...	...	...	...

6. Knowledge and behaviour indicators

	Can identify two prevention methods and reject three misconceptions (%) (15–24)		Had sex before age 15 (%) (15–19)		Reported higher-risk sex in the last year (%) (15–24)		Used a condom the last time they had higher-risk sex, of those who had high-risk sex in the last year (%) (15–24)		Year
Country	Female	Male	Female	Male	Female	Male	Female	Male	
South & South-East Asia									
Afghanistan	...	...	...	...	...	...	...	...	...
Bangladesh **	...	...	...	...	...	...	...	...	...
Bhutan	...	...	...	...	...	...	...	...	...
Brunei Darussalam	...	...	...	...	...	...	...	...	...
Cambodia	37	...	1	...	1	...	...	...	2000 d
India	21 x	17 x	...	...	2	12	51	59	2001 a
Indonesia	7	...	...	...	...	...	...	...	2000 c
Iran (Islamic Republic of)	...	...	...	...	...	...	...	...	...
Lao People's Dem. Rep.	...	...	...	...	...	...	...	...	...
Malaysia	...	...	...	...	...	...	...	...	...
Maldives	...	...	...	...	...	...	...	...	...
Myanmar **	...	...	...	...	...	...	...	...	...
Nepal	...	...	9	20	...	...	...	...	2001 d
Pakistan	...	...	...	...	...	...	...	...	...
Philippines	...	...	1 d,v	...	...	...	...	...	2000 c
Singapore	...	...	...	...	...	...	...	...	...
Sri Lanka	...	...	...	...	...	...	...	...	...
Thailand	...	...	...	...	...	...	...	...	...
Viet Nam	25	...	...	...	...	...	...	...	2000 c
Eastern Europe & Central Asia									
Armenia	7	8	1	1	0	69	0	44	2000 d
Azerbaijan	2	...	1 f,y	...	...	...	...	...	2000 c
Belarus	...	...	...	...	...	...	...	...	...
Bosnia and Herzegovina	...	...	...	...	...	...	...	...	2000 c
Bulgaria	...	...	...	...	...	...	...	...	...
Croatia	...	...	...	...	...	...	...	...	...
Czech Republic	...	...	...	...	...	...	...	...	...
Estonia	...	...	...	...	...	...	...	...	...
Georgia	...	...	3	...	...	...	...	...	1999 f
Hungary	...	...	...	...	...	...	...	...	...
Kazakhstan	...	...	1	6	27	78	32	65	1999 d
Kyrgyzstan	...	...	...	...	...	...	...	...	...
Latvia	...	...	...	...	...	...	...	...	...
Lithuania	...	...	...	...	...	...	...	...	...
Poland	...	...	...	...	...	...	...	...	...
Republic of Moldova	19	...	...	...	...	...	...	...	2000 c
Romania	...	...	3	12	...	...	...	...	1999 f
Russian Federation	...	...	...	...	...	...	...	...	...
Slovakia	...	...	...	...	...	...	...	...	...
Tajikistan	...	...	...	...	...	...	...	...	2000 c
Turkmenistan	...	...	0	...	...	...	...	...	2000 d
Ukraine	...	...	...	...	...	...	...	...	2000 c
Uzbekistan	3	...	...	...	...	...	...	...	2000 c
Western Europe									
Albania	0	...	...	...	...	...	...	...	2000 c
Austria	...	...	...	...	...	...	...	...	...
Belgium	...	...	...	...	...	...	...	...	...
Denmark	...	...	...	...	...	...	...	...	...
Finland	...	...	...	...	...	...	...	...	...
France	...	...	...	...	...	...	...	...	...
Germany	...	...	...	...	...	...	...	...	...
Greece	...	...	...	...	...	...	...	...	...
Iceland	...	...	...	...	...	...	...	...	...
Ireland	...	...	...	...	...	...	...	...	...
Italy	...	...	...	...	...	...	...	...	...
Luxembourg	...	...	...	...	...	...	...	...	...
Malta	...	...	...	...	...	...	...	...	...
Netherlands	...	...	...	...	...	...	...	...	...
Norway	...	...	...	...	...	...	...	...	...
Portugal	...	...	...	...	...	...	...	...	...

Country	1. Estimated number of people living with HIV: Adults and children, end 2003		Adults and children, end 2001		Adults (15–49), end 2003	
	Estimate	[low estimate - high estimate]	Estimate	[low estimate - high estimate]	Estimate	[low estimate - high estimate]
Serbia and Montenegro	10,000	[3,400 - 20,000]	10,000	[3,400 - 20,000]	10,000	[3,300 - 20,000]
Slovenia	<500	[<1,000]	<500	[<1,000]	<500	[<1,000]
Spain	140,000	[67,000 - 220,000]	130,000	[65,000 - 210,000]	130,000	[66,000 - 220,000]
Sweden	3,600	[1,200 - 6,900]	3,400	[1,100 - 6,600]	3,500	[1,200 - 6,900]
Switzerland	13,000	[6,500 - 21,000]	12,000	[6,000 - 20,000]	13,000	[6,400 - 21,000]
The former Yugoslav Republic of Macedonia	<200	[<400]	<200	[<400]	<200	[<400]
United Kingdom	32,000	[16,000 - 52,000]	24,000	[12,000 - 38,000]	31,000	[15,000 - 51,000]
North Africa & Middle East	**480,000**	**[200,000 - 1,400,000]**	**340,000**	**[130,000 - 910,000]**	**460,000**	**[190,000 - 1,300,000]**
Algeria	9,100	[3,000 - 18,000]	6,800	[2,200 - 14,000]	9,000	[3,000 - 18,000]
Bahrain	<600	[200 - 1,100]	<500	[<1,000]	<600	[200 - 1,100]
Cyprus	...	...	...	...	...	...
Egypt	12,000	[5,000 - 31,000]	11,000	[3,600 - 22,000]	12,000	[5,000 - 30,000]
Iraq	<500	[<1,000]	...	...	<500	[<1,000]
Israel	3,000	[1,500 - 4,900]	...	...	3,000	[1,500 - 4,900]
Jordan	600	[<1,000]	600	[<1,000]	<500	[<1,000]
Kuwait	...	...	...	...	...	...
Lebanon	2,800	[700 - 4,100]	2,000	[400 - 2,500]	2,800	[700 - 4,000]
Libyan Arab Jamahiriya	10,000	[3,300 - 20,000]	...	...	10,000	[3,300 - 20,000]
Morocco	15,000	[5,000 - 30,000]	...	...	15,000	[5,000 - 30,000]
Oman	1,300	[500 - 3,000]	1,000	[300 - 2,100]	1,300	[500 - 2,900]
Qatar	...	...	...	...	...	...
Saudi Arabia	...	...	...	...	...	...
Sudan	400,000	[120,000 - 1,300,000]	320,000	[110,000 - 890,000]	380,000	[120,000 - 1,200,000]
Syrian Arab Republic	<500	[300 - 2,100]	...	...	<500	[300 - 2,100]
Tunisia	1,000	[400 - 2,400]	600	[200 - 1,200]	1,000	[400 - 2,300]
Turkey	...	...	...	...	...	...
United Arab Emirates	...	...	...	...	...	...
Yemen	12,000	[4,000 - 24,000]	...	...	12,000	[4,000 - 24,000]
North America	**1,000,000**	**[520,000 - 1,600,000]**	**950,000**	**[490,000 - 1,500,000]**	**990,000**	**[510,000 - 1,600,000]**
Canada	56,000	[26,000 - 86,000]	49,000	[24,000 - 79,000]	55,000	[25,000 - 85,000]
United States of America	950,000	[470,000 - 1,600,000]	900,000	[450,000 - 1,500,000]	940,000	[460,000 - 1,500,000]
Caribbean	**430,000**	**[270,000 - 760,000]**	**400,000**	**[270,000 - 650,000]**	**410,000**	**[260,000 - 720,000]**
Bahamas	5,600	[3,200 - 8,700]	5,200	[3,300 - 8,300]	5,200	[3,100 - 8,400]
Barbados	2,500	[700 - 9,200]	2,500	[800 - 7,300]	2,500	[700 - 9,100]
Cuba	3,300	[1,100 - 6,600]	3,200	[1,100 - 6,500]	3,300	[1,100 - 6,400]
Dominican Republic	88,000	[48,000 - 160,000]	90,000	[52,000 - 150,000]	85,000	[47,000 - 150,000]
Haiti	280,000	[120,000 - 600,000]	260,000	[130,000 - 500,000]	260,000	[120,000 - 560,000]
Jamaica	22,000	[11,000 - 41,000]	15,000	[7,700 - 28,000]	21,000	[11,000 - 40,000]
Trinidad and Tobago	29,000	[11,000 - 74,000]	26,000	[11,000 - 59,000]	28,000	[10,000 - 72,000]
Latin America	**1,600,000**	**[1,200,000 - 2,100,000]**	**1,400,000**	**[1,100,000 - 1,800,000]**	**1,600,000**	**[1,200,000 - 2,000,000]**
Argentina	130,000	[61,000 - 210,000]	120,000	[59,000 - 200,000]	120,000	[61,000 - 200,000]
Belize	3,600	[1,200 - 10,000]	2,900	[1,100 - 7,200]	3,500	[1,200 - 9,800]
Bolivia	4,900	[1,600 - 11,000]	4,200	[1,300 - 9,000]	4,800	[1,600 - 9,400]
Brazil	660,000	[320,000 - 1,100,000]	630,000	[310,000 - 1,000,000]	650,000	[320,000 - 1,100,000]
Chile	26,000	[13,000 - 44,000]	25,000	[12,000 - 42,000]	26,000	[13,000 - 43,000]
Colombia	190,000	[90,000 - 310,000]	130,000	[61,000 - 210,000]	180,000	[90,000 - 300,000]
Costa Rica	12,000	[6,000 - 21,000]	11,000	[5,500 - 19,000]	12,000	[6,000 - 20,000]
Ecuador	21,000	[10,000 - 38,000]	20,000	[9,700 - 36,000]	20,000	[10,000 - 34,000]
El Salvador	29,000	[14,000 - 50,000]	24,000	[12,000 - 43,000]	28,000	[14,000 - 46,000]
Guatemala	78,000	[38,000 - 130,000]	69,000	[34,000 - 110,000]	74,000	[36,000 - 120,000]
Guyana *	11,000	[3,500 - 35,000]	11,000	[4,300 - 30,000]	11,000	[3,300 - 33,000]
Honduras	63,000	[35,000 - 110,000]	51,000	[29,000 - 90,000]	59,000	[33,000 - 100,000]
Mexico	160,000	[78,000 - 260,000]	150,000	[74,000 - 250,000]	160,000	[78,000 - 260,000]
Nicaragua	6,400	[3,100 - 12,000]	5,800	[2,700 - 10,000]	6,200	[3,000 - 10,000]
Panama	16,000	[7,700 - 26,000]	11,000	[5,500 - 19,000]	15,000	[7,500 - 25,000]
Paraguay	15,000	[7,300 - 25,000]	10,000	[5,000 - 17,000]	15,000	[7,300 - 24,000]
Peru	82,000	[40,000 - 140,000]	53,000	[26,000 - 88,000]	80,000	[39,000 - 130,000]
Suriname	5,200	[1,400 - 18,000]	4,100	[1,300 - 13,000]	5,000	[1,400 - 18,000]
Uruguay	6,000	[2,800 - 9,700]	5,600	[2,700 - 9,500]	5,800	[2,800 - 9,400]
Venezuela	110,000	[47,000 - 170,000]	73,000	[35,000 - 120,000]	100,000	[47,000 - 160,000]
Global Total	**37,800,000**	**[34,600,000 - 42,300,000]**	**34,900,000**	**[32,000,000 - 39,000,000]**	**35,700,000**	**[32,700,000 - 39,800,000]**

	1. Estimated number of people living with HIV (continued)							
	Adults (15–49), end 2001		Adults (15–49) rate (%) end 2003		Adults (15–49) rate (%) end 2001		Women (15–49), end 2003	
Country	Estimate	[low estimate - high estimate]	Estimate	[low estimate - high estimate]	Estimate	[low estimate - high estimate]	Estimate	[low estimate - high estimate]
Serbia and Montenegro	10,000	[3,300 - 20,000]	0.2	[0.1 - 0.4]	0.2	[0.1 - 0.4]	2,000	[700 - 3,900]
Slovenia	<500	[<1,000]	<0.1	[<0.2]	<0.1	[<0.2]	...	...
Spain	130,000	[64,000 - 210,000]	0.7	[0.3 - 1.1]	0.6	[0.3 - 1.0]	27,000	[13,000 - 44,000]
Sweden	3,300	[1,100 - 6,500]	0.1	[0.0 - 0.2]	0.1	[0.0 - 0.2]	900	[300 - 1,800]
Switzerland	12,000	[5,900 - 20,000]	0.4	[0.2 - 0.6]	0.4	[0.2 - 0.6]	3,900	[1,900 - 6,400]
The former Yugoslav Republic of Macedonia	<200	[<400]	<0.1	[<0.2]	<0.1	[<0.2]	...	...
United Kingdom	23,000	[11,000 - 37,000]	0.1	[0.1 - 0.2]	0.1	[<0.2]	7,000	[3,400 - 11,000]
North Africa & Middle East	**320,000**	**[130,000 - 860,000]**	**0.2**	**[0.1 - 0.6]**	**0.2**	**[0.1 - 0.5]**	**220,000**	**[70,000 - 690,000]**
Algeria	6,800	[2,200 - 13,000]	0.1	[<0.2]	<0.1	[<0.2]	1,400	[500 - 2,700]
Bahrain	<500	[<1,000]	0.2	[0.1 - 0.3]	0.1	[0.0 - 0.2]	<500	[<1,000]
Cyprus	...	...	...	...	...	...	...	...
Egypt	11,000	[3,600 - 21,000]	<0.1	[<0.2]	<0.1	[<0.2]	1,600	[500 - 3,200]
Iraq	...	...	<0.1	[<0.2]	...	...	...	...
Israel	...	...	0.1	[0.1 - 0.2]	...	...	...	...
Jordan	<500	[<1,000]	<0.1	[<0.2]	<0.1	[<0.2]	...	...
Kuwait	...	...	...	...	...	...	...	...
Lebanon	2,000	[400 - 2,400]	0.1	[0.0 - 0.2]	0.1	[<0.2]	<500	[<1,000]
Libyan Arab Jamahiriya	...	...	0.3	[0.1 - 0.6]	...	...	...	...
Morocco	...	...	0.1	[0.0 - 0.2]	...	...	...	...
Oman	1,000	[300 - 2,000]	0.1	[0.0 - 0.2]	0.1	[0.0 - 0.2]	<500	[<1,000]
Qatar	...	...	...	...	...	...	...	...
Saudi Arabia	...	...	...	...	...	...	...	...
Sudan	300,000	[100,000 - 840,000]	2.3	[0.7 - 7.2]	1.9	[0.7 - 5.2]	220,000	[66,000 - 690,000]
Syrian Arab Republic	...	...	<0.1	[<0.2]	...	...	<200	[<1,000]
Tunisia	500	[200 - 1,100]	<0.1	[<0.2]	<0.1	[<0.2]	<500	[<1,000]
Turkey	...	...	...	...	...	...	...	...
United Arab Emirates	...	...	...	...	...	...	...	...
Yemen	...	...	0.1	[0.0 - 0.2]	...	...	...	...
North America	**940,000**	**[480,000 - 1,500,000]**	**0.6**	**[0.3 - 1.0]**	**0.6**	**[0.3 - 1.0]**	**250,000**	**[130,000 - 400,000]**
Canada	48,000	[24,000 - 79,000]	0.3	[0.2 - 0.5]	0.3	[0.2 - 0.5]	13,000	[6,400 - 21,000]
United States of America	890,000	[440,000 - 1,500,000]	0.6	[0.3 - 1.1]	0.6	[0.3 - 1.0]	240,000	[120,000 - 390,000]
Caribbean	**380,000**	**[260,000 - 610,000]**	**2.3**	**[1.4 - 4.1]**	**2.2**	**[1.5 - 3.5]**	**200,000**	**[120,000 - 370,000]**
Bahamas	4,900	[3,200 - 8,000]	3.0	[1.8 - 4.9]	3.0	[1.9 - 4.8]	2,500	[1,500 - 4,200]
Barbados	2,500	[800 - 7,300]	1.5	[0.4 - 5.4]	1.5	[0.5 - 4.4]	800	[200 - 3,100]
Cuba	3,200	[1,100 - 6,300]	0.1	[<0.2]	0.1	[<0.2]	1,100	[400 - 2,100]
Dominican Republic	87,000	[51,000 - 150,000]	1.7	[0.9 - 3.0]	1.8	[1.1 - 3.1]	23,000	[13,000 - 41,000]
Haiti	240,000	[130,000 - 460,000]	5.6	[2.5 - 11.9]	5.5	[2.8 - 10.4]	150,000	[66,000 - 320,000]
Jamaica	14,000	[7,500 - 27,000]	1.2	[0.6 - 2.2]	0.8	[0.4 - 1.6]	10,000	[5,500 - 20,000]
Trinidad and Tobago	26,000	[11,000 - 57,000]	3.2	[1.2 - 8.3]	3.0	[1.3 - 6.8]	14,000	[5,200 - 36,000]
Latin America	**1,400,000**	**[1,000,000 - 1,800,000]**	**0.6**	**[0.5 - 0.8]**	**0.5**	**[0.4 - 0.7]**	**560,000**	**[420,000 - 730,000]**
Argentina	120,000	[59,000 - 200,000]	0.7	[0.3 - 1.1]	0.7	[0.3 - 1.1]	24,000	[12,000 - 39,000]
Belize	2,800	[1,100 - 6,900]	2.4	[0.8 - 6.9]	2.1	[0.8 - 5.2]	1,300	[400 - 3,600]
Bolivia	4,000	[1,300 - 7,900]	0.1	[0.0 - 0.2]	0.1	[0.0 - 0.2]	1,300	[400 - 2,500]
Brazil	620,000	[300,000 - 1,000,000]	0.7	[0.3 - 1.1]	0.6	[0.3 - 1.1]	240,000	[120,000 - 400,000]
Chile	25,000	[12,000 - 41,000]	0.3	[0.2 - 0.5]	0.3	[0.2 - 0.5]	8,700	[4,300 - 14,000]
Colombia	120,000	[61,000 - 200,000]	0.7	[0.4 - 1.2]	0.5	[0.3 - 0.8]	62,000	[30,000 - 100,000]
Costa Rica	11,000	[5,400 - 18,000]	0.6	[0.3 - 1.0]	0.6	[0.3 - 0.9]	4,000	[2,000 - 6,600]
Ecuador	19,000	[9,500 - 32,000]	0.3	[0.1 - 0.5]	0.3	[0.1 - 0.5]	6,800	[3,400 - 11,000]
El Salvador	24,000	[12,000 - 39,000]	0.7	[0.3 - 1.1]	0.6	[0.3 - 1.0]	9,600	[4,700 - 16,000]
Guatemala	65,000	[32,000 - 110,000]	1.1	[0.6 - 1.8]	1.1	[0.5 - 1.7]	31,000	[15,000 - 51,000]
Guyana *	11,000	[4,000 - 28,000]	2.5	[0.8 - 7.7]	2.5	[0.9 - 6.4]	6,100	[1,900 - 19,000]
Honduras	48,000	[27,000 - 84,000]	1.8	[1.0 - 3.2]	1.6	[0.9 - 2.8]	33,000	[19,000 - 59,000]
Mexico	150,000	[74,000 - 250,000]	0.3	[0.1 - 0.4]	0.3	[0.1 - 0.4]	53,000	[26,000 - 87,000]
Nicaragua	5,500	[2,700 - 9,100]	0.2	[0.1 - 0.3]	0.2	[0.1 - 0.3]	2,100	[1,000 - 3,400]
Panama	11,000	[5,400 - 18,000]	0.9	[0.5 - 1.5]	0.7	[0.3 - 1.1]	6,200	[3,100 - 10,000]
Paraguay	10,000	[5,000 - 17,000]	0.5	[0.2 - 0.8]	0.4	[0.2 - 0.6]	3,900	[1,900 - 6,400]
Peru	51,000	[25,000 - 84,000]	0.5	[0.3 - 0.9]	0.4	[0.2 - 0.6]	27,000	[13,000 - 44,000]
Suriname	4,000	[1,300 - 12,000]	1.7	[0.5 - 5.8]	1.3	[0.4 - 4.1]	1,700	[500 - 6,100]
Uruguay	5,500	[2,700 - 9,100]	0.3	[0.2 - 0.5]	0.3	[0.2 - 0.5]	1,900	[900 - 3,200]
Venezuela	71,000	[35,000 - 120,000]	0.7	[0.4 - 1.2]	0.6	[0.3 - 0.9]	32,000	[16,000 - 53,000]
Global Total	**32,900,000**	**[30,200,000 - 36,700,000]**	**1.1**	**[1.0 - 1.2]**	**1.0**	**[0.9 - 1.1]**	**17,000,000**	**[15,800,000 - 18,800,000]**

	1. Estimated number of people living with HIV (continued)					
	Women (15–49), end 2001		Children (0–14), end 2003		Children (0–14), end 2001	
Country	**Estimate**	**[low estimate - high estimate]**	**Estimate**	**[low estimate - high estimate]**	**Estimate**	**[low estimate - high estimate]**
Serbia and Montenegro	2,000	[700 - 3,900]	...	...	...	...
Slovenia	...	...	...	...	...	...
Spain	26,000	[13,000 - 43,000]	...	...	...	...
Sweden	900	[300 - 1,700]	...	...	...	...
Switzerland	3,600	[1,800 - 5,900]	...	...	...	...
The former Yugoslav Republic of Macedonia	...	...	...	...	...	...
United Kingdom	5,000	[2,500 - 8,200]	...	...	...	...
North Africa & Middle East	**170,000**	**[62,000 - 480,000]**	**21,000**	**[6,300 - 72,000]**	**16,000**	**[5,400 - 48,000]**
Algeria	800	[300 - 1,600]	...	...	...	...
Bahrain	<200	[<400]	...	...	...	...
Cyprus	...	...	...	...	...	...
Egypt	1,200	[400 - 2,300]	...	...	...	...
Iraq	...	...	...	...	...	...
Israel	...	...	...	...	...	...
Jordan	...	...	...	...	...	...
Kuwait	...	...	...	...	...	...
Lebanon	<500	[<1,000]	...	...	...	...
Libyan Arab Jamahiriya	...	...	...	...	...	...
Morocco	...	...	...	...	...	...
Oman	<200	[<400]	...	...	...	...
Qatar	...	...	...	...	...	...
Saudi Arabia	...	...	...	...	...	...
Sudan	170,000	[59,000 - 470,000]	21,000	[6,000 - 72,000]	16,000	[5,200 - 48,000]
Syrian Arab Republic	...	...	...	...	...	...
Tunisia	<200	[<400]	...	...	...	...
Turkey	...	...	...	...	...	...
United Arab Emirates	...	...	...	...	...	...
Yemen	...	...	...	...	...	...
North America	**190,000**	**[100,000 - 310,000]**	**11,000**	**[5,600 - 17,300]**	**11,000**	**[5,500 - 17,200]**
Canada	12,000	[5,900 - 20,000]	...	...	...	...
United States of America	180,000	[88,000 - 300,000]	...	...	...	...
Caribbean	**180,000**	**[120,000 - 310,000]**	**22,000**	**[11,000 - 48,000]**	**22,000**	**[12,000 - 42,000]**
Bahamas	2,500	[1,600 - 4,000]	<200	[<400]	<200	[<400]
Barbados	800	[300 - 2,400]	<200	[<400]	<200	[<400]
Cuba	1,000	[300 - 2,000]	...	...	...	...
Dominican Republic	23,000	[13,000 - 39,000]	2,200	[1,100 - 4,400]	2,100	[1,100 - 4,100]
Haiti	140,000	[71,000 - 260,000]	19,000	[7,900 - 45,000]	18,000	[8,700 - 39,000]
Jamaica	7,200	[3,700 - 14,000]	<500	[<1,000]	<500	[<1,000]
Trinidad and Tobago	13,000	[5,600 - 28,000]	700	[300 - 2,100]	600	[300 - 1,500]
Latin America	**480,000**	**[360,000 - 640,000]**	**25,000**	**[20,000 - 41,000]**	**24,000**	**[19,000 - 40,000]**
Argentina	23,000	[11,000 - 37,000]	...	...	...	...
Belize	1,000	[400 - 2,500]	<200	[<400]	<200	[<400]
Bolivia	1,100	[300 - 2,100]	...	...	...	...
Brazil	230,000	[110,000 - 380,000]	...	...	...	...
Chile	8,000	[3,900 - 13,000]	...	...	...	...
Colombia	40,000	[20,000 - 65,000]	...	...	...	...
Costa Rica	3,500	[1,700 - 5,700]	...	...	...	...
Ecuador	6,200	[3,000 - 10,000]	...	...	...	...
El Salvador	7,700	[3,800 - 13,000]	...	...	...	...
Guatemala	27,000	[13,000 - 45,000]	...	...	...	...
Guyana *	6,100	[2,300 - 16,000]	600	[200 - 2,000]	700	[200 - 1,900]
Honduras	27,000	[15,000 - 47,000]	3,900	[2,000 - 7,800]	3,200	[1,600 - 6,200]
Mexico	49,000	[24,000 - 80,000]	...	...	...	...
Nicaragua	1,800	[900 - 2,900]	...	...	...	...
Panama	4,100	[2,000 - 6,700]	...	...	...	...
Paraguay	2,700	[1,300 - 4,400]	...	...	...	...
Peru	16,000	[8,000 - 27,000]	...	...	...	...
Suriname	1,300	[400 - 3,900]	<200	[<800]	<200	[<800]
Uruguay	1,800	[900 - 2,900]	...	...	...	...
Venezuela	23,000	[11,000 - 37,000]	...	...	...	...
Global Total	**15,700,000**	**[14,600,000 - 17,400,000]**	**2,100,000**	**[1,900,000 - 2,500,000]**	**2,000,000**	**[1,800,000 - 2,300,000]**

	2. AIDS deaths				3. Orphans due to AIDS			
	Deaths in adults and children, end 2003		Deaths in adults and children, end 2001		Orphans (0–17), living 2003		Orphans (0–17), living in 2001	
ountry	Estimate	[low estimate - high estimate]	Estimate	[low estimate - high estimate]	Estimate	[low estimate - high estimate]	Estimate	[low estimate - high estimate]
erbia and Montenegro	<100	[<200]	<100	[<200]	...	...	...	...
lovenia	<100	[<200]	<100	[<200]	...	...	...	...
pain	<1000	[<2,000]	<1000	[<2,000]	...	...	...	...
weden	<100	[<200]	<100	[<200]	...	...	...	...
witzerland	<200	[<400]	<200	[<400]	...	...	...	...
he former Yugoslav Republic of Macedonia	<100	[<200]	<100	[<200]	...	...	...	...
nited Kingdom	<500	[<1,000]	<500	[<1,000]	...	...	...	...
orth Africa & Middle East	**24,000**	**[9,900 - 62,000]**	**17,000**	**[7,500 - 40,000]**				
lgeria	<500	[<1,000]	<500	[<1,000]	...	...	...	...
ahrain	<200	[<400]	<200	[<400]	...	...	...	...
yprus	...	...	...	...	...	...	...	...
gypt	700	[200 - 1,600]	<500	[<1,000]	...	...	...	...
aq	...	...	...	...	...	...	...	...
srael	...	...	...	...	...	...	...	...
ordan	<200	[<400]	<200	[<400]	...	...	...	...
uwait	...	...	...	...	...	...	...	...
ebanon	<200	[<400]	<200	[<400]	...	...	...	...
ibyan Arab Jamahiriya	...	...	...	...	...	...	...	...
lorocco	...	...	...	...	...	...	...	...
man	<200	[<400]	<200	[<400]	...	...	...	...
atar	...	...	...	...	...	...	...	...
audi Arabia	...	...	...	...	...	...	...	...
udan	23,000	[8,700 - 61,000]	16,000	[6,800 - 39,000]	...	...	...	...
yrian Arab Republic	<200	[<400]	...	...	...	...	...	...
unisia	<200	[<400]	<200	[<400]	...	...	...	...
urkey	...	...	...	...	...	...	...	...
nited Arab Emirates	...	...	...	...	...	...	...	...
emen	...	...	...	...	...	...	...	...
orth America	**16,000**	**[8,300 - 25,000]**	**16,000**	**[8,300 - 25,000]**				
anada	1,500	[740 - 2,500]	1,500	[740 - 2,500]	...	...	...	...
nited States of America	14,000	[6,900 - 23,000]	14,000	[6,900 - 23,000]	...	...	...	...
aribbean	**35,000**	**[23,000 - 59,000]**	**32,000**	**[22,000 - 50,000]**				
ahamas	<200	[<400]	<200	[<400]	...	...	...	...
arbados	<200	[<400]	<200	[<400]	...	...	...	...
uba	<200	[<400]	<200	[<400]	...	...	...	...
ominican Republic	7,900	[4,700 - 13,000]	7,000	[4,200 - 12,000]	...	...	...	...
aiti	24,000	[12,000 - 47,000]	22,000	[13,000 - 40,000]	...	...	...	...
Jamaica	900	[500 - 1,600]	<500	[<1,000]	...	...	...	...
Trinidad and Tobago	1,900	[900 - 4,100]	1,500	[800 - 2,900]	...	...	...	...
atin America	**84,000**	**[65,000 - 110,000]**	**63,000**	**[50,000 - 81,000]**				
Argentina	1,500 ***	[1,400 - 3,000] ***	1,500 ***	[1,400 - 3,000] ***	...	...	...	...
Belize	<200	[<400]	<200	[<400]	...	...	...	...
Bolivia	<500	[<1,000]	<500	[<1,000]	...	...	...	...
Brazil	15,000 ***	[14,000 - 22,000] ***	14,600 ***	[13,000 - 20,000] ***	...	...	...	...
Chile	1,400	[700 - 2,500]	800	[400 - 1,500]	...	...	...	...
Colombia	3,600 ***	[2,200 - 6,000] ***	3,300 ***	[2,000 - 5,800] ***	...	...	...	...
Costa Rica	900	[400 - 1,600]	800	[400 - 1,400]	...	...	...	...
Ecuador	1,700	[800 - 3,600]	1,600	[700 - 3,200]	...	...	...	...
El Salvador	2,200	[1,000 - 4,100]	2,000	[1,000 - 3,800]	...	...	...	...
Guatemala	5,800	[2,900 - 10,000]	4,900	[2,400 - 8,400]	...	...	...	...
Guyana *	1,100	[500 - 2,600]	1,300	[600 - 2,700]	...	...	...	...
Honduras	4,100	[2,300 - 7,200]	3,100	[1,700 - 5,500]	...	...	...	...
Mexico	5,000 ***	[4,500 - 10,000] ***	4,200 ***	[4,000 - 9,000] ***	...	...	...	...
Nicaragua	<500	[<1,000]	<500	[<1,000]	...	...	...	...
Panama	<500	[<1,000]	<200	[<400]	...	...	...	...
Paraguay	600	[300 - 1,000]	<500	[<1,000]	...	...	...	...
Peru	4,200	[2,100 - 7,300]	3,700	[1,800 - 6,400]	...	...	...	...
Suriname	<500	[<1,000]	<500	[<1,000]	...	...	...	...
Uruguay	<500	[<1,000]	<500	[<1,000]	...	...	...	...
Venezuela	4,100	[1,900 - 8,000]	2,600	[1,200 - 5,300]	...	...	...	...
Global Total	**2,900,000**	**[2,600,000 - 3,300,000]**	**2,500,000**	**[2,300,000 - 2,800,000]**	**15,000,000**	**[13,000,000 - 18,000,000]**	**11,500,000**	**[10,000,000 - 14,000,000]**

	4. HIV prevalence (%) in young pregnant women (15–24) in capital city		5. HIV prevalence (%) in groups with high-risk behaviour in capital city						6. Knowledge and behaviour indicators	
			Injecting drug users		Sex workers		Men who have sex with men		Know a healthy-looking person can have HIV (%) (15–24)	
Country	**Year**	**Median**	**Year**	**Median**	**Year**	**Median**	**Year**	**Median**	**Female**	**Male**
Serbia and Montenegro	...	...	...	...	...	...	...	...	...	...
Slovenia	...	...	...	...	...	...	1999	1.7	...	...
Spain	...	...	...	...	...	...	...	...	...	...
Sweden	...	...	...	...	...	...	...	...	...	...
Switzerland	...	...	...	...	...	...	...	...	...	...
The former Yugoslav Republic of Macedonia	...	...	...	...	...	...	...	...	...	
United Kingdom	...	...	...	...	...	...	...	...	...	...
North Africa & Middle East										
Algeria	...	...	...	...	...	...	...	...	...	...
Bahrain	...	...	...	...	...	...	...	...	...	...
Cyprus	...	...	...	...	...	...	...	...	...	...
Egypt	...	...	...	...	...	...	...	...	...	...
Iraq	...	...	...	...	...	...	...	...	...	...
Israel	...	...	...	...	...	...	...	...	...	...
Jordan	...	...	...	...	...	...	...	...	...	...
Kuwait	...	...	...	...	...	...	...	...	...	...
Lebanon	...	...	...	...	...	...	...	...	...	...
Libyan Arab Jamahiriya	...	...	...	...	...	...	...	...	...	...
Morocco	...	...	...	...	...	...	...	...	...	...
Oman	...	...	...	...	...	...	...	...	...	...
Qatar	...	...	...	...	...	...	...	...	...	...
Saudi Arabia	...	...	...	...	...	...	...	...	...	...
Sudan	...	...	...	...	...	...	...	...	...	...
Syrian Arab Republic	...	...	...	...	...	...	...	...	...	...
Tunisia	...	...	...	...	...	...	...	...	...	...
Turkey	...	...	...	...	...	...	...	...	...	...
United Arab Emirates	...	...	...	...	...	...	...	...	...	...
Yemen	...	...	...	...	...	...	...	...	...	...
North America										
Canada	...	...	...	...	...	...	...	...	...	...
United States of America	...	...	...	...	...	...	...	...	...	...
Caribbean										
Bahamas	...	...	...	...	...	...	...	...	...	...
Barbados	...	...	...	...	...	...	...	...	...	...
Cuba	...	...	...	...	...	...	...	...	91	...
Dominican Republic	...	...	...	...	1999	3.5	...	...	92	91
Haiti	...	...	...	...	...	...	...	...	68	78
Jamaica	...	...	...	...	...	...	...	...	...	...
Trinidad and Tobago	...	...	...	...	...	...	...	...	95	...
Latin America										
Argentina	...	...	2001	44.3	...	...	2001	24.3	...	...
Belize	...	...	...	...	...	...	...	...	...	...
Bolivia	...	...	...	...	...	...	...	...	64	74
Brazil	...	...	...	...	...	...	...	...	...	...
Chile	...	...	...	...	...	...	...	...	...	...
Colombia	...	...	...	...	...	...	...	...	82	...
Costa Rica	...	...	...	...	...	...	...	...	...	...
Ecuador	...	...	...	...	2002	14.0	...	...	58 w	...
El Salvador	...	...	...	...	2002	4.0	2002	17.7	68	...
Guatemala	...	...	...	...	2002	3.3	2002	11.5	...	...
Guyana *	...	...	...	...	...	...	...	...	84	...
Honduras	...	...	...	...	2002	8.1	2002	8.2	81	90
Mexico	...	...	...	...	1999	0.3	...	...	...	...
Nicaragua	...	...	...	...	2002	0.0	2002	9.3	73 z	...
Panama	...	...	...	...	2002	1.8	2002	10.6	...	...
Paraguay	...	...	...	...	...	...	...	...	...	...
Peru	...	...	...	...	...	...	2002	22.0	72	...
Suriname	...	...	...	...	...	...	...	...	70	...
Uruguay	...	...	...	...	...	...	...	...	...	...
Venezuela	...	...	...	...	...	...	...	...	78	...
Global Total										

6. Knowledge and behaviour indicators

	Can identify two prevention methods and reject three misconceptions (%) (15–24)		Had sex before age 15 (%) (15–19)		Reported higher-risk sex in the last year (%) (15–24)		Used a condom the last time they had higher-risk sex, of those who had high-risk sex in the last year (%) (15–24)		Year
Country	**Female**	**Male**	**Female**	**Male**	**Female**	**Male**	**Female**	**Male**	
Serbia and Montenegro	...	...	...	...	...	...	...	...	...
Slovenia	...	...	...	...	...	...	...	...	...
Spain	...	...	...	...	...	...	...	...	...
Sweden	...	...	...	...	...	...	...	...	...
Switzerland	...	...	...	...	...	...	...	...	...
The former Yugoslav Republic of Macedonia	...	...	...	...	...	...	...	...	...
United Kingdom	...	...	...	...	...	...	...	...	...
North Africa & Middle East									
Algeria	...	...	...	...	...	...	...	...	...
Bahrain	...	...	...	...	...	...	...	...	...
Cyprus	...	...	...	...	...	...	...	...	...
Egypt	...	...	...	...	...	...	...	...	...
Iraq	...	...	...	...	...	...	...	...	...
Israel	...	...	...	...	...	...	...	...	...
Jordan	...	...	...	...	...	...	...	...	...
Kuwait	...	...	...	...	...	...	...	...	...
Lebanon	...	...	...	...	...	...	...	...	...
Libyan Arab Jamahiriya	...	...	...	...	...	...	...	...	...
Morocco	...	...	...	...	...	...	...	...	...
Oman	...	...	...	...	...	...	...	...	...
Qatar	...	...	...	...	...	...	...	...	...
Saudi Arabia	...	...	...	...	...	...	...	...	...
Sudan	...	...	...	...	...	...	...	...	...
Syrian Arab Republic	...	...	...	...	...	...	...	...	...
Tunisia	...	...	...	...	...	...	...	...	...
Turkey	...	...	...	0	...	...	...	...	1998 d
United Arab Emirates	...	...	...	...	...	...	...	...	...
Yemen	...	...	...	...	...	...	...	...	...
North America									
Canada	...	...	...	...	...	...	...	...	...
United States of America	...	...	...	...	...	...	...	...	...
Caribbean									
Bahamas	...	...	...	...	...	...	...	...	...
Barbados	...	...	...	...	...	...	...	...	...
Cuba	52	...	...	...	...	...	...	...	2000 c
Dominican Republic	...	...	13	18	16	49	...	...	2002 d
Haiti	14	24	12	28	59	93	19	30	2000 d
Jamaica	...	...	...	...	...	...	...	...	...
Trinidad and Tobago	33	...	...	...	...	...	...	...	2000 c
Latin America									
Argentina	...	...	...	...	...	...	...	...	...
Belize	...	...	...	...	...	...	...	...	...
Bolivia	22 c,x	...	5	15	...	...	...	...	1998 d
Brazil	...	...	...	...	...	...	...	...	...
Chile	...	...	...	...	...	...	...	...	...
Colombia	...	...	10	...	49	...	29	...	2000 d
Costa Rica	...	...	...	...	...	...	...	...	...
Ecuador	...	...	7	...	...	...	...	...	2001 f
El Salvador	...	...	...	...	...	...	...	...	1998 f
Guatemala	...	...	7	15	...	...	...	...	2002 f
Guyana *	36	...	...	...	...	...	...	...	2000 c
Honduras	...	...	13	19	...	...	...	...	2001 f
Mexico	...	...	...	...	...	...	...	...	...
Nicaragua	...	...	11	...	10	...	17	...	2001 d
Panama	...	...	...	...	...	...	...	...	...
Paraguay	...	...	...	...	...	...	...	...	...
Peru	...	...	5	...	29	...	19	...	2000 d
Suriname	27	...	...	...	...	...	...	...	2000 c
Uruguay	...	...	...	...	...	...	...	...	...
Venezuela	...	...	...	...	...	...	...	...	2000 c
Global Total									

Annex:

HIV/AIDS estimates and data, end 2003 and end 2001

The estimates and data provided in the following tables relate to the end of 2003 and the end of 2001 unless stated otherwise. These estimates have been produced and compiled by UNAIDS/WHO. They have been shared with national AIDS programmes for review and comments, but are not necessarily the official estimates used by national governments. For countries where no recent data were available, country-specific estimates have not been listed in the table. In order to calculate regional totals, older data or regional models were used to produce minimum estimates for these countries.

The estimates are given in rounded numbers. However, unrounded numbers were used in the calculation of rates and regional totals, so there may be minor discrepancies between the regional/global totals and the sum of the country figures.

The general methodology and tools used to produce the country-specific estimates in the table have been described in a series of papers in Sexually Transmitted Infections 2004, 80 (Suppl 1). The estimates produced by UNAIDS/WHO are based on methods and on parameters that are informed by advice given by the UNAIDS Reference Group on HIV/AIDS Estimates, Modelling and Projections.

This group is made up of leading researchers in HIV and AIDS, epidemiology, demography and related areas. The Reference Group assesses the most recent published and unpublished work drawn from research studies in different countries. It also reviews advances in the understanding of HIV epidemics, and suggests methods to improve the quality and accuracy of the estimates.

Based on suggestions from the Reference Group, new software has been developed to model the course of HIV epidemics and their impact. These changes in procedures and assumptions have resulted in improved estimates of HIV and AIDS for 2003. To allow readers to assess recent trends in the epidemic, we also present end-2001 estimates developed using the same methodology and data as for the end-2003 estimates.

The new estimates in this report are presented together with ranges, called 'plausibility bounds'. These bounds reflect the certainty associated with each of the estimates. The wider the bounds, the greater the uncertainty surrounding an estimate. The extent of uncertainty depends mainly on the type of epidemic, and the quality, coverage and consistency of a country's surveillance system. A full description of the methods used to develop plausibility bounds can be found in Sexually Transmitted Infections 2004, 80 (Suppl 1).

Adults in this report are defined as men and women aged 15–49 years. This age range captures those in their most sexually active years. While the risk of HIV infection continues beyond 50 years, the vast majority of people who will become infected are likely to have done so by this age.

Since population structures differ greatly from one country to another, especially for children and older adults, the restriction of 'adults' to 15–49-year-olds has the advantage of making different populations more comparable. This age range was used as the denominator in calculating the adult HIV prevalence proportion. It is also consistent with previous estimates.

Notes on specific indicators listed in the table

1. Estimated number of people living with HIV, end-2003 and end-2001

These estimates include all people with HIV infection, whether or not they have developed symptoms of AIDS, alive at the end of 2003 and the end of 2001. For countries marked with one asterisk (*) a population-based survey with HIV prevalence measurement will be conducted in the near future. For countries marked with two asterisks (**), new surveillance has been conducted recently but the results were not available for inclusion in the estimation process. For some countries where sufficient data from the last six years were not available, no estimates have been made.

Adults and children

Estimated number of adults and children living with HIV at the end of 2003 and 2001. Children are defined as those aged 0–14 years.

Adults (15–49 years)

Estimated number of adults living with HIV at the end of 2003 and 2001.

Adult (15–49 years) prevalence proportion (%)

To calculate the adult HIV prevalence proportion, the estimated number of adults living with HIV at the end of 2003 was divided by the 2003 adult population (aged 15–49) and similarly for 2001.

Women (15–49 years)

Estimated number of women (aged 15–49) living with HIV at the end of 2003 and 2001.

Children (0–14 years)

Estimated number of children under age 15 living with HIV at the end of 2003 and 2001.

2. AIDS deaths

Adults and children

Estimated number of adults and children who died of AIDS during 2003 and 2001. Estimates and ranges marked with three asterisks (***) have been informed by data from vital registration systems.

3. Orphans due to AIDS

Orphans (0–17 years) currently living

Estimated number of children aged 0-17 years as of end-2003 who have lost one or both parents to AIDS.

4. Plausibility bounds for the above indicators

Depending on the reliability of the data available, there may be more or less uncertainty surrounding each estimate. While a measure of uncertainty applies to all estimates, in this report the plausibility bounds are presented for the following estimates:

- Estimated number of adults (15–49 years) and children (0–14 years) living with HIV at the end of 2003 and 2001
- Estimated number of adults (15–49 years) living with HIV at the end of 2003 and 2001
- Estimated number of women (15–49 years) living with HIV at the end of 2003 and 2001
- Estimated number of children (0–14 years) living with HIV at the end of 2003 and 2001
- Estimated number of AIDS deaths in adults (15–49 years) and children (0–14 years) during 2003 and 2001
- Orphans (0–17 years) due to AIDS in 2003 and 2001

5. HIV prevalence proportion (%) in young pregnant women (15–24 years) in capital city, antenatal clinic sites

These indicators are taken from the 2001 United Nations General Assembly Special Session on HIV/AIDS, and give a reasonable estimate of relatively recent trends over time in HIV infection in countries with generalized epidemics (prevalence over 1%) that are predominantly heterosexually driven. The number of pregnant women attending antenatal clinics (ANC) aged 15–24 years whose test results were positive is divided by the number of pregnant women aged

15–24 years who had an HIV test. The median of the capital city sites and year of the last report are included.

6. HIV prevalence proportion (%) among specific populations at higher risk of HIV exposure in capital cities

These indicators are recommended for reporting against the goals of the 2001 United Nations General Assembly Special Session on HIV/AIDS in countries with low-level epidemics (prevalence under 1%; prevalence in specific populations at higher risk below 5%) or concentrated HIV epidemics (prevalence under 1%; prevalence in specific populations at higher risk above 5%). Most of these data are from routine sentinel surveillance. For each of the populations the table gives the year of the most recent report and the median for the surveillance sites in the capital city. The specific populations at higher risk of HIV exposure in the tables include:

- Injecting drug users
- Sex workers
- Men who have sex with men

7. Knowledge and behaviour indicators

Before 2000, the definition of 'high-risk-sex' varied between surveys and thus the values presented should be considered as indicative of the risk level in the respective countries. Attempts have been made to present standardized results, but the values given should not be used to compare risk levels between countries.

The sources are denoted as follows: 'a' Behavioural Surveillance Surveys (FHI[U31]), 'b' Botswana AIDS Impact Survey ([U32]2001), 'c' Multi-Indicator Cluster Survey (UNICEF[U33]), 'd' Demographic and Health Survey, 'e' Survey of Youth and Adolescent Reproductive Health and Sexual Behaviours in Mozambique (INJAD, 2001[U34]); 'f' Reproductive Health Survey (CDC[U35]). For indicators derived from an additional survey, the year of the survey is denoted as follows: 'v' 1998, 'w' 1999, 'x' 2000, 'y' 2001, 'z' 2002.

Know that a healthy-looking person can have the AIDS virus (%) (15–24 years)

Percentage of 15–24-year-old respondents (female and male) who know that a healthy-looking person can be infected with the AIDS virus.

Can identify two prevention methods and reject three misconceptions (%) (15-24 years)

Percentage of 15–24-year-old respondents (female and male) who could identify two ways a person could avoid getting the AIDS virus (using a condom and avoiding multiple partners) and reject three misconceptions (know that a healthy-looking person can have the AIDS virus and two local misconceptions, such as that mosquito bites can transmit AIDS virus).

Had sex before age 15 (%) (15-19 years)

Percentage of 15–19-year-old respondents (female and male) who reported having sex before the age of 15.

Reported higher-risk sex (15-24) in the last year (%)

Proportion of 15–24-year-old respondents who had sex with a non-marital, non-cohabiting partner in the last 12 months[U36], of all respondents reporting sexual activity in the last 12 months.

Used a condom the last time they had higher-risk sex, of those who had high-risk sex in the last year (%) (15-24)

Percentage of 15–24-year-old respondents who say they used a condom the last time they had sex with a non-marital, non-cohabiting partner, of those who have had sex with such a partner in the last 12 months.

Year

Year of the survey in which knowledge and behavioural data was collected.

References

Chapter 1 – Overcoming AIDS: the 'Next Agenda'

Policy Project (2004). Coverage of selected services for HIV/AIDS prevention and care in low and middle income countries in 2003. (in press).

Chapter 2 – A global overview of the AIDS epidemic

Box: Women: increasingly infected by HIV

Dunkle et al. (2004). Gender-based violence, relationship power, and risk of HIV infection among women attending antenatal clinics in South Africa. *Lancet*, 363:1415–21.

UNDP (2003). *Regional human development report: HIV/AIDS and development in South Asia*. New York. Available at www.undp.org.np/publications/reghdr2003

Remainder of chapter

Dhaka (2003). HIV in Bangladesh: is time running out? National AIDS/STD Programme of the Directorate General of Health Services, Ministry of Health and Family Welfare, Government of the People's Republic of Bangladesh.

French K (2004). *Report for UNAIDS scenarios for Africa: the future of the HIV/AIDS epidemic in China, India, Russia and Eastern Europe*. London, Department of Infectious Disease Epidemiology, Imperial College, March.

Girault et al. (2004). HIV, STIs, and sexual behaviours among men who have sex with men in Phnom Penh, Cambodia.

Gisselquist et al. (2002). *International Journal of STD & AIDS*, 13:657–66.

Lydié N et al. (2004). Mobility, sexual behaviour and HIV infection in an urban population in Cameroon. *Journal of Acquired Immune Deficiency Syndrome*, 35(1).

Lurie M et al. (2003). Who infects whom? HIV-1 concordance and discordance among migrant and non-migrant couples in South Africa. *AIDS*, 17(15).

Schmid G et al. (2004). Transmission of HIV-1 infection in sub-Saharan Africa and effect of elimination of unsafe injections. *Lancet*, 363.

Stover, J (2004). *STI*, 80(Suppl. 1).

VanLandingham M, Trujillo L (2002). Recent changes in heterosexual attitudes, norms and behaviors among unmarried Thai men: a qualitative analysis. *International Family Planning Perspectives*, 28(1):6–15.

Chapter 3 – The impact of AIDS on people and societies

Box: Women more vulnerable to HIV than men

Cambodian National Institute of Statistics/Orc International (2000). *Cambodia demographic and health survey 2000: preliminary report*. Available at www.childinfo.org/MICS2/natlMICSrepz/Cambodia/PRELIMrj.pdf

Glynn et al. (2001). Why do young women have a much higher prevalence of HIV than young men? A study in Kisumu, Kenya and Ndola, Zambia. *AIDS*, 15(Suppl. 4):S51–60.

HelpAge International and International HIV/AIDS Alliance (2003). Forgotten families: older people as carers of orphans and vulnerable children. Brighton, United Kingdom.

Human Rights Watch (2003). Policy paralysis: a call for action on HIV/AIDS-related human rights abuses against women and girls in Africa. New York, Human Rights Watch USA. Available at http://www.hrw.org/reports/2003/africa1203/africa1203.pdf

Maman S, Mbwambo J K, Hogan N M et al. (2002). HIV-positive women report more lifetime partner violence: findings from a voluntary counseling and testing clinic in Dar es Salaam, Tanzania. American Journal of Public Health, 92(8): 1331–7.

UNICEF (2003). *Africa's orphaned generations, 2003.* New York.

WHO (2001). *Violence against women and HIV/AIDS: setting the research agenda.* Meeting report, 23–25 October 2000. Geneva. Available at whqlibdoc.who.int/hq/2001/WHO_FCH_GWH_01.08.pdf

Xu et al. (2000). HIV-1 seroprevalence, risk factors, and preventive behaviors among women in northern Thailand. *Journal of Acquired Immune Deficiency Syndrome*, 25(4):353–9.

Remainder of chapter

Adams A (1993). Food insecurity in Mali: exploring the role of the moral economy. *Institute for Development Studies Bulletin*, 24(4):41.

Akintola O, Quinlan T (2003). *Report of the scientific meeting on empirical evidence for the demographic and socioeconomic impact of HIV/AIDS*. Durban, 26–28 March.

Asingwire N (1996). *AIDS and agricultural production: its impact and implications for community support in ACORD programme areas, Mbabara district*. Consultancy report, cited in Mutangadura G B. 2000. *Household welfare impacts of mortality of adult females in Zimbabwe: Implications for policy and program development.* Paper presented at The AIDS and Economics Symposium (IAEN Network). Durban, 7–8 July.

Bachmann M O, Booysen F L R (2003). Health and socioeconomic impact of HIV/AIDS on South African households: cohort study. *BioMedCentral*, 3(14).

Badcock-Walters P (2001). The impact of HIV/AIDS on education in KwaZulu-Natal. Durban, KZNDEC Provincial Education Development Unit.

Badcock-Walters P, Desmond C, Wilson D, Heard W (2003). Educator mortality in-service in KwaZulu-Natal: a consolidated study of HIV/AIDS impact and trends. Paper presented to Demographics and Socio-Economic Conference. Durban, 28 March.

Barnett T, Whiteside A (2002). *AIDS in the 21st century: disease and globalization.* New York, Macmillan.

Baylies C (2002). The impact of AIDS on rural households in Africa: a shock like any other? Development and Change 33(4):611–632.

Beegle K (2003) Labor effects of adult mortality in Tanzanian households. World Bank Policy Research Working Paper 3062. Washington, May.

Bell C, Devarajan S, Gersbach H (2003). The long-run economic costs of AIDS: theory and application to South Africa, June draft. University of Heidelberg, World Bank.

Bennell P, Hyde K, Swainson N (2002). *The impact of the HIV/AIDS epidemic on the education sector in sub-Saharan Africa: A synthesis of findings and recommendations of three country studies.* University of Sussex, February.

Bollinger L, Stover J (1999). The economic impact of AIDS in Kenya. The Futures Group International in collaboration with: Research Triangle Institute (RTI). The Centre for Development and Population Activities (CEDPA).

Cohen D (2002). Human capital and the HIV epidemic in sub-Saharan Africa. Geneva, UNDP.

Food and Agriculture Organization (2001). The impact of HIV/AIDS on food security. FAO: Committee on World Food Security, Twenty-seventh Session, Rome, 28 May–1 June 2001.

Food and Agriculture Organization (2003a). *Measuring impacts of HIV/AIDS on rural livelihoods and food security*. Rome.

Food and Agriculture Organization (2003b). *Mitigating the impact of HIV/AIDS on food security and rural poverty.* Rome.

Food and Agriculture Organization (2003c). *State of food insecurity in the world 2003* (summary). Rome.

Food Economy Group (2001). *Food economy baseline training and assessment in Siavonga district, Zambia.* April.

Goliber T J (2000). Exploring the implications of the HIV/AIDS epidemic for educational planning in selected African countries: the demographic question. New York, World Bank, AIDS Campaign Team for Africa (ACT). Available at wbln0018.worldbank.org/HDNet/HDdocs.nsf/0/9631986c0c414a8085256a33004f1e23?OpenDocument

Gould B, Huber U (2002). HIV/AIDS, poverty and schooling in Tanzania and Uganda. British Society for Population Studies meeting on Poverty and Well-being in HIV/AIDS affected African countries. London, 8 January. Available at www.socstats.soton.ac.uk/choices/Gould%20Paper.doc

Gregson S, Waddell H, Chandiwana S (2001). School education and HIV control in sub-Saharan Africa: from discord to harmony? 3 March 2001. Available at www.zimaids.co.zw/hae/webfiles/Electronic%20Versions/SchooleducationandHIVcontrolfromdiscord.doc

Harris A M, Schubert J G (2001). Defining "Quality" in the midst of HIV/AIDS: ripple effects in the classroom. 44th annual meeting of the Comparative and International Education Society, Washington, March. Available at www.zimaids.co.zw/hae/webfiles/Electronic%20Versions/Defining%20Quality%20In%20the%20midst%20of%20HIV%20.doc

Harvey P (2003). *HIV/AIDS: what are the implications for humanitarian action? A literature review.* London, Overseas Development Institute. Available at http://www.aidsalliance.org/_res/reports/CAA_Cambodia.pdf

Hunter S, John Williamson (1997). *Children on the brink: strategies to support HIV/AIDS.* Washington, USAID.

Liese B, Blanchet N, Dussault G (2003). The human resource crisis in health services in sub-Saharan Africa. Washington, World Bank.

Lisk F (2002). Labour market and employment implications of HIV/AIDS. Working Paper 1. ILO Programme on HIV/AIDS and the World of Work. Geneva.

Lundberg M, Over M, Mujinja P (2000). Sources of financial assistance for households suffering an adult death in Kagera, Tanzania. Paper. World Bank.

Malaney P (2000). The impact of HIV/AIDS on the education sector in southern Africa. CAER II Discussion Paper. Boston. Available at www.hiid.harvard.edu/caer2/htm/content/papers/paper81/paper81.htm

Malawi Institute of Management/UNDP (2002). The impact of HIV/AIDS on human resources in the public sector in Malawi.

Mutangadura G B (2000). Household welfare impacts of mortality of adult females in Zimbabwe: Implications for policy and program development. Paper presented at The AIDS and Economics Symposium (IAEN Network). Durban, 7–8 July.

Nalugoda F et al. (1997). HIV infection in rural households, Rakai District, Uganda. *Health Transition Review*, 7 (Suppl. 2): 127–140.

Ogden J, Esim S (2003). *Reconceptualizing the care continuum for HIV/AIDS: Bringing carers into focus.* (desk review draft). International Center for Research on Women.

Pitayanon S, Kongsin S, Janjareon W S (1997). The economic impact of HIV/AIDS mortality on households in Thailand. In: Bloom D, Godwin P, eds. *The economics of HIV and AIDS: the case of South and South East Asia.* Delhi, Oxford University Press, 66.

Porter K, Zaba B (2004). The empirical evidence for the impact of HIV on adult mortality in the developing world: data from serological studies. *AIDS.*

Rugalema G (1998). It is not only the loss of labour: HIV/AIDS, loss of household assets and household livelihood in Bukoba district, Tanzania. Paper presented at the East and Southern Africa Regional Conference on Responding to HIV/AIDS: Development Needs of African Smallholder Agriculture. Harare, 8–10 June.

Rugalema G (2000). Coping or struggling? A journey into the impact of HIV/AIDS in Southern Africa. *Review of African Political Economy*, 86:537–545.

Sackey J, Raparla T (2000). *Namibia: the development, impact of HIV/AIDS—selected issues and options*. World Bank Report No. 22046 –NA.

SADC FANR Vulnerability Assessment Committee (2003). Towards identifying impacts of HIV/AIDS on food security in Southern Africa and implications for response: findings from Malawi, Zambia and Zimbabwe. Harare, SADC.

Sauerborn R, Adams A, Hien M (1996). Household strategies to cope with the economic costs of illness. *Social Science & Medicine*, 43(3):291–301.

Steinberg M, Johnson S, Schierhout S, Ndegwa D (2002). *Hitting home: how households cope with the impact of the HIV/AIDS epidemic*. Cape Town, Henry J Kaiser Foundation & Health Systems Trust. October.

Swaziland Ministry of Education (1999). Impact assessment of HIV/AIDS on the education sector. In *Education International* (2001) "Education in the Era of HIV/AIDS" Dossier of Education International Magazine, December 2001 edition.

Tawfik L, Kinoti S (2001). The impact of HIV/AIDS on the health sector sub-Saharan Africa: the issue of human resources. USAID: Support for Analysis and Research in Africa Project USAID, Bureau for Africa, Office of Sustainable Development, October.

Timaeus I, Jassen M (2003). Adult mortality in sub-Saharan Africa: evidence from the demographic and health surveys. Paper presented to Conference on Empirical Evidence for the Demographic and Socio-Economic Impact of AIDS. Durban, 26–28 March.

Topouzis D (2003). Addressing the impact of HIV/AIDS on ministries of agriculture: focus on eastern and southern Africa. Rome, FAO/UNAIDS.

UNAIDS Central Executive Board, CEB/2003/HLCP/CRP.27 (2003). Organizing the UN Response to the Triple Threat of Food Insecurity, Weakened Capacity for Governance and AIDS, particularly in Southern and Eastern Africa. Geneva.

UNDP (2001). *HIV/AIDS: implications for poverty reduction*. New York.

UNDP (2002). *Conceptual shifts for sound planning: towards an integrated approach for HIV/AIDS and poverty*. Concept paper. UNDP Regional Project on HIV and Development. August.

UNDP (2003). *Disease, HIV/AIDS and capacity implication: a case of the public education sector in Zambia*. Research paper 2. February.

UNESCO (2000). The Dakar framework for action, education for all: meeting our collective commitments. World Education Forum. Dakar, 26–28 April.

UNESCO (2002). *EFA global monitoring report, 2002: is the world on track?* Paris. Available at http://www.unesco.org/education/efa/monitoring/monitoring_2002.shtml

United Nations (2001). United Nations Millennium Development Goals [webpage]. http://www.un.org/millenniumgoals/)

United Nations Conference on Trade and Development (2002). *The least developed countries report 2002: escaping the poverty trap*. Geneva.

United Nations Population Division (2003). *The HIV/AIDS epidemic and its social and economic implications*. New York. September.

USAID Report to Congress (2002). USAID'S Expanded Response to HIV/AIDS. June.

Villareal M (2003). Mitigating the impact of HIV/AIDS on food security and rural poverty. Food and Agriculture Organization, HIV/AIDS Programme.

Wiggins S (2003). Lessons from the current food crisis in Southern Africa. The forum for food security in Southern Africa and other initiatives. Scott Drimie and Micheal Lafon. IFAS/HSRC/SARPN, June.

World Bank (1999). *Confronting AIDS: Public Priorities in a Global Epidemic*, revised ed. New York, Oxford University Press.

Yamano T, Jayne T S (2002). Measuring the impacts of prime-age adult death on rural households in Kenya. Tegemeo Working Paper 5. Tegemeo Institute of Agricultural Policy and Development, Nairobi, Kenya. October 2002.

Yuan J et al. (2002). *The Socioeconomic Impact of HIV/AIDS in China*. UN Theme Group on HIV/AIDS in China, August.

Focus – AIDS and orphans: a tragedy unfolding

Beckerman K (2002). Mothers, orphans and prevention of paediatric AIDS. *Lancet*, 359:1168–1169.

Bell C, Devarajan S, Gerbach H (2003). *The long-run economic costs of AIDS: theory and an application to South Africa*. Washington, World Bank.

Deininger K, Garcia M, Subbarao K (2003). AIDS-induced orphanhood as a systemic shock: magnitude, impact and program interventions in Africa. *World Development*, 31(7):1201–1220.

Family Health International (2002). Results of the orphans and vulnerable children head of household baseline survey in four districts in Zambia. (draft).

Foster G (2002). Understanding community responses to the situation of children affected by AIDS: lessons for external agencies. Geneva, UNRISD.

Monasch R, Snoad N (2003). The situation of orphans in a region affected by HIV/AIDS. A review of population-based household surveys from 40 countries in sub-Saharan Africa.

Stein J (2003). Sorrow makes children of us all: a literature review on the psycho-social impact of HIV/AIDS on children. Cape Town, Centre for Social Science Research Working Paper 47. Cape Town.

UNAIDS (2003). *Progress report on the global response to the HIV/AIDS epidemic 2003*. Geneva.

UNICEF (2003). *Africa's orphaned generations, 2003*. New York.

UNICEF et al. (2004). Draft framework for the protection, care and support of orphans and vulnerable children living in a world with HIV/AIDS. New York.

USAID (2004). Monks as change agents for HIV/AIDS care and support. Success stories. Available at www.fhi.org/en/HIVAIDS/Publications/SuccessStories.htm.

Williamson J (2004). *A family is for life*. (draft). Washington, USAID/the Synergy Project.

Chapter 4 – Bringing comprehensive HIV prevention to scale

Box: Prevention needs of girls and women

Helene A et al. (2002). Clients of female sex workers in Nyanza province, Kenya. *Sexually transmitted diseases*, 29(8): 444–452.

UNFPA (2002). Strategy for prevention [webpage]. http://www.unfpa.org/hiv/2002update/1d2.htm

WHO (2003). Integrating gender into HIV/AIDS programmes: expert consultation 3-5 June 2002, Geneva. WHO/International Center for Research on Women (ICRW). Available at http://www.who.int/hiv/pub/prev_care/Gender_hivaidsreviewpaper.pdf

Remainder of chapter

AFEW (2003). HIV prevention and health promotion in prisons: Russian Federation [webpage]. AIDS Foundation East-West (AFEW). http://www.afew.org/english/projects_prison_rus.php

Alary M et al. (2002). Decline in the prevalence of HIV and sexually transmitted diseases among female sex workers in Cotonou, Benin, 1993–1999. *AIDS*, 16(3):463–470.

All-Party Parliamentary Group on AIDS (2003). *Migration and HIV: improving lives in Britain. An inquiry into the impact of the UK nationality and immigration system on people living with HIV.* London, All-Party Parliamentary Group on AIDS. Available at http://www.appg-aids.org.uk/Publications/Migration%20and%20HIV%20Improving%20Lives.pdf

Amirkhanian Y A, Kelly J A, Kabakchieva E, McAuliffe T L, Vassileva S (2003). Evaluation of a social network HIV prevention intervention program for young men who have sex with men in Russia and Bulgaria. *AIDS Education & Prevention*, 15(3):205–20.

Betts S C, Peterson D J, Huebner A J (2003). Zimbabwean adolescents' condom use: what makes a difference? Implications for intervention. *Journal of Adolescent Health*, 33(3):165–71.

Braithwaite R, Arriola K (2003). Male prisoners and HIV prevention: a call for action ignored. *American Journal of Public Health*, 93(5):759–763.

Brussa L (2002). Migrant sex workers in Europe: STI/HIV prevention, health and human rights, *Research for Sex Work*, 5.

Burrows D (2003). *HIV prevention among injecting drug users in transitional and developing countries.* (draft). UNAIDS Best Practice Report.

CDC (2002). Fact sheet for public health personnel: male latex condoms and sexually transmitted diseases [webpage]. http://www.cdc.gov/hiv/pubs/facts/condoms.htm

CDC (2003). Advancing HIV prevention: new strategies for a changing epidemic—United States 2003. *MMWR Weekly*. Available at www.cdc.gov/mmwr/preview/mmwrhtml/mm5215a1.htm

Cohen J (2003). Two hard-hit countries offer rare success stories. *Science*, 19.

Colby D (2003). HIV knowledge and risk factors among men who have sex with men in Ho Chi Minh City, Vietnam. *Journal of Acquired Immune Deficiency Syndrome*, 32(1):80–85. Available at www.thebody.com/cdc/news_updates_archive/2003/mar17_03/vietnam_msm_aids.html

Dabis F, Ekpini E R (2002). HIV-1/AIDS and maternal and child health in Africa. *Lancet*, 359(9323):2097–2104.

De Groot A et al. (1999). *Women in prisons: the impact of HIV.* HIV Education Prisons Project. June.

Drummond M (2002). *Return on investment in needle and syringe programs in Australia.* Commonwealth of Australia. ISBN 0 642 821178.

Elizabeth Glaser Pediatric AIDS Foundation (2003). Elizabeth Glaser Pediatric AIDS Foundation [webpage]. http://www.pedaids.org/

Foss A, Vickerman P, Heise L, Watts C H (2003). Shifts in condom use following microbicide introduction: should we be concerned? *AIDS*, 17:1227–1237.

Ghys P et al. (2002). Increase in condom use and decline in HIV and sexually transmitted disease among female sex workers in Abijan, Côte d'Ivoire, 1991–1998. *AIDS*, 16(2):251–258.

Ghys P et al. (2003). Best of AIDS 2003, *AIDS* 17(Suppl. 4):S121–122.

Global HIV Prevention Working Group (2003). *Access to HIV prevention: closing the gap*. Available at http://www.kff.org/hivaids/200305-index.cfm

Goyer K (2003). *HIV/AIDS in South African prisons*, Monograph 79, February 2003, Institute for Security Studies.

Hamers F, Downs A (2003). HIV in central and Eastern Europe. *Lancet*, 361:1035–1044.

Haour-Knipe M (2002). HIV-infected migrants in Europe: missing out on the benefits of early care. *A&M News*, 4:3–4.

Hauri A M , Armstrong G L, Hutin Y J (2004). The global burden of disease attributable to contaminated injections given in health care settings. *International Journal of STD & AIDS*,15:7–16.

Hitchcock L, Fransen B (1999). Preventing HIV infection: lessons from Mwanza and Rakai. *Lancet*, 353:513–514.

Human Rights Watch (1998). Just die quietly: domestic violence and women's vulnerability to HIV in Uganda.

Human Rights Watch (2003). Ravaging the vulnerable. *Abuses against persons at high risk of HIV infection in Bangladesh*. Human Rights Watch Report, August. Available at www.hrw.org

ILO/IPEC (2002). Unbearable to the human heart: child trafficking and action to eliminate it. Geneva.

INCB (2003). *Report of the International Narcotics Control Board for 2003*. Vienna.

International Centre for Prison Studies (2003). World prison brief: prison brief for South Africa [webpage]. London, Kings College. Available at http://www.kcl.ac.uk/depsta/rel/icps/worldbrief/africa_records.php?code=45

International Lesbian and Gay Association (2002). World Legal Survey, Updated 21.07/02. Available at www.ilga.org/Information/legal_survey/Summary%20information/

IOM (2003). *World migration 2003: managing migration— challenges and responses for people on the move*. Geneva.

IOM/UNAIDS/UNDP (2002). *HIV/AIDS prevention and care programmes for mobile populations in Africa: an inventory*. Geneva.

Jürgens R (2003). HIV/AIDS prevention for drug dependent persons within the criminal justice system. Paper presented at the Commission on Narcotic Drugs Ministerial Segment: Ancillary Meeting on HIV/AIDS and Drug Abuse. Vienna, 16 April.

Kamali A et al. (2003). Sydromic management of sexually transmitted infections and behaviour change interventions on transmission of HIV-1 in rural Uganda: a community randomised trial. *Lancet*, 361:645–652.

Kerrigan D et al. (2003). Environmental-structural factors significantly associated with consistent condom use among female sex worker in the Dominican Republic. *AIDS*, 17 (3):415–423.

Levi G C, Vitória M A (2002). Fighting against AIDS: the Brazilian experience. *AIDS*, 16(18):2373–83.

Lowe D (2002). *Perceptions of the Cambodian 100 per cent condom use program.* (draft report). Washington, Policy Project, the Futures Group. Available at www.nswp.org/safety/CUP-REPORT.DOC.

Lurie et al. (2003). The impact of migration on HIV-1 transmission in South Africa. *Sexually Transmitted Diseases*, 30(2): 149–156.

Malinowska-Sempruch K, Hoove, J, Alexandrova A (2003). *Unintended consequences: drug policies fuel the HIV epidemic in Russia and Ukraine*. New York, International Harm Reduction Development Program/OSI. Available at http://www.harm-reduction.org/pub_files/unintended_consequences.pdf

Manjunath J, Thappa D, Jaisankar T (2002). Sexually transmitted diseases and sexual lifestyles of long-distance truck drivers: A clinico-epidemiological study in south India. *International Journal of STD & AIDS*, 13:612–617.

Mathur M, Kumta S, Setia M et al. (2002). An experience of MSM surveillance in a tertiary care center in Mumbai. Abstract no. TuPeG568. Barcelona, XIV International Conference on AIDS.

Merson M H, Dayton J M, O'Reilly K (2000). Effectiveness of HIV prevention interventions in developing countries. *AIDS*, 14 (Suppl. 2):S68–84.

Ministry of Health (2003). National estimates of adult HIV infection. Ministry of Health of the Republic Of Indonesia Directorate General of Communicable Disease Control and Environmental Health.

Ministry of Health/UN Theme Group (2003). A joint assessment on HIV/AIDS prevention, treatment and care in China. Geneva.

NACO (2003). National baseline general population behavioural surveillance survey (BSS). New Delhi, Ministry of Health.

Norman L R (2003). Predictors of consistent condom use: a hierarchical analysis of adults from Kenya, Tanzania and Trinidad. *International Journal of STD/AIDS*, 14(9):584–90.

Ostrow et al. (2002). Attitudes towards highly active antiretroviral therapy are associated with sexual risk taking among HIV-infected and uninfected homosexual men. *AIDS*, 16(5):775–80.

Policy Project (2004). *Coverage of selected services for HIV/AIDS prevention and care in low- and middle-income countries in 2003.* (in press).

Population Report Volume XXVII (1999). Number 1, April. Available at http://www.infoforhealth.org/pr/h9/h9chap1_1.shtml

Riehman K S (1996). Injecting drug use and AIDS in developing countries: determinants and issues for policy consideration. New York, World Bank Policy Research Department. Available at http://www.worldbank.org/aids-con/confront/backgrnd/riehman/indexp6.htm.

Shelton J D et al. (2004). Partner reduction is crucial for balanced 'ABC' approach to HIV prevention. *British Medical Journal*, 328(10).

Singh S, Darroch J E, Bankole A (2003). *A, B and C in Uganda: the roles of abstinence, monogamy and condom use in HIV decline*. Washington, The Alan Guttmacher Institute. Available at http://www.synergyaids.com/documents/UgandaABC.pdf

Stover H, Ossietzky C (2001). *An overview study: assistance to drug users in European prisons.* The United Kingdon, European Monitoring Centre for Drugs and Drug Addiction. ISBN 1 902114035.

Stover J, Walker N, Garnett G P et al. (2002). Can we reverse the HIV/AIDS pandemic with an expanded response. *Lancet*, 360:73–77. Available at http://www.ncbi.nlm.nih.gov/entrez/query.fcgi?cmd=Retrieve&db=PubMed&dopt=Citation&list_uids=12114060

Strathdee S A, Vlahov D (2001). The effectiveness of needle exchange programs: a review of the science and policy. *AIDScience*, 1(16). Available at http://www.aidscience.org/Articles/aidscience013.asp.

Suarez T P, Kelly J A, Pinkerton S D et al. (2001). Influence of a partner's HIV serostatus, use of highly active antiretroviral therapy, and viral load on perceptions of sexual risk behavior in a community sample of men who have sex with men. *Journal of Acquired Immune Deficiency Syndrome*, 28(5):471–7.

Ukwuani F A, Tsui A O, Suchindran C M. (2003). Condom use for preventing HIV infection/AIDS in sub-Saharan Africa: a comparative multilevel analysis of Uganda and Tanzania. *Journal of Acquired Immune Deficiency Syndrome*, 34(2): 203–13.

UNAIDS and Ministry of Public Health, Thailand (2000). Evaluation of the 100% condom programme in Thailand. UNAIDS Case Study. Available at http://www.unaids.org/html/pub/publications/irc-pub01/jc275-100pcondom_en_pdf.pdf

UNAIDS (2002). *Report on the global HIV/AIDS epidemic, July 2002.* Joint United Nations Programme on HIV/AIDS, Geneva. Available at http://www.unaids.org/html/pub/Global-Reports/Barcelona/BRGlobal_AIDS_Report_en_pdf.pdf

UNAIDS (2003). Progress Report on the Global Response to HIV/AIDS, 2003. Geneva.

UNDP (2001). Mobile populations and HIV vulnerability: inventory of organizations. Bangkok. UNDP South East Asia HIV and Development Programme. Available at http://www.hiv-development.org/publications/Inventory.htm

UNDP (2001a). Regional Update—Sri Lanka [webpage]. UNDP HIV and Development Programme. http://www.hivanddevelopment.org/regionalupdate/srilanka/index.asp

UNFPA (2003). *Prevention of HIV transmission to pregnant women, mothers and their children (PMTCT).* Inputs for the Bangkok Report. Geneva.

UNFPA/UNAIDS (2004). Myths, perceptions, and fears: addressing condom use barriers (in print).

Valdiserri R O (2003). The roots of HIV/AIDS complacency: implications for policy development. Conference paper for international policy dialogue on HIV/AIDS, organized by the government of Poland, Health Canada, UNAIDS, Open Society Institute and Canadian International Development Agency. Warsaw. Available at http://www.ceehrn.lt/EasyCEE/sys/files/Roots%20of%20HIV%20AIDS%20Complacency_Valdiserri.doc

Walker N, Schwartlander B, Bryce J (2002). Meeting international goals in child survival and HIV/AIDS. *Lancet*, 360 (9329):284–9.

Weinhardt L S, Carey M P, Johnson B, Bickam N L (1999). Effects of HIV counselling and testing on sexual risk behavior: a meta-analytic review of published research 1985–1997. *American Journal of Public Health*, 89(9):1397–1404.

Weir S, Pailman C, Mahlalela X, Coetzee N, Meidany F, Boerma J T (2003). From people to places: focusing AIDS prevention efforts where it matters most. *AIDS*, 17(6):685–903.

WHO/UNAIDS (1997). The female condom: an information pack. Geneva.

WHO (2002). Blood and Clinical Technology: Progress 2000-2001. WHO/BCT/02.10. Geneva.

WHO (2002a). Regional Office for Africa 2002: HIV/AIDS Epidemiological Surveillance Update for the WHO African Region.

WHO (2003). Educate, motivate, recruit and retain blood donors from low risk populations [webpage]. http://www.who.int/bct/Main_areas_of_work/BTS/Blood%20Donors.htm

WHO (2003a). Saving mothers, saving families: the MTCT-plus initiative: perspectives and practice in antiretroviral treatment. Case Study. Geneva. Available at http://www.who.int/hiv/pub/prev_care/pub40/en/

WHO (2003b). Strategy for the prevention of HIV infections in infants in Europe. (draft).

Wolffers I, van Beelen N (2003). Public health and human rights of sex workers. *Lancet*, 361, 7:1981.

Wu Z et al. (2002). Diffusion of HIV/AIDS knowledge, positive attitudes, and behaviors through training of health professionals in China. Available at http://aids.cdc.gov.tw/EN/international02.asp?sno=75

Xu F et al. (2000). HIV-1 seroprevalence, risk factors, and preventive behaviors among women in Northern Thailand. *Journal of Acquired Immune Deficiency Syndrome*, 25(4):353–359.

Focus – HIV and young people: the threat for today's youth

Cohen A (2003). *Beyond slogans: Lessons of Uganda's experience of ABC and HIV/AIDS*. New York, Alan Guttmacher Institute.

Cowan F (2002). Adolescent reproductive health interventions. *Sexually Transmitted Infections*, 78:315–318.

Family Health International (2003). *MTV: 'Staying Alive' 2002. A global HIV mass media campaign*. Available at www.fhi.org/en/Youth/Youthnet/Pubications/YouthIssuesPapers.htm

Global HIV Prevention Working Group Report (2003). *Access to HIV prevention: closing the gap*.

Glynn J R et al. (2001). The study group on heterogeneity of HIV epidemics in African cities. Why do young women have a much higher prevalence of HIV than young men? A study in Kisumu, Kenya and Ndola, Zambia. *AIDS*, 15 (Suppl. 4): S51–60.

Greene M, Rasekh Z, Amen K-H (2002). *In this generation: sexual & reproductive health policies for a youthful world*. Washington, Population Action International. Available at www.populationaction.org/resources/publications/InThisGeneration

Kirby D (2002). The impact of schools and school programmes upon adolescent sexual behavior. *Journal of Sexual Research*, 39:27–33.

Luke N, Kurz K (2002). *Cross-generational and transactional sexual relations in sub-Saharan Africa*. Washington, AIDSmark. Available at www.icrw.org/docs/crossgensex_Report_902pdf

Lopez V (2002). *HIV/AIDS and young people. A review of the state of the epidemic and its impact on world youth*. (unpublished report). Geneva, UNAIDS.

Manzini N (2001). Sexual initiation and childbearing among adolescents in KwaZulu Natal. *Reproductive Health Matters*, 9(17):44–52.

Obasi A et al. (2003). *Mema Kwa Vijana. A randomised controlled trial of an adolescent sexual and reproductive health intervention programme in rural Mwanza, Tanzania. Intervention and Process Indicators*.

Pisani E (2003). *The epidemiology of HIV at the start of the 21st century: reviewing the evidence*. Geneva, UNICEF.

Population Reference Bureau (2003). HIV/AIDS Demographics, Africa.

Rhodes T et al. (2002). *Behavioural risk factors in HIV transmission in Eastern Europe and Central Asia*. (unpublished draft). Geneva, UNAIDS.

UNAIDS (2003). *AIDS epidemic update*. Geneva.

UNDP (2003). *Ukraine human development report special edition 2003*. Kiev.

UNFPA (2003). *The state of the world population, 2003. Making one billion count: investing in adolescents' health rights*. New York.

UNICEF/UNAIDS/WHO (2002). *Young people and HIV/AIDS. Opportunity in crisis*. New York.

United Nations (2003). *Facing the future together.* Report of the United Nations Secretary-General's Task Force on Women, Girls and HIV/AIDS in Southern Africa.

WHO/Progress in Reproductive Health Research (2000). *Sex and youth— misperceptions and risk.* Available at http://www.who.int/reproductive-health/hrp/progress/53/news53_1.en.html

Chapter 5 – Treatment, care and support for people living with HIV

Box: Treatment and care for women and girls

Center for Health and Gender Equity (2004). Gender, AIDS, and ARV Therapies: ensuring that women gain equitable access to drugs within U.S. funded treatment initiatives. Available at http://www.genderhealth.org/pubs/TreatmentAccessFeb2004.pdf.

Farzadegan H, Hoover D, Astemborski J et al. (1998). Sex differences in HIV-1 viral load and progression to AIDS. *Lancet*, 352:1510–1514.

Fleischman J (2004). Breaking the cycle: ensuring equitable access to HIV treatment for women and girls. Washington, Center for Strategic and International Studies. Available at http://www.csis.org/africa/0402_breakingcycle.pdf

Project Inform (2001). Women and AIDS at twenty. *Project Inform Perspective*, August. Available at http://www.projinf.org/pub/33/women.html

Remainder of chapter

De Cock K M, Chaisson R E (1999). Will DOTS do it? A reappraisal of tuberculosis control in countries with high rates of HIV infection. *International Journal of Tuberculosis and Lung Disease*, 3:457–65.

Dummett H (2003). *African manufacturers gear up for generic ARV production.* World Markets Analysis, 11 November 2003, World Markets Research Centre.

Family Health International (2001). Tuberculosis control in high HIV prevalent areas. A strategic framework. Arlington.

Farmer P, Leandre F, Mukherjee J S et al. (2001). Community-based treatment of advanced HIV disease: Introducing DOT-HAART. *Bull World Health Organ*, 79.

Garbus L (2003a). *HIV/AIDS in Ethiopia.* Country AIDS Policy Analysis Project. San Francisco, University of California. AIDS Policy Research Center.

Garbus L (2003b). *HIV/AIDS in Malawi.* Country AIDS Policy Analysis Project. San Francisco, University of California. AIDS Policy Research Center.

Garbus L (2003c). *HIV/AIDS in Zambia.* Country AIDS Policy Analysis Project. San Francisco, University of California. AIDS Policy Research Center.

Garbus L, Marseille E (2003). *HIV/AIDS in Uganda.* Country AIDS Policy Analysis Project. San Francisco, University of California. AIDS Policy Research Center.

Global Fund to Fight AIDS, Tuberculosis and Malaria (2003). *Annual Report 2003.* Geneva.

Moatti J P et al. (2003). Antiretroviral treatment for HIV infection in developing countries: an attainable new paradigm. *Nature Medicine*, 9(12).

Mpiima S et al. (2003). *Increased demand for VCT services driven by introduction of HAART in Masaka District, Uganda.* Poster presentation to the Second IAS Conference on HIV Pathogenesis and Treatment, Paris, 13–17 July.

Médecins sans Frontières (2004). *Briefing Note, MSF Campaign for Access to Essential Medicines*. February.

Ogden J, Esim S (2003). *Reconceptualizing the care continuum for HIV/AIDS: bringing carers into focus*. International Center for Research on Women.

Piyaworawong S et al. (2003). Responding to tuberculosis and HIV epidemic in a general health service setting, Chiang Rai, Thailand. 3rd Global TB/HIV Working Group Meeting. Montreux, 4–6 June. Available at www.who.int/gtb/TBHIV/montreux_june03/presentations/wed/piyaworawang_Thailand.pdf

Project Inform (2001). Women and AIDS at Twenty. *Project Inform Perspective*, August. Available at http://www.projinf.org/pub/33/women.html

Ramsay S (2003). Leading the way in African home-based palliative care: free oral morphine has allowed expansion of home-based palliative care in Uganda. *Lancet*, 362(9398):29.

Raviglione M C (2003). The TB epidemic from 1992 to 2002. *Tuberculosis*, 83(1–3). Proceedings from the 4th World Congress on Tuberculosis, 3–5 June 2002. Available at www.who.int/gtb/publications/refsubject.html.

UNAIDS (2000). *Caring for the carers: managing stress in those who care for people with HIV/AIDS*. Best Practice Collection. Geneva.

UNAIDS (2003). *Where there's a will there's a way: nursing and midwifery champions in HIV/AIDS care in Southern Africa*. Best Practice Collection. Geneva.

UNAIDS (2003a). *Stepping back from the edge: The pursuit of antiretroviral therapy in Botswana, South Africa and Uganda*. Best Practice Collection. Geneva.

WHO (2002). *Community health approach to palliative care for HIV/AIDS and cancer patients in Africa*. Progress Report of WHO Joint Project Cancer and HIV/AIDS Programmes, August.

WHO (2003a). *Access to antiretroviral treatment and care: the experience of the HIV Equity Initiative, Cange, Haiti*. Perspectives and Practice in Antiretroviral Treatment, May.

WHO (2003b). *Public health approaches to expand antiretroviral treatment*. (draft).WHO/HIV, 07 May.

WHO (2003c). *WHO calls for widespread free access to anti-TB drugs for people living with HIV*. WHO Press Release 15 July 2003.

WHO (2003d). *Technical and operational recommendations for emergency scale up of ART in resource-limited settings*. Report from the WHO/UNAIDS Consultation, Lusaka, Zambia, November.

WHO (2003e). Approaches to the management of HIV/AIDS in Cuba. Perspectives and practice in antiretroviral treatment. (draft). October.

WHO (2004). Antiretroviral drugs and the prevention of mother-to-child transmission of HIV infection in resource-constrained settings, recommendations for use, 2004 Revision. Available at http://www.who.int/3by5/publications/documents/en/pmtct_2004.pdf

WHO (2004a). Report on the "lessons learnt" workshop on the six ProTEST pilot projects in Malawi, South Africa and Zambia. (document in preparation). Durban, 3–6 February 2003. Geneva.

WHO (2004b). The Interim Policy on Collaborative TB/HIV Activities. Geneva, WHO/HTM/TB.

World Bank (2003). World Development Indicators. April.

Chapter 6 – Financing the response to AIDS

Box: The care economy

Ogden J, Esim S (2003). *Reconceptualizing the care continuum for HIV/AIDS: bringing carers into focus*. (desk review draft). International Center for Research on Women. October.

Steinberg M, Johnson S, Schierhout S, Ndegwa D (2002). *Hitting home: how households cope with the impact of the HIV/AIDS epidemic.* Cape Town, Henry J Kaiser Foundation & Health Systems Trust. October.

UN Population Division (2003). *The HIV/AIDS epidemic and its social and economic implications. New York.*

UNDP (2003). *Regional human development report: HIV/AIDS and development in South Asia.* New York. Available at www.undp.org.np/publications/reghdr2003

UNDP (2003a). *The socio-economic impact of HIV/AIDS in Viet Nam: a preliminary note.* Available at http://www.undp.org.vn/undp/docs/2003/seimpact/seimpacte.pdf

Remainder of chapter

Boyce J (2002). Africa's debt: who owes whom? Working Paper Series N. 48. Amherst, University of Massachusetts, Political Economy Research Institute.

Cashel J (2003). *AIDS and the World Bank.* Transcript of interview with Dr Debrework Zewdie of the World Bank, 29 April. IAEN Global Dialogue Series. Available at http://www.iaen.org/globdial/zewdie/index.php

Cashel J, Rivers B (2003). Transcript of interview with Dr Richard Feacham, Executive Director of The Global Fund to Fight AIDS, Tuberculosis and Malaria, 14 March. Available at http://www.iaen.org

The Futures Group (2003). *Funding required for the response to AIDS in Eastern Europe and Central Asia.* Report prepared for UNAIDS and the World Bank.

Global Business Coalition on HIV/AIDS (2001). *Business action on HIV/AIDS—a blueprint.*

Global Fund to Fight AIDS, Tuberculosis and Malaria (2003). *Annual Report 2002/2003. Geneva.*

Global Fund to Fight AIDS, Tuberculosis and Malaria (2004). *Progress Report,* 14 January 2004. Geneva.

Global Fund to Fight AIDS, Tuberculosis and Malaria (2004a). *Update: Resource Mobilization and Resource Needs,* 14 January 2004. Geneva.

Global HIV Prevention Working Group (2003). *Access to HIV prevention: closing the gap.* Available at: www.gatesfoundation.org or www.kaisernetwork.org

Graydon T R (2000). Medicaid and the HIV/AIDS epidemic in the United States. *Health care financing review* 22(1): 117–122.

Gutiérrez J P et al. (2004). Achieving the WHO/UNAIDS antiretroviral treatment '3 by 5' goal: what will it cost? *Lancet* (in press).

Hardstaff P (2003). *Treacherous conditions: how IMF and World Bank policies tied to debt are undermining development.* London, World Development Movement.

Hickey A (2003). *What are provincial health departments allocating for HIV/AIDS from their own budgets?* Budget Brief No. 135. IDASA, South Africa.

Hickey A (2004). *New allocations for ARV treatment: an analysis of 2004/5 national budget from an HIV/AIDS perspective.* The Institute for Democracy in South Africa, AIDS Budget Unit.

Hickey A, Ndlovu N, Guthrie T (2003). *Budgeting for HIV/AIDS in South Africa: report on intergovernmental funding flows for an integrated response in the social sector.* IDASA, South Africa. Available at www.bis.idasact.org.za

International AIDS Vaccine Initiative (2003). Slide presentation at AIDS Vaccine 2003 Conference, 18 September 2003.

Inter-American Development Bank (2003). *Resources required to fight HIV/AIDS in Latin America and the Caribbean.* Report prepared for the IDB by the *Instituto Nacional de Saluda Publica* (INSP), Mexico and The Futures Group.

IRIN (2004). Transcript of interview with Dr. Ndwapi Ndwapi, director of the Princess Marina Hospital Antiretroviral Programme in Botswana, *IRIN PlusNews*, 11 March.

Kimalu P (2002). *Debt relief and health care in Kenya.* WIDER Discussion Paper No. 2002/65. Finland, United Nations University.

Martin G (2003). *A comparative analysis of the financing of HIV/AIDS programmes in Botswana, Lesotho, Mozambique, Swaziland and South Africa.* Human Sciences Research Council, South Africa, October 2003.

Ogden J, Esim S (2003). *Reconceptualizing the care continuum for HIV/AIDS: bringing carers into focus.* International Center for Research on Women.

Oxfam (2002). Debt relief and the HIV/AIDS crisis in Africa: does the heavily indebted poor country (HIPC) initiative go far enough? Oxfam Briefing Paper 25.

UNAIDS (2003). *Report on the State of HIV/AIDS Financing.* UNAIDS/PCB (14)/03 Conference Paper 2a. Geneva.

UNAIDS (2003a). *Progress on the Development of a Global Resource Mobilization Strategy for HIV/AIDS*, UNAIDS/PCB (14)/03 Conference Paper 2b. Geneva.

UNAIDS (2003b). *Stepping back from the edge: vision, activism and risk-taking in pursuit of antiretroviral therapy.* Best Practice Collection. Geneva.

UNAIDS (2003c). *Progress report on the global response to the HIV/AIDS epidemic, 2003.* UNAIDS, Geneva.

UN/MOH China (2003). *Joint assessment of HIV/AIDS treatment and care in China.* Ministry of Health and UN Theme Group on HIV/AIDS in China, 1 December.

WHO (2000). *Health systems: improving performance.* World Health Report. Geneva.

WHO (2001). *Mental health: new understanding, new hope.* World Health Report. Geneva.

World Bank (2003). *Sustainable development in a dynamic world: transforming institutions, growth and quality of life.* The World Development Report 2003. New York.

World Bank/IMF/IDA (2003). *HIPC Initiative—statistical update, 2003.* Available at www.worldbank.org/hipc/

Chapter 7 – National responses to AIDS: more action needed

Box: The gender factor within national AIDS responses

IRIN (2003). Women's coalition on HIV/AIDS launched [webpage]. UN Office for the Coordination of Humanitarian Affairs, Integrated Regional Information Networks (IRIN). www.aegis.com/news/irin/2003/IR030627.html

Mingat A, Bruns B (2002). Achieving education for all by 2015: simulation results for 47 low-income countries. Washington, World Bank, Human Development Network, Africa Region and Education Department. Available at www1.worldbank.org/education/pdf/EFA%20Complete%20Draft.pdf

NWMI (2003). Global population policy update [webpage]. Network of Women in Media, India (NWMI). http://www.nwmindia.org/resources/research/global_pop_policy.htm (accessed 5 March 2004).

UNDP (2003). Gender equality [webpage]. UNDP Cambodia Country Office. http://www.un.org.kh/undp/index.asp?page=gender/pge.asp (accessed 5 March 2004).

UNESCO (2002). *EFA global monitoring report, 2002: is the world on track?* Paris. Available at http://www.unesco.org/education/efa/monitoring/monitoring_2002.shtml

UNESCO (2003). *EFA global monitoring report, 2003–2004: gender and education for all—the leap to equality.* Paris. Available at portal.unesco.org/education/ev.php?URL_ID=23023&URL_DO=DO_TOPIC&URL_SECTION=201

United Nations (2001). United Nations millennium development goals [webpage]. www.un.org/millenniumgoals/

Remainder of chapter

Cape Argus (2003). Eskom pledges R5m to provide HIV training to medics. *Cape Argus*, 1 May 2003, Cape Town.

Development Gateway (2003). Muslim religious leaders in Mali join the fight against AIDS [webpage]. www.psi.org/news/0703d.html (accessed 8 September 2003).

Elsey H, Kutengule P (2003). *AIDS mainstreaming: a definition, some experiences and strategies.* Durban, University of Natal, Health Economics and AIDS Research Division (HEARD). Available at www.und.ac.za/und/heard/papers/DFID%20mainstreaming%20report_Jan031.pdf

FAO/Government of Zambia (2003). Draft TCP Proposal: strengthening institutional capacity in mitigating AIDS impact on the agricultural sector in Zambia. Lusaka.

GRI (2003). *Reporting guidance on AIDS: a GRI resource document.* Amsterdam. Available at http://www.globalreporting.org/guidelines/HIV/hivaids.asp

International AIDS Alliance (2002). *Participation in the Global Fund: a review paper.* London. Available at www.aidsalliance.org/_docs/_languages/_eng/_content/_3_publications/download/Policy/NGO%20Participation.pdf

IOM (2003). Migration for Development in Africa (MIDA). Available at www.iom.int/MIDA/

Kaiser Daily AIDS Report (2003). Indian Prime Minister Calls for 'Undelayed Response' to AIDS at Indian AIDS Convention, 28 July. Available at www.thebody.com/kaiser/2003/jul28_03/india_aids.html

Lauring H (2002). Action needed on brain drain. Globaleyes. Available at http://manila.djh.dk/global/stories/storyReader$98

Lenton C, Hawkins K, Jani R (2003). *Evaluation of targeted interventions in reduction of HIV transmission in five states in India.* London, Department for International Development (DFID).

Lubben M et al. (2002). Reproductive health and health sector reform in developing countries: establishing a framework for dialogue. *Bulletin of the World Health Organization,* 80(8):667–74.

Mpanju-Shumbusho W (2003). Presentation by Winnie Mpanju-Shumbusho, Director, Strategy and Partnerships, AIDS Department, WHO. Planning Workshop for Increasing Access to Care and Treatment for PLWHA, Harare, 7–10 June.

Piot P (2003). *AIDS: The need for an exceptional response to an unprecedented crisis.* Presidential Fellows Lecture, Washington. Available at http://www.unaids.org/html/pub/Media/Speeches02/Piot_WorldBank_20Nov03_en_pdf.pdf

SELA (2003). Brazilian Intervention [webpage]. Latin America Economic System (SELA). lanic.utexas.edu/~sela/AA2K3/ENG/docs/Coop/south/Di16.htm

Thomson A (2003). Medical exodus saps South Africa's war on AIDS. *Reuters AlertNet*, 3 February.

UNAIDS (2003). *Coordination of national responses to AIDS: guiding principles for national authorities and their partners.* Available at www.unaids.org/html/pub/UNA-docs/coordination_national_responses_pdf.pdf

UNAIDS (2003a). *Partenariat entre le gouvernement et le secteur privé pour la lutte contre le Sida.* Republique of Cameroon, Yaoundé, UNAIDS Cameroon/National AIDS Control Programme.

UNAIDS (2003b). *Progress report on the global response to the AIDS epidemic*, 2003. Geneva.

UNAIDS (2003c). *Stepping back from the edge: vision, activism and risk-taking in pursuit of antiretroviral therapy.* Best Practice Collection. Geneva.

UNAIDS/Ministry of Health (2003). *Joint assessment on AIDS prevention, treatment and care in China.* UN Theme Group on AIDS/Ministry of Health, Republic of China, Beijing.

UNDP (2002). *Introducing governance into AIDS programmes: People's Republic of China, Lao PDR and Viet Nam.* UNDP South-East Asia HIV and Development Programme, Bangkok. Available at www.hiv-development.org/publications/introducing-Governance.htm

USAID et al. (2003). *The level of effort in the national response to AIDS: the AIDS Program Effort Index (API)—the 2003 Round.* Washington, Futures Group International.

WHO (2003). Human capacity-building plan for scaling up AIDS treatment [web page]. http://www.who.int/3by5/publications/documents/capacity_building/en/index.html (accessed 6 January 2004).

WHO/UNAIDS (2003). *Second generation HIV surveillance: lessons learned in 8 countries.* (in press). Geneva.

Focus – AIDS and conflict: a growing problem worldwide

Cavaljuga S (2002). Federation of Bosnia and Herzegovina, in HIV prevention and care among mobile groups in the Balkans. Rome, IOM.

Hankins C, Friedman S, Zafar T et al. (2002). Transmission and prevention of HIV and sexually transmitted infections in war settings: implications for current and future armed conflicts. *AIDS*, 16:2245–2252.

IASC (2003). Interagency Agency Task Force on HIV in Emergency Settings (2003). May.

International Rescue Committee (2001). Mortality in Eastern Democratic Republic of Congo. May.

Kaiser R, Spiegel P, Salam P et al. (2002). *HIV seroprevalence and behavioural risk factor survey in Sierra Leone.* Report, Centers for Disease Control and Prevention. Atlanta, April.

Lubbers R (2003). HIV and refugees. Misperceptions and new approaches. UNHCR Press statement.

McGinn T et al. (2001). Forced migration and transmission of HIV and other sexually transmitted infections: policy and programmatic responses. HIV InSite Knowledge Base Chapter 2001. Available at http://hivinsite.ucsf.edu/

Norwegian People's Aid (2002). *Prevention of mother-to-child transmission of HIV program.* Progress Report. (unpublished report).

Salama P, Laurence B, Nolan M L (1999). Health and human rights in contemporary humanitarian crises: is Kosovo more important than Sierra Leone? *British Medical Journal*, 319:1569–1571.

Smith A (2002). HIV and emergencies: analysis and recommendations for practice. Humanitarian Practice Network. ODI.

Spiegel P (2003). HIV surveillance in situations of forced migration. (currently submitted for publication). Presented at Workshop on Fertility and Reproductive Health in Humanitarian Crises, Roundtable on the Demography of Forced Migration/Committee on Population, The National Academies of Science, Washington, 23–24 October 2002.

Spiegel P, de Jong E (2003). HIV and refugees/returnees. Mission to Luanda, Angola. 30 March–3 April 2003. UNHCR.

Spiegel P, Nankoe A (2004). UNHCR, HIV/AIDS and refugees: lessons learned. *Forced Migration Review*, 19:21–23.

Strathdee S A, Zafar T, Brahmbhatt H, ul Hassan S (2002). Higher level of needle sharing among injection drug users in Lahore, Pakistan, in the aftermath of the US-Afghan war. Presented at XIV International Conference on AIDS, Barcelona, July.

UNAIDS/UNHCR (2003). HIV and STI prevention and care in Rwandan refugee camps in The United Republic of Tanzania. Geneva.

Focus – The essential role of people living with AIDS

Horizons Program (2002). *Greater involvement of PLHA in NGO service delivery: findings from a four-country study*. Washington, Population Council. Available at http://www.popcouncil.org/pdfs/horizons/plha4cntrysum.pdf

Manchester J (2003). *Hope, involvement and vision: reflections on positive women's activism around HIV*. (in press).

Senterfitt W (1998). The Denver Principles: the original manifesto of the PWA self-empowerment movement. *Being Alive*, May 1998. Available at http://www.aegis.com/pubs/bala/1998/Ba980509.html

Uganda AIDS Commission/UNAIDS (2003). The Uganda HIV/AIDS partnership. Draft partnership information note 31/07/03. Kampala.

UNAIDS (2003). *Stepping back from the edge: vision, activism and risk-taking in pursuit of antiretroviral therapy*. Best Practice Collection. Geneva.

UNDP (2003). *Ukraine and HIV/AIDS: time to act*. Ukraine Human Development Report Special Edition. Kiev.

WHO (2003). *Treating 3 million by 2005. Making it happen: the WHO strategy*. Geneva. Available at http://www.who.int/3by5/publications/documents/isbn9241591129/en/

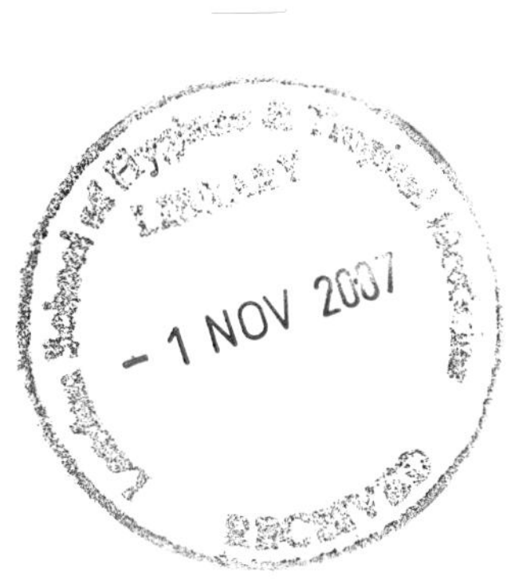

Notes

Notes